# STRATEGIC MARKETING FOR HEALTH CARE ORGANIZATIONS

T0338116

# STRATEGIC MARKETING FOR HEALTH CARE ORGANIZATIONS

## Building a Customer-Driven Health System

### SECOND EDITION

**PHILIP KOTLER**
**ROBERT J. STEVENS**
**JOEL SHALOWITZ**

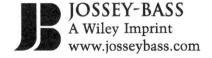

JOSSEY-BASS
A Wiley Imprint
www.josseybass.com

This edition first published 2021
© 2021 John Wiley & Sons, Inc.

*Edition History*
John Wiley & Sons, Inc. (1e, 2008)

The right of Philip Kotler, Robert J. Stevens, Joel Shalowitz to be identified as the author(s) of this work and has been asserted in accordance with law.

*Registered Office(s)*
John Wiley & Sons, Inc., 111 River Street, Hoboken, NJ 07030, USA

*Editorial Office*
111 River Street, Hoboken, NJ 07030, USA

For details of our global editorial offices, customer services, and more information about Wiley products visit us at www.wiley.com.

Wiley also publishes its books in a variety of electronic formats and by print-on-demand. Some content that appears in standard print versions of this book may not be available in other formats.

*Library of Congress Cataloging-in-Publication Data*
Names: Kotler, Philip, author. | Shalowitz, Joel, 1953- author. | Stevens, Robert J. (Robert John), 1955- author.
Title: Strategic marketing for health care organizations: building a customer-driven health system / Philip Kotler, Joel Shalowitz, and Robert J. Stevens.
Description: 2nd edition. | San Francisco, CA : Jossey-Bass, [2020] | Includes bibliographical references and index.
Identifiers: LCCN 2020024726 (print) | LCCN 2020024727 (ebook) | ISBN 9781118355831 (paperback) | ISBN 9781118448304 (adobe pdf) | ISBN 9781118448410 (epub)
Subjects: MESH: Marketing of Health Services—methods | Consumer Behavior | United States
Classification: LCC RA410.56 (print) | LCC RA410.56 (ebook) | NLM W 74 AA1 | DDC 362.1068/8—dc23
LC record available at https://lccn.loc.gov/2020024726
LC ebook record available at https://lccn.loc.gov/2020024727

Cover image: © Ariel Skelley / Getty Images, © JohnnyGreig / Getty Images © OsakaWayne Studios / Getty Images, © Dean Mitchell / Getty Images
Cover design: Wiley

Set in 10.5/12.5pts Times New Roman by Integra Software Services Pvt. Ltd, Pondicherry, India
SKY10023539_011821

To our nine grandchildren, Jordan, Jamie, Ellie, Abby, Olivia, Sam, Dante, Sapphire, and Shaina
— Philip Kotler

To Elizabeth & Derek, Anne & Andy, and Rob
— Robert J. Stevens

To the next generation: Parker Gordon Spivack, Chase Ryan Spivack, and Hanna Eleanor Bunce Shalowitz
— Joel Shalowitz

# CONTENTS

# PREFACE

The value of U.S. health care needs improvement. We spend more on health care, as a share of the economy, than any other member country in the Organization for Economic Co-operation and Development (OECD). Regrettably, we also have the lowest life expectancy and highest suicide rate among any of the other 37 OECD members. The U.S. has the highest[1]:

- Chronic disease burden
- Obesity rate that is two times higher than the OECD average
- Number of hospitalizations from preventable causes
- Rate of avoidable deaths

U.S. health care quality varies significantly among different regions of the country and even within some counties. Sixty percent of U.S. consumers have a chronic condition and 40% have two or more. Health costs are highly variable, and in spite of recent regulations, health care pricing remains a mystery. It is difficult to know in advance what a hernia operation or a knee replacement will actually cost. Consumer out-of-pocket costs continue to rise, and Gallup polls show that 70% of consumers have a negative view of the U.S. health care system.[2]

We believe that health care leaders can address these problems and increase value by being customer and market-driven. Marketing is both a philosophy and a set of tools. As a philosophy, it calls for serving and meeting the needs of different customers while satisfying organizational requirements. As a set of tools, marketing helps stakeholders understand market and individual customer needs, develop quality products and services, price them correctly, make them convenient and easily accessible, and inform and communicate their offerings to target markets.

The first edition of this book was written as a traditional marketing text with many health care examples. Feedback from students and instructors led us to change the emphasis for the second edition and focus on how marketing solves real-life health care problems. In the first chapter of the new edition, we begin by explaining how marketing can create health care value, and we compare the transaction view of marketing with the customer relationship view. Principal marketing concepts are described in Chapter 2 and are applied to a marketing plan for an innovative, market-driven orthopedic practice.

Chapter 3 describes how market opportunities can be exploited and threats can be avoided through marketing research and a comprehensive analysis of the health care environment. Chapter 4 focuses on consumer demand for health care, consumer marketing psychology and health care behavior, and the three most important environmental forces affecting consumers.

Chapters 5 through 8 explore strategic marketing for physician practices, hospitals, health technology companies, and biopharma companies. Each of the chapters begins with an evaluation of market data, identification and analysis of environmental forces, a review of stakeholder behavior in response to market trends, and an explanation of marketing tools being used to innovatively solve health care problems.

Chapter 9 explains how social cause marketing improves public health. It illustrates how social marketing tools increase availability of safe water, motivate consumers to make healthier lifestyle decisions, and contribute to reducing HIV/AIDs infection. As this preface is being written, the world is struggling with the Covid-19 pandemic. Social marketing can be used to increase the effectiveness of current protocols like physical distancing, wearing a mask, contact tracing, and help to support supply chains and economic performance.

At the end of each chapter, there are exercises or mini case studies that students can use to apply various health care marketing tools. Examples are developing an environmental analysis for a health care organization, getting people to exercise, a channels analysis of a truck-stop primary care practice, exploring how a rural hospital increased customer loyalty, developing a positioning for a new health IT sleep app, and evaluating biopharma marketing ethics in relation to the opioid epidemic.

In summary, we wrote this book to serve the needs of those who will be, or are, working in health care: physicians and other clinicians, medical researchers, hospital administrators, public health workers, health technology and biopharma managers, among others. Ideally, readers will learn to market products and services that are aligned with customer needs. Our hope is that this book will give you the marketing concepts and tools that will enable you to be even more effective in your chosen field and make a strong contribution to the health of our nation.

*July 2020*

Philip Kotler
*Glencoe, Illinois*

Robert J. Stevens
*Durham, North Carolina*

Joel Shalowitz
*Glencoe, Illinois*

# ACKNOWLEDGMENTS

We would like to acknowledge the following for their contributions to our book: Tal Lassiter, Randy Ely, Elizabeth Bell, Mark G. Rubin, Dorothea Bonds, Holli Salls, Joel Lee, Christopher Kane, Monica Horvath, Abhi Sindhwani, Alison Bechtel, Austin Raper, Jessica Behrendsen, Laura Cunningham, Gilbert Mott, Richard Freeman, Alison Smith, Tim Harlin, George Luke, Fred Navarro, Elizabeth Upton, Jessica Krupka, and the late Sal Novin. We would also like to acknowledge the many Elon University students who offered feedback on numerous drafts. Last but not least, we want to thank Wiley editors Darren Lalonde, Ethan Lipson, Monica Rogers, Christina Weyrauch, Liz Wingett, Daniel Finch, Patricia Rossi, Purvi Patel, Seth Schwartz, and the late Andy Pasternack for their fine editorial help in guiding and producing this book.

# THE AUTHORS

**PHILIP KOTLER** is the S.C. Johnson Distinguished Professor of International Marketing at the Kellogg School of Management, Northwestern University (Emeritus). He has been honored as one of the world's leading marketing thinkers. He received his MA in economics (1953) from the University of Chicago and his PhD in economics (1956) from the Massachusetts Institute of Technology (MIT). He has received honorary degrees from 22 foreign universities. He is the author of over 150 articles and 80 books, including *Marketing Management, Principles of Marketing, Marketing for Hospitality and Tourism, Strategic Marketing for Nonprofit Organizations, Social Marketing, Winning at Innovation, The Marketing of Nations,* and *Advancing the Common Good.* His research covers strategic marketing, consumer marketing, business marketing, professional services marketing, and e-marketing. He has been a consultant to IBM, Merck, General Electric, AT&T, Bank of America, Motorola, Ford, and others.

**ROBERT J. STEVENS** is President of Health Centric Marketing Services, a health care marketing research and strategy firm. He teaches health care marketing as an adjunct instructor at the Love School of Business at Elon University. Previous adjunct teaching positions were with the Gillings School of Global Health and the Kenan-Flagler School of Business at the University of North Carolina–Chapel Hill, and with the Owen Graduate School of Management at Vanderbilt University. Stevens received a BA from Colgate University, an MA in English from Duke University, and an MBA from the Kellogg School of Management, Northwestern University. Before starting Health Centric, he held health care marketing positions with a consumer packaged goods company, a health care system, a physician staffing and billing company, and a physician information systems company.

**JOEL SHALOWITZ** was a professor and director of the Health Industry Management Program at the Kellogg School of Management, Northwestern University for 28 years, where he taught courses on US and international health care systems and conducted executive education courses for health care organizations. In addition to his business school teaching, for 30 years Dr. Shalowitz taught the core health care systems course for Northwestern University's MPH degree program, where he has been a professor of preventive medicine. Since 2006 he has also taught courses in Northwestern's Master's Program in Healthcare Quality and Patient Safety. As a board-certified internist, he practiced medicine and was managing partner of a primary care medical group with six locations in north and northwest Chicago.

He has extensive international health care experience, including three Fulbright awards: the Schulich Business School at York University in Toronto; Keio University Medical School in Tokyo; and the Scuola Superiore Sant'Anna in Pisa. Dr. Shalowitz is currently an Affiliate Professor, Institute of Management, Scuola Superiore Sant'Anna, and Senior Fellow at ETLA, the Research Institute of the Finnish Economy.

He received his bachelor's and MD degrees from Brown University, and he completed his internal medicine residency and MBA degree at Northwestern. Honors have included election to Sigma Xi, Beta Gamma Sigma, Fellowship in the American College of Physicians, and teaching awards.

His third book, *The US Healthcare System: Origins, Organization and Opportunities*, was released in September 2019. In conjunction with that book, he is the author of the daily health care blog www.HealthcareInsights.MD.

# CHAPTER

# THE ROLE OF MARKETING IN HEALTH CARE ORGANIZATIONS

## LEARNING OBJECTIVES

In this chapter, we will address the following questions:

1. What are the major areas in health care in which marketing is regularly applied and practiced?
2. What is the purpose of marketing thinking and planning in health care organizations?
3. What are the major concepts, tools, and skills in marketing?
4. How is marketing normally organized in health care organizations?

## OVERVIEW: MARKETING IS PERVASIVE IN HEALTH CARE

Readers might find it strange to hear that marketing plays an important and pervasive role in the health care marketplace. They are probably aware of the marketing efforts of pharmaceutical and medical device companies to sell their branded products and services. But what about hospitals, nursing homes, hospices, physician practices, health plans, rehabilitation centers, and other health care organizations? After all, don't people get sick on their own?

These organizations, for the most part, didn't think about marketing until the early 1970s. But today we see a great deal of marketing taking place in health care organizations. Consider the following facts:

- Virtually every hospital uses its website to tout its facilities and services. Some hospitals run community health programs. Some hospital CEOs appear on talk shows. All of these efforts go toward building their brand.

- Health plans develop insurance products and use marketing tools to vie with other companies in promoting themselves to employers and their employees.

- New physicians seeking to open their own practices use marketing to help determine good locations, attractive office designs, and practice styles that will attract and retain new patients.

- The American Cancer Society, American Heart Association, and other health associations turn to social marketing to encourage more people to adopt healthier life styles, like quitting smoking, cutting down on saturated fats in their diet, and increasing exercise.

These illustrations demonstrate one side of marketing, namely the use of influential advertising and selling to attract and retain customers. But marketing tasks and tools go beyond developing a stream of persuasive messages. Consider the following:

## FOR EXAMPLE

**Two Vignettes**

A hospital is considering adding a sports medicine program to its portfolio of services. Before deciding whether to launch such a program, it plans to do market research to gauge the size of the community need, discover which competitors already offer such a program, consider how it will organize and deliver the program, understand how to price its various services, and determine how profitable the program is likely to be.

Walgreens is opening store-based clinics to provide basic health care services, such as measuring blood pressure, providing vaccinations, and treating such common conditions as sore throats, ear infections, and colds. Key marketing tasks it must perform include deciding which stores will have this service, setting prices, and, most important, determining how physician customers will view this service as possible competition.

From these examples, we recognize that many health sector participants are trying to solve their problems by relying on marketing tools and concepts. Readers who already work in the health care field may recognize some of these tasks as the realm of epidemiology; however, the discipline of marketing is much broader. The American Marketing Association offers the following definition: *Marketing is an organizational function and a set of processes for creating, communicating, and delivering value to customers and for managing customer relationships in ways that benefit the organization and its stakeholders.*

While value is the fundamental concept underlying modern marketing, value is also now the central focus of health care. The Affordable Care Act, enacted in 2010, linked reimbursements to improved clinical performance. Value-based payment holds health care providers accountable for both the cost and quality of care they provide. It attempts to reduce inappropriate care and to identify and reward the best-performing providers. It makes sense to expand the use of marketing to manage health care since value is their common goal.

Marketing takes place when at least one party to a potential transaction thinks about the means of achieving desired responses from other parties. Marketing takes place when:

- a physician designs an office and trains their staff to enhance the customer experience

- a hospital develops a state-of-the-art cancer center in a location with a growing population of seniors

- a health plan adds free exercise, weight-loss, and smoking cessation benefits to reduce long-term hospitalization costs

- a pharmaceutical firm hires more salespeople to gain physician acceptance and preference for a new drug

- the American Medical Association lobbies Congress to gain support for a new bill

- the Centers for Disease Control and Prevention (CDC) runs a campaign to get more people to get an annual flu shot

- a health information technology firm automates manual tasks for a health plan to improve accuracy and lower costs.

A marketer may aim to secure various responses including a purchase of a product or service; increased awareness, interest, or preference toward an offering or supplier; a change in behavior; or a higher level of customer loyalty.

## THE ELEMENTS OF MARKETING THOUGHT

In this section, we introduce the purpose of marketing, some important marketing concepts and skills, and how marketing is organized in health care organizations. We will discuss these topics in greater depth in the following chapters.

### The Purpose of Marketing

There are two quite different opinions about marketing's purpose. One might be called the *transaction view*, which says that its aim is to get an order or make a sale. Marketing's role is, therefore, to use sales skills and advertising to sell more "stuff."[1] The focus is on doing everything possible to stimulate a transaction.

The other opinion about marketing can be called the *customer relationship-building and loyalty view*. Here the focus is more on the customer and less on the particular product or service. The marketer aims to serve the customer in such a way that they will be satisfied and come back for more services or products. In fact, the marketer hopes that loyalty will be sufficiently high that the customer will recommend the seller to others. For example, we know that a physician who develops an excellent service reputation will attract many new patients as a result of word-of-mouth recommendations. Also, as patients experience new medical needs and problems, they will return to the same physician for treatment and advice.

Some marketers question the use of terms such as *consumer* and *patient*. The traditional view of a consumer or patient is that of someone who is passively consuming something, but today's consumers are also producers. With respect to health care products and services, they are actively sending messages about their experiences, creating new uses, providing new findings from the web and other resources to their physicians, and lobbying for more and better benefits. Predicting this current environment, Peter Drucker, the noted management consultant, viewed marketing as playing the role of serving as the customer's agent or representative.

In fact, more organizations are moving from the transaction view to the relationship view of marketing, in a shift from Old Marketing to New Marketing. In this environment, the New Marketer's job is to create a long-term, trusted, and valued relationship with customers, which means getting the whole organization to think about and serve customers and their interests. For instance, hospitals that have built a pervasive marketing culture will usually financially outperform those that see themselves simply as selling visits, tests, and services, one at a time.

### Marketing Uses a Set of Concepts

The first question a health care organization must ask is, who is potentially interested in the kind of products or services that we offer or plan to offer? Examples include young women and obstetric services, older adults and bypass surgery services, and diabetics and portable blood sugar testing devices. We can summarize the customer-focused marketing philosophy with the acronym CCDV: The aim of marketing is to *create, communicate, and deliver value*. It is not value just because the supplier believes they are giving value, but true value must be perceived by the customer. One job of the marketer is to turn invisible value into perceived value.

Very few organizations try to serve the entire market, preferring instead to distinguish different groups (segments) that make up a market. This distinguishing process is called *market segmentation*. The organization will then consider which market segments it can serve best in light of the segments' needs and the organization's capabilities. We call the chosen segment the *target market*. We can extend CCDV into CCDVT, with the "T" standing for a *target market*. Instead of an organization generating general value, it aims to generate specific value for a well-defined target market.

If a nursing home decides to serve a high-income market, it must create, communicate, and deliver the value expected by high-income families, with the price set high enough to cover the extra costs of better facilities and services. Finally, we need to further extend the expression to CCDVTP, with the "P" standing for *profitably*. The marketing aim is to *create, communicate, and deliver value to a target market profitably*. Even a nonprofit organization must earn revenues in excess of expenses in order to sustain and continue its charitable mission.

To help their firms prepare a valued offering, marketers have long used a tools framework known as the marketing mix: *product, price, place*, and *promotion*, or the 4Ps (Figure 1.1). The organization decides on a product (its features, benefits, styling, packaging), its price (including list price as well as rebate and discount programs), its place (namely, where it is available and its distribution strategies), and the promotion mix (such as customer word-of-mouth, personal selling, and public relations).

It turns out that the 4Ps are already present in the CCDVTP formulation. Creating value is very much about developing an excellent *product* and appropriate *price*. Communicating value involves *promotion*. Delivering value requires an understanding about *place*. CCDVTP is a more active way to state the 4Ps. Some critics have also proposed adding more Ps (*people, passion, process*, and so on).

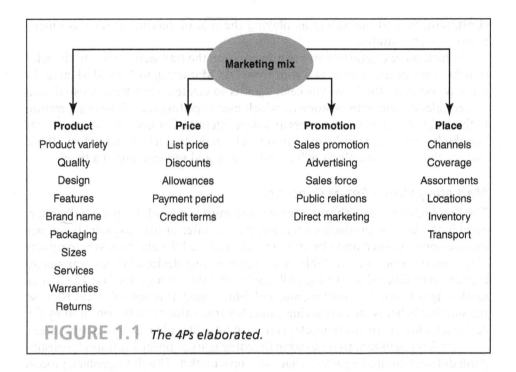

| | | | |
|---|---|---|---|
| **Product** | **Price** | **Promotion** | **Place** |
| Product variety | List price | Sales promotion | Channels |
| Quality | Discounts | Advertising | Coverage |
| Design | Allowances | Sales force | Assortments |
| Features | Payment period | Public relations | Locations |
| Brand name | Credit terms | Direct marketing | Inventory |
| Packaging | | | Transport |
| Sizes | | | |
| Services | | | |
| Warranties | | | |
| Returns | | | |

FIGURE 1.1 *The 4Ps elaborated.*

Marketers recognize that the 4Ps represent the set of the seller's decisions, not the buyer's decisions. Part of the transition from the Old Marketing to the New Marketing involves marketers looking at everything from the buyer's or consumer's point of view. For a consumer to be interested in an offering, the consumer must have *awareness* of the offering and find it *acceptable*, *available* at the right time and place, and *affordable*. Professor Jagdish Sheth calls these attributes the "4As of marketing."[2]

We introduce one final concept—positioning. An organization or company positions itself to be the place of choice for its target market. A hospital might position itself as having the most advanced medicine or the best patient service, or being the most efficient hospital. Good positioning requires looking at how to best implement the 4As of that target market. We refer to these steps of *segmentation*, *targeting*, and *positioning* by the acronym STP.

Combining this concept with those just described, we now have a more robust model of marketing strategy: first segment, next target, then position, determine the 4As, and finally set the appropriate 4Ps.

When we say that marketing's purpose is to create value for the customer and profits (or margins for nonprofits) for the organization and its stakeholders, we don't mean that the organization should give customers everything that they want.

Customers may really desire to have free products and services. Google offers internet search, docs, calendars, and other services at no charge, but Google collects and sells customer data to generate revenue. Customer desires and needs must correspond with the mission or purpose of the organization. For example, a rehabilitation hospital does not need to open a cardiac bypass program just because some of its patients have heart disease. A further problem arises when the customer wants something that is not in their best interest. For example, a patient may request an antibiotic to treat a cold or ask for a narcotic for nonmedical reasons.

### The Main Skills of Marketing

Marketers rely on seven traditional skills: marketing research, product design, distribution, pricing, customer loyalty, positioning, and promotion. Effective marketing must start with marketing research, which in turn consists of other skills. Suppose a hospital is planning to build a second facility in one of several neighboring communities. It clearly needs to conduct systematic marketing research to find which site is the most promising. The marketing research will use both secondary and primary data. Secondary data come from existing sources and yield information about such factors as the population's size, age, income, and education distribution as well as land costs and transportation resources. Primary data come from making firsthand observations in each community by hosting focus groups to gather consumer reactions to different proposals, conducting in-depth interviews with specific community members, undertaking surveys to get a more accurate picture of customer attitudes and needs, and, finally, applying statistical techniques to draw insights from the data. By combining primary and secondary data, the hospital hopes that some neighboring community will emerge as the best target market to be served by a second facility.

Product design is the second marketing skill. Suppose a manufacturer of hospital beds wants to design a product that patients can more easily adjust on their own. It will assign a product team to design the new bed, consisting of an engineer, a designer, and a marketer. The marketer will supply some preliminary data about how patients feel about different features of a hospital bed, including functions, colors, and general design appearance. After the design is developed, the marketer might test it with a number of patients.

Although we are talking about designing a physical product, the same principles apply to a service. Many people complain about their experience in hospital emergency departments (EDs), including long waiting times, crowded facilities, and uneven customer service. Marketers are increasingly studying how to improve the ED experience. This is because hospital administrators realize that it is the place in which patients often experience their first encounter with the institution and it influences their probability of choosing the hospital for future care.

The third traditional skill of marketers is distribution. Marketers have to choose places in which their products and services will be readily accessible and available to the customers. Marketers have learned to work with different types of wholesalers, jobbers, brokers, retailers, and transportation companies. This knowledge is very useful in activities ranging from pharmaceutical channel distribution to setting up a regional or national chain of in-store medical clinics.

Pricing is the fourth traditional skill of marketers. Marketers have gained much of their experience through setting prices and adjusting them for different markets and in different circumstances. They are guided by both internal constraints (such as their companies' production cost structure) as well as the realities of the marketplace (such as price elasticity of demand). In the realm of health insurance, the marketplace also demands flexibility to customize the product, with an attendant set of fixed and optional services and their varied prices.

The fifth traditional skill is improving customer loyalty. There is a statistical correlation between loyalty and an organization's financial performance. Many health care organizations give special attention to customer satisfaction. Satisfaction reporting is required by Centers for Medicare & Medicaid Services (CMS) to receive reimbursement, but satisfaction does not correlate with financial performance. Loyalty is measured by the Net Promoter Score (NPS), and it is based on a customer's experience with a product and its organization. Marketers find opportunities to improve experience and loyalty by working closely with operations, finance, and human resources managers as well as clinical staff.

The sixth traditional skill of marketers is positioning. Strategic positioning determines how the market thinks and feels about the product or the organization. An effective positioning statement includes the target, the frame of reference, the primary benefit, and key differentiating attributes. Positioning strategy is used to guide the development of all of the marketing mix strategies: product, price, channels, and promotion. Marketers use innovative ideas to meet customer needs, and the acid test for a new idea is usually "Is it supported by our positioning strategy?" Either the idea is supported and accepted, or it is not supported and not used, or the positioning strategy is reviewed and possibly modified.

Promotion is the seventh traditional skill of marketers. Promotion is the skill used last because if a product is poorly designed, priced too high, or difficult to buy, then promotion does not matter. Promotion can be divided by personal and non-personal communication. An example of personal communication is customer word-of-mouth. Health care buying is based on a combination of emotion, analysis, and trust. Having a personal recommendation from a friend or family member is powerful. Selling is another example of personal communication. For example, the General Electric (GE) Medical Products division uses a well-trained sales force to sell sophisticated diagnostic imaging equipment to hospitals. This equipment is expensive, so hospitals must be convinced not only that they need this technology, but also that they should purchase it from GE. GE's professional sales force will need to explain the benefits of buying this equipment and the GE brand promise to justify its higher cost. GE also needs to hire, train, compensate, motivate, and evaluate hundreds of skilled professional salespeople.

Advertising, public relations, and social media communications are effective non-personal health care communications tools. Marketers have extensive experience in working with ad agencies in designing messages, choosing media, setting budgets, and evaluating outcomes of advertising campaigns. The marketer must advise the organization about the best media mix to use—television, online, print, outdoor, and others—to reach a particular target market. Sales promotion is another promotion skill that uses wide-ranging incentives to stimulate trial or purchase of a product or service. For example, the ultimate goal of local community health leaders may be to have 100% of residents get a flu shot. The leaders may test different marketing stimuli to increase vaccinations such as offering a free booklet on staying fit, a coupon for other health services, more convenient hours, or a chance to win a gift card.

The seven marketing skills are represented and implemented through a strategic marketing plan. A marketing plan consists of a situation analysis of the market and product, annual goals and objectives, overall targeting and positioning strategies, marketing mix strategies including the 4Ps, and marketing management measures like monthly revenue, market share, and spending tracking. Chapter 2 explains how health care marketing plans organize and manage collective marketing ideas, strategies, results, and the plans are developed and used in an organization.

### How Marketing is Organized in Health Care

Formal marketing positions—such as marketing researchers, sales managers, and advertising managers—have existed in pharmaceutical firms, medical device firms, and medical supply firms for many years. It wasn't, however, until 1975 that a U.S. hospital appointed a head of marketing. The Evanston Hospital in Evanston, Illinois (now NorthShore University HealthSystem), appointed Dr. John McLaren, a physician, to be its vice president of marketing.

As more hospitals began to appoint a marketing manager, two title variations emerged: director of marketing and vice president of marketing. The director of marketing typically provides and orchestrates marketing-related activities and resources. The vice president of marketing performs these activities and also works with the other hospital executives in developing policies and strategies. Importantly, the vice president of marketing also represents the voice of the customer (VOC) in management and board meetings.

When hospitals first started appointing marketing heads, the public relations (PR) person on the staff often objected on the grounds that they were doing the marketing. The PR person's job was to generate good news about the hospital and defend it against bad news. Hospital CEOs soon realized, however, that PR and marketing have quite different roles and skills, although there is some overlap.

PR managers are trained in communication skills and work closely with media (editors, journalists) and occasionally with government officials, although the latter contacts are often handled by public affairs officers. Marketing people, on the other hand, are trained in economic analysis and the social sciences to understand and analyze markets and customer choice behavior. Marketers use the tools detailed earlier to provide estimates of a defined market's size and its needs, preferences, perceptions, and readiness to respond to alternative offers. Marketers develop strategies and tactics for serving the target market in a way that will meet the organization's mission.

Today the marketing departments in health care organizations may be staffed with a marketing researcher or analyst, an advertising and sales promotion manager, a sales force director, product managers, and market segment managers. Even when there are no specific marketing department positions dedicated to the functions of product development, pricing, communication, and distribution, these functions are carried out by other managers in the organization.

## CHAPTER SUMMARY

Marketing plays an important role in helping participants in the health care system create, communicate, and deliver value (CCDV) to their respective target markets. Modern marketers start with the customers rather than with the products or services. They are more interested in building a lasting relationship than in securing a single transaction. Their aim is to create a high level of loyalty so that customers return and recommend the organization, service, or product to others.

Marketers have used many traditional skills, including marketing research, product design, distribution, pricing, customer loyalty, positioning, and promotion. These skills are collected and organized through a strategic health care marketing plan. These plans are structured for a one-year period, and they are continually updated and modified based on feedback and effectiveness.

## DISCUSSION QUESTIONS

1. You are the president of a 100-bed hospital that has a public relations person and a development officer but no marketer. Do you need a marketer? How would this person's role differ from the others? Make an argument pro and con for hiring a marketer.

2. The governor of your state believes that more state funds need to be invested in preventing illness and accidents. He hires you as a social marketer with the mandate to raise consciousness about healthier life styles and to focus on two causes that will have the highest impact. How would you approach this assignment and what would you suggest?

3. You head the marketing department for a medical device firm whose sales department reports not to you but to a vice president of sales. Do you think that the vice president of sales and the sales force should report to you, or is it better to run marketing and sales as separate departments? What are the likely problems? What are the arguments for and against combining the departments?

# CHAPTER

## 2

# DEVELOPING A STRATEGIC HEALTH CARE MARKETING PLAN

**LEARNING OBJECTIVES**

In this chapter we will address the following questions:

1. Why is strategic marketing planning important to a health care organization?
2. What are the steps for preparing and implementing a marketing plan?
3. What is the role of evidence and data in supporting marketing strategies?
4. How would a new physician practice complete a strategic marketing plan?

## HOW NOT TO DEVELOP A MARKETING PLAN

The marketing strategy meeting had been a complete disaster. Mack, the president of PhyInfo, a physician information system company, had been anxiously awaiting new ideas for increasing revenue. Revenue growth had always been the top priority for this entrepreneurial health IT company. Mack started PhyInfo on a shoestring 10 years ago with his business partner, and they were both high-energy sales people. Now the stakes were higher because PhyInfo had just gone public with an IPO. Top management was consumed with Wall Street analysts and striving to reach quarterly earnings forecasts.

Ken had recently been hired as the first PhyInfo marketing director. He had come from another successful publicly-traded physician management company, so expectations for his "marketing magic" were very high. He had spent his first few weeks meeting with management and learning how the company operated. Like many entrepreneurial businesses, the PhyInfo culture emphasized action and tactics—but not data, strategies, or planning. Several managers mentioned that the pervasive company approach was "Shoot from the hip."

The first ever PhyInfo strategic marketing plan was based on extensive secondary marketing research. Ken independently analyzed these data and information to develop broad product, pricing, channels, and promotion strategies. The plan was over 50 pages, and when it was finally ready, he called a meeting with Mack and the four vice presidents. Ken was proud of his plan, and he was looking forward to coming up with tactics to implement the approved strategies.

The presentation began with a detailed explanation of the situation analysis. After 10 minutes, Mack interrupted and told Ken he knew the situation and to move on to the marketing that would result in more profits. Ken started outlining the product, pricing, and channels strategies, but Mack interrupted again and said all of these strategies were unnecessary. He had expected new advertising and sales tactics, but Ken did not have those details. At that point, Mack pronounced the meeting a complete waste of time and left the room. What had gone wrong?

## CHECKLIST FOR AN EFFECTIVE STRATEGIC MARKETING PLAN

Plan implementation failure is common, but it can be avoided. Effective marketing planning is consensus-based and is an iterative, not linear, process. Ken would have been more successful if he had not worked independently but had followed the marketing planning steps developed by Calkins.[1]

*Step 1: Build a cross-functional team*

This step is required to create shared ownership of marketing strategy development and implementation. All employees influence marketing whether or not their job title includes the word "marketing." Operations is usually the leading management function in health care service organizations, and its dominance may prompt rivalries with other departments. In health care businesses, competitive rifts between sales departments and marketing departments are common. An individual whose name is on the cover page of a marketing plan, however, is unlikely to criticize it. Inviting a range of department managers to participate in developing the plan is not only good politics, but their different perspectives bring value to the process. Ideas and assumptions that seem straightforward to a staff manager may actually be more complex from the perspective of a line manager.

After forming a cross-disciplinary team, the first activity is to brainstorm the contents of the plan at completion. The vision and details will likely change, but it helps to have a sense of the finished document and the big picture at the start of planning. Achieving buy-in from a range of departments may seem unnecessary, as it did to Ken, based on the "silo mentality" common among many organizations. Information represents power, and sharing information risks losing power. PhyInfo leadership was from the independent and self-reliant sales culture. Corporate teamwork and consensus-building was not a company value or supported by employee incentives.

### Step 2: *Check the foundation and long-term business direction*

Ken would have benefited from clearly understanding the PhyInfo vision and positioning. Entrepreneurial organizations usually do not have formal vision statements describing a sense of purpose and future achievements. Having a strategic positioning statement defining what the brand means is even more unlikely. Talking to company leaders about these ideas, however, could have helped Ken. For example, one of his marketing channel strategies was to create alliances with regional health IT dealers to sell a basic version of the PhyInfo system. This idea had been considered by PhyInfo in the past but was soundly rejected. Mack and the vice presidents had no interest in modifying the sales territory management structure even though it had weaknesses.

### Step 3: *Clarify the goals and objectives*

Understanding what company leadership wants to achieve over the course of the next year is very important. Be clear about organizational goals before writing a marketing plan. Ken should have confirmed the company's short-term financial targets, given to senior management by the investment community, before he began the marketing plan. Importantly, he also should have consulted with the regional sales vice presidents about their quarterly sales targets and quotas. Marketing support is crucial to sales planning and reaching revenue objectives.

### Step 4: *Conduct a comprehensive analysis*

This step involves understanding changes in market trends, needs, and competitors. Dumping data into a document without analysis does not add value. Ken reviewed, analyzed, and showed a wide range of data in his situation analysis.

Mack was impatient, however, because he intuitively already knew this information and he expected high-performing tactics. The situation analysis should have emphasized specific changes in market opportunities and threats that could lead directly to increased revenue.

*Step 5: Recommend the most important strategies and tactics*

This is the critical planning step because it focuses on how the value of the business will be increased. The most important strategic initiatives should be selected from the many possible options based on the data in Steps 1 through 4. Strategy is sacrificed because many initiatives are available and resources are always limited. Is it better to invest in building customer awareness, generating product trial, or increasing repeat purchases? Other examples of marketing strategies are increasing market share, changing pricing, and building stronger brand relationships with current customers. Tactics support specific strategies and include specific programs, actions, and activities. The budgeted investment in tactics should have a positive return-on-investment (ROI). For example, assume that $1 million is budgeted for advertising. In order to achieve a positive ROI, the advertising needs to result in profits in excess of $1 million based on incremental product sales.

*Step 6: Check the numbers*

Develop a rough profit and loss pro forma based on the plan assumptions. Explain how the strategies and tactics will deliver the financial results. If the financial objectives seem unlikely to be achieved, review the plan elements and make adjustments.

*Step 7: Sell the plan*

Your plan will not be implemented if key decision-makers and cross-functional groups do not support it. Do not underestimate the time needed to accomplish this step. Informally share the plan goals and objectives, strategies, and tactics with senior managers. Ask for their feedback, probe to ensure that they understand your ideas, and proactively address their questions and concerns. Political sensitivity is important to identify those individuals who seem to agree with your ideas but actually do not. A comment like "That was interesting" has been found to be code for "I have no confidence in the idea." After senior management agrees to the plan, communicate with the larger team to both inform them and enlist their support.

*Step 8: Execute and track progress*

Developing a marketing plan is useless unless it is executed. Communicating and delegating clear actions and schedules is needed to implement the plan. Each strategy should include regular measurements to gauge progress in reaching scheduled objectives. If milestones and schedules are missed, early course corrections need to be made.

## HOW DOES A STRATEGIC MARKETING PLAN ADD VALUE TO A HEALTH CARE ORGANIZATION?

The foundation of a strategic marketing plan is rooted in market needs. It is a repository for all of the organization's marketing ideas, objectives, strategies, and tactics. An organization's marketing department is primarily responsible for analyzing the environment and directing marketing strategy. The marketing department is also charged with building relationships with other internal departments, driving management consensus, and maintaining the marketing plan document.

Marketing plans in health care organizations also vary in detail and scope. A basic plan emphasizing marketing tactics for a hospital telehealth service may be 20 pages in length, while a comprehensive nationwide plan for a new cardiac stent may be over 300 pages. Tactics may be emphasized over strategies. Measuring marketing results of tactics are often overlooked. Calculating the ROI for advertising spending will determine if that tactic was effective. Marketing planning in some health care organizations can be an annual event with little bearing on actual marketing activity throughout the year. Conversely, a marketing plan for an over-the-counter cold and flu product may be implemented and modified daily. Every time a new marketing initiative is recommended by someone in the organization, the acid-test for acceptance of the idea is based on one question: is it on strategy? The answer is always found in the strategic marketing plan.

Health care organizations sometimes blur the differences among marketing plans, business plans, and strategic plans. A business plan is comprehensive and considers all management functions of the business: finance, operations, facilities, real estate, human resources, marketing, and others. Business plans typically have a three- to five-year time horizon, and the marketing section of a business plan is less detailed than a marketing plan.

Strategic plans fall between marketing plans and business plans. A strategic plan usually begins with examining the capacity of the organization or the product. The primary goal is to increase or decrease operating capacity in specific areas. For example, if a hospital is using 60% of its bariatric surgery capacity, a strategic plan could focus on increasing capacity to 85%. Strategic plans include environmental and market data, but the perspective is from the organization or the product and not the customer or market. A strategic plan point of view is "inside looking out." Strategic plans are usually prepared every two to five years.

Marketing plans focus on the customer and have an "outside looking in" perspective. The marketing plan is detailed and forces organizational clarity. It is accessible, dynamic, and is updated in real-time to incorporate environmental, market, customer, and competitive changes. Unlike business and strategic plans that are used to guide companies and organizations, marketing plans are used to manage individual products or product lines. An academic medical center will have a strategic plan for the institution, and the cancer and heart services lines will each have their respective marketing plans.

Additionally, a health care marketing plan provides a point of connection between data and action. For example, an analysis of ED wait times shows that most waiting patients present with low-acuity health problems. These data and other evidence may be used to support the development of a no-appointment primary care clinic in a separate building adjacent to the ED. This clinic—staffed with a nurse practitioner or physician assistant—would reduce ED waiting time and have lower costs and prices than an ED.

The scope of a strategic marketing plan is one year and is especially appropriate for the dynamic changes in the health care environment. An example of a strategic health care marketing plan is outlined next.

## STRATEGIC HEALTH CARE MARKETING PLAN OUTLINE

I. Executive Summary
- Define the most important marketing goal over the next 12 months
- What is the primary impediment blocking the goal?
- What is the marketing solution that will remove the impediment?

II. Situation Analysis
- A. Market Summary
  1. Total available market
  2. Market segmentation
  3. Competition
  4. Market opportunities and threats
- B. Product Summary
  1. Product description
  2. Value proposition
  3. Product results
  4. Product strengths and weaknesses
- C. Primary Marketing Challenges

III. Marketing Goals and Objectives
- A. Goal and Objective #1—Often financial
- B. Goal and Objective #2
- C. Goal and Objective #3

IV. Overall Strategies
- A. Target Market Strategy
- B. Marketing Research Strategy
- C. Positioning Strategy

V.  Marketing Mix Strategies and Tactics
    A.  Product Strategy and Tactics
        1.  Tactic # 1
        2.  Tactic # 2
    B.  Pricing Strategy and Tactics
        1.  Tactic # 1
        2.  Tactic # 2
    C.  Channels Strategy and Tactics
        1.  Tactic # 1
        2.  Tactic # 2
    D.  Promotion Strategy and Tactics
        1.  Tactic # 1
        2.  Tactic # 2
VI.  Implementation and Controls
    A.  Plan Performance Tracking
    B.  Revenue, Spending, and Market Share Measures

## A STRATEGIC HEALTH CARE MARKETING PLAN EXAMPLE

Each marketing plan concept will now be explained. Examples of concepts in this chapter are from Shoulder Shop marketing plan, an orthopedic physician practice plan. This plan was developed as an academic exercise by a team of public health graduate students including an orthopedic surgeon.[2] Importantly, plan concepts and strategies for actual plans need to be supported by data and evidence.

### I. Executive Summary

This summary is written after the plan has been completed. Its objective is to concisely explain the organization's most important strategic marketing goal, the impediment to reaching the goal, and the solution to removing the impediment. Your selection of the primary marketing goal is based on the most important marketing problem facing the organization. The goal should be achievable, specific, and insightful. For example, "Increasing Shoulder Shop's net income" is vague. A more specific goal explains how you intend to increase revenue: "Reach breakeven for this new service in 12 months by developing a value network with other providers." Second, explain what factors make the goal that you selected the primary goal for the year. Use evidence and data to support your conclusions.

Next, identify the most important impediment that blocks the goal. The impediment should be actionable. You should be able to remove it with your solution. For example, "The economy is in a recession" or "Management cannot make a decision" are not actionable impediments. "A non-existing pipeline of referral sources" is an actionable impediment for Shoulder Shop, and it can be acted upon by understanding and then exceeding the expectations of referral sources.

Finally, offer a solution to the proposed problem that will result in the achievement of your goal. The solution explains the actions you will take to remove your impediment. The solution has three parts. First, outline the strategy of your solution. It may involve strategic marketing tools such as segmentation, targeting, positioning, distribution, promotion, product development, or others.

For example, "Provide innovative orthopedic shoulder services with (1) above average quality measures, (2) proven preventive and rehabilitation outcomes, and (3) a higher value/cost ratio than competitors" will help Shoulder Shop reach its goal. Justify your solution over other possible solutions, but do not provide excessive tactical details. Second, add a fact-based argument *against* your solution that covers the potential disadvantages of the proposed solution. This section identifies the potential downside risk in your solution that management may be considering. Finally, mount a *counter-argument* that shows how the disadvantages described in the argument can be overcome or ignored.

## SHOULDER SHOP—EXECUTIVE SUMMARY

The most important marketing goal in the first 12 months is to reach sales revenue and profit projections. Revenue for the first year of operations is estimated to be $1 million. The practice is expected to be cash flow positive beginning in month 10. Annual revenue is expected to grow 25% in year 2 and 20% in year 3. The forecast for the 10 most frequent shoulder procedures in the local market is 59,000. Shoulder Shop will need 590 procedures (10% of total procedures) to meet its goal.

Shoulder Shop is a new product, and the primary impediment blocking the goal is building awareness and generating trial. The marketing solution that will remove this impediment is targeting orthopedic shoulder referral sources, especially primary care physicians.

The strategy to add new customers is to build relationships with referral sources and communicate Shoulder Shop benefits and points of differentiation. The second step is to retain new customers. Shoulder Shop's most important point of differentiation is delivering a customer-centric experience. This strategy is expected to create customer loyalty and lead to a high level of financial performance.

## II. Situation Analysis

The situation analysis of a strategic health care marketing plan is often misunderstood. Many marketers view the situation analysis as a repository of all market and product data and information. Only data and information relevant to the plan goals and strategies is needed.

### A. Market Summary

1. *Total available market*: A *market* is the set of all actual and potential buyers of a market offer. The size of a market hinges on the number of buyers who might exist for a particular market offer. The *potential market* is the set of people who profess a sufficient level of interest in a market offer. The *available* market also requires that people have the necessary interest, income, and ability to access the product offer. Describe your total available market (TAM) in a short paragraph and quantify the size of the TAM based on evidence.

## SHOULDER SHOP—TOTAL AVAILABLE MARKET

This TAM consists of two different markets. The first is consumers who reside within 30 minutes of the practice, participate in sports, and are willing to spend money to prevent and treat shoulder injuries. There is an estimated 300,000 consumers in this TAM. The second TAM is referral sources for these consumers that include physical therapists, primary care physicians, and Workers' Compensation insurance companies, among others. There are an estimated 400 referral sources in this TAM.

2. *Market segmentation*: A market segment consists of a group of customers who share a similar set of needs and wants. Examples of two different segments of health insurance consumers are those who want low-cost premiums and others who want generous health care benefits. Marketers do not create segments. Their task is to identify segments and decide which to target. Common segmentation variables are: geographic, demographic, psychographic, behavioral, buying criteria, resource level, and buying process.

Not all segmentations are practical for every product. For example, aspirin buyers could be segmented into consumers with blond hair and consumers with brunette hair. Of course, hair color is not relevant to the purchase of aspirin. If all aspirin customers consume the same number of tablets each month, believe that every aspirin brand is essentially the same, and would pay only one price, any type of aspirin buyer market segmentation would have little value. Market segments must rate favorably on five key criteria to be useful:

### Market Segment Criteria

1. Measurable: The size, purchasing power, and characteristics of the segment can be measured.
2. Substantial: The segment is large and profitable enough to serve.
3. Accessible: The segment can be effectively reached and served.
4. Differentiable: The segments are conceptually distinguishable and respond differently to marketing mix elements and programs. If two segments respond similarly to an offer, they are not separate segments.
5. Actionable: Effective programs can be formulated to attract and serve the segment.

Marketers are increasingly combining several variables in an effort to recognize smaller segments to better define target groups. This has led some market researchers to advocate a seven-step needs-based market segmentation approach:[3]

## Steps in the Segmentation Process

| | |
|---|---|
| 1. Needs-based segmentation | Group customers into segments based on similar needs and benefits sought by customers to solve a particular consumption problem. |
| 2. Segment identification | For each needs-based segment, determine which demographics, lifestyles, and usage behaviors make the segment distinct and identifiable (actionable). |
| 3. Segment attractiveness | Using predetermined segment attractiveness criteria (such as market growth, competitive intensity, and market access), determine the overall attractiveness of each segment. |
| 4. Segment profitability | Determine segment profitability by estimating segment revenue and costs to serve. |
| 5. Segment positioning | For each segment, create a value proposition and the product-price positioning strategy based on that segment's unique customer needs and characteristics. |
| 6. Segment "acid-test" | Create segment storyboards to test the attractiveness of each segment's positioning strategy through consumer research. |
| 7. Marketing mix strategy | Expand segment positioning strategy to include all aspects of the marketing mix: product, price, promotion, and place. |

## SHOULDER SHOP—MARKET SEGMENTATION

*End-user consumer segmentation*

The arthroscopic shoulder surgery end-user consumer market can be divided into three segments. Each segment is expected to contribute to 30% of Shoulder Shop annual revenue.

1. Young athletes: Segment size = 130,000. Age 15 to 25, men and women, involved in sporting activities with extreme overhead activity such as swimming, tennis, pitching, and weightlifting. *Psychographics*: Segment is emotionally "invincible" until they become physically incapacitated.

2. Injured workers: Segment size = 28,000. This population includes laborers performing everyday activities such as washing walls, hanging curtains, masonry, and landscaping. A typical segment member in the local market is an Hispanic male, age 20 to 50. *Psychographics*: Segment tends to delay treatment for physical injury until it substantially impairs work performance.

3. Older adult athletes: Segment size = 140,000. Men and women, age 45 to 70, who are increasingly active and susceptible to shoulder injuries such as rotator cuff tears and shoulder instability related athletic performance that is subject to aging and weakening shoulder structures. This segment has aged physically but has not fully accepted the need to modify physical performance expectations.

*Referral source segmentation*

An analysis of orthopedic physician procedures indicates that 95% of end-users seek orthopedic care based on a referral and the remaining 5% are self-referred. Primary care physicians are forecast to represent 85% of total referrals; and the remaining 15% of referrals will be from Workers' Compensation plans, health and fitness clubs, sports teams, and attorneys specializing in representing injured clients. The primary care physician segment will be further analyzed by medical specialty, size of group, location, affiliation with Shoulder Shop, and referral volume.

3. *Competition*: It is important to understand the strengths, weaknesses, positioning, and apparent strategy of competitors. This information allows you to monitor product differentiation and to anticipate competitor moves. Table 2.1 is a useful tool to summarize an analysis of your most important competitors.

"Competition" can be broadly considered as any product that can be used as a substitute. Substitutes include similar organizations such as two pediatric practices in the same ZIP code. Losing weight and exercise are important to managing adult-onset Type 2 diabetes. A yoga studio may be considered a competitor to a spin or a Pilates studio for members of the Type 2 diabetes market. Identify com-

TABLE 2.1 **Strategic Competitor Analysis Grid**

| Competitor | Market Share Estimate | Strengths | Weaknesses | Positioning | Apparent Strategy |
|---|---|---|---|---|---|
| 1. | | | | | |
| 2. | | | | | |
| 3. | | | | | |

petitors by asking consumers about their potential exercise choices. Organizations offering a new product frequently think they have no competition. The first company to market an electronic health record did not have another software product competitor, but they did compete with traditional paper-based medical records.

## SHOULDER SHOP—COMPETITION: ANALYSIS BASED ON THE STRATEGIC COMPETITOR GRID

Orthopedic surgeon competitors were identified for our market area using the American Academy of Orthopedic Surgeons (AAOS) database. A total of 36 board-certified orthopedic surgeons are in our target market area. The population is approximately 363,000. Therefore, there are 9.9 orthopedic surgeons per 100,000 population.

Although the density of orthopedic surgeons in the target market exceeds the national estimate of 6.2 per 100,000 population, rapid growth in the target market and a fixed number of orthopedic surgeons has resulted in a relative decline in orthopedic surgeon availability. Additionally, the density data do not account for our shoulder subspecialty. According to AAOS data, fewer than 4% of orthopedic surgeons designate a shoulder subspecialty.

4. *Market opportunities and threats*: Market opportunities and threats are identified through analyzing health care environmental trends and how they affect market participants. The six trends are demographic, economic, social-cultural, natural, technological, and political-legal. The nine participants are consumers, providers, payers, employers, government, professional associations, health care advocacy groups, health care suppliers, and competitors. Environmental trends and market participants are fully explained in Chapter 3.

A market opportunity is an area of buyer need and interest in which there is a high probability that the organization can profitably satisfy that need. There are three main sources of market opportunities. The first is provide more of a product that is in short supply. An example during the current, ongoing Covid-19 pandemic is providing face masks, toilet paper, and lounge wear. A second source is adding a benefit to an existing product based on consumer suggestions. Another Covid-19 example is moving gym-based exercise classes from indoor to outdoor locations. A third approach is to ask consumers to imagine an ideal version of the offering and ask them to chart their steps in acquiring, using, and disposing of the product. The third source often leads to a totally new product. Creating alternative travel experiences using virtual reality technology, expert native tour guides, combined with the food and beverage of the area of travel is an opportunity for home-based travel during the pandemic.[4]

Next, the organization applies market opportunity analysis (MOA) to determine the attractiveness and success probability of each opportunity by asking the following five questions:[5]

1. Can the benefits involved in the opportunity be articulated to a defined target market?

2. Can the target market(s) be located and reached with cost-effective communication channels?

3. Does the organization have access to the capabilities and resources needed to deliver the customer benefits?

4. Can the organization deliver the benefits better than any actual or potential competitor?

5. Will the financial rate of return meet or exceed the company's threshold for investments?

## SHOULDER SHOP—MARKET OPPORTUNITY ANALYSIS

The best market opportunity facing Shoulder Shop is in the upper-left cell (#1) of the Opportunity Matrix. The opportunity in the lower-right cell (#4) is too minor to consider. The opportunities in the upper-right cell (#2) and the lower-left cell (#3) should be monitored for attractiveness and success probability.

1. The increase in national rates of rotator cuff repair over the last decade has been dramatic, particularly for arthroscopic assisted repair (the focus of Shoulder Shop).

2. There is a slow-growing payer preference for capitated, bundled orthopedic services and pricing.

3. An academic medical center has expressed interest in acquiring Shoulder Shop in two years.
4. Payers may be interested in an innovative orthopedic surgical outcome measure.

### Opportunity Matrix

|  |  | Success Probability | |
|---|---|---|---|
|  |  | **High** | **Low** |
| **Attractiveness** | **High** | 1 | 2 |
|  | **Low** | 3 | 4 |

Answer the questions and then create an opportunity matrix to compare the different marketing opportunities.

An environmental threat is a challenge posed by an unfavorable external trend or development that would lead, in the absence of defensive marketing action, to lower sales or profit. Threats should be classified according to seriousness and probability of occurrence. Major threats require the development of contingency plans that spell out changes the organization can make if necessary.

## SHOULDER SHOP—MARKET THREAT ANALYSIS

The threats in the upper-left cell of the Threat Matrix are major since they can seriously hurt Shoulder Shop and they have a high probability of occurrence. To deal with them, the practice needs contingency plans that spell out changes it can make before or during the threat. The threats in the lower-right cell are very minor and can be ignored. The threats in the upper-right and lower-left cells need to be monitored carefully in the event that they grow more serious.

1. Blue Cross Blue Shield, the largest practice payer, is about to require additional quality and outcomes reporting. This will necessitate a substantial investment in health information technology.
2. The Medicare percentage of payers is expected to increase rapidly, and practice reimbursement will decrease. The market has been acclaimed by *Sunset* magazine as a new prime retirement location.

3. Several higher acuity procedures require inpatient hospitalization, and health systems near the practice have not decided if they will offer privileges to Shoulder Shop physicians.
4. Tennis, golf, bowling, and swimming are becoming less popular and so will reduce shoulder injuries.

**Threat Matrix**

|  |  | Success Probability | |
| --- | --- | --- | --- |
|  |  | **High** | **Low** |
| **Seriousness** | **High** | 1 | 2 |
|  | **Low** | 3 | 4 |

### B. Product Summary

1. *Product description*: This section briefly explains the different components of the product in two or three short paragraphs. For example, it could describe the physical product if there is a physical element, the service product, and how the physical and service components relate to each other. The purpose of this section is to succinctly describe the product offering as you would to a new acquaintance at a party.

## SHOULDER SHOP—PRODUCT DESCRIPTION

This new practice will provide a single site, niche, subspecialty orthopedic surgery clinic focusing on prevention, evaluation, surgery, and rehabilitation of the shoulder. The on-site facilities include a state-of-the-art ambulatory surgery center, physical medicine and rehabilitation services, Workers' Compensation evaluation services, and a chronic pain management clinic. Specific surgical procedures include:

- arthroscopic rotator cuff repair
- open rotator cuff repair
- arthroscopic acromioplasty
- total shoulder replacement
- resection of distal clavicle for arthritis
- manipulations and arthroscopic releases for frozen shoulder
- arthroscopic stabilization for dislocation
- open stabilization for dislocation
- operative fixation of clavicle fractures
- operative fixation of proximal humeral fracture.

2. *Value proposition*: The value proposition consists of the whole cluster of benefits the organization promises to deliver. The value proposition is a statement about the resulting experience customers will gain from the organization's market offering and from their relationship with the organization itself. The brand must represent a promise about the total experience customers can expect. Whether the promise is kept depends on the organization's ability to manage its customer experiences.[6] Your plan value proposition should be aimed at a specific target market, be differentiated from competitors, and supported by every product and service touch point between your organization and your customers.

## SHOULDER SHOP—VALUE PROPOSITION

There are two target markets and two distinct value propositions.

*Value proposition for referral sources*
Shoulder Shop delivers orthopedic services using a team-based approach. This approach, similar to the collaborative delivery model used by the Mayo Clinic, is patient-centered, includes all of the clinicians involved in a particular case, and focuses on clear two-way communication. Participants are primary care physicians, physiatrists, occupational therapists, physical therapists, massage therapists, and Workers' Compensation coordinators. A much sought after fellowship training site will be offered for subspecialized post-graduate surgical training in the managementof shoulder disorders.

*Value proposition for consumers*
Delivering a customer experience that exceeds expectations is the essence of the Shoulder Shop value proposition. Each customer will have a personal health coach. The coach will be the customer contact for all clinical, scheduling, and billing services. Additionally, pain-free operative recoveries will be offered using an innovative catheter-based regional anesthetic technique providing 7 to 10 days of analgesia, extending into the rehabilitation phases of the postoperative period.

3. *Product results*: Product volume and revenue data over the past three years are summarized. Begin by collecting these data and building a table that includes indices showing the percentage change from year to year for each data point. Use these data to analyze the trends and summarize conclusions.

# SHOULDER SHOP—PRODUCT RESULTS

*(Shoulder Shop is a new product and does not yet have product results. The example of product results below, from an established orthopedic practice shown as "The Practice," illustrates patient visit volume.)*

The Practice received patient referrals from 47% of total referral sources in the primary market.

The Practice had referrals from 42 different referral sources in the past year. There are 90 total orthopedic referral sources in the primary market. The Practice received referrals from 63% of physiatrists and 61% of internal medicine doctors and only 30% of fitness centers.

### 2019 Referral Sources

| Referral source | Referred Patients to The Practice | Number of Referral Market Sources | Referral Market Share |
|---|---|---|---|
| Internal medicine | 11 | 18 | 61% |
| Physiatrists | 5 | 8 | 63% |
| Urgent care centers | 3 | 8 | 38% |
| Fitness centers | 6 | 20 | 30% |
| Family medicine | 17 | 36 | 47% |
| **Total** | **42** | **90** | **47%** |

New patient visit volume in 2019 is the highest in three years.

There were 110 new patients in 2019 compared to 94 in 2016, a 17% increase. This reverses the 28% slide in new patients from 2015 to 2016. This change is the result of adding a new physician to The Practice in early 2017.

### New Patient Visits

| New Visits | 2019 | Index vs. Yr. Ago | 2016 | Index vs. Yr. Ago |
|---|---|---|---|---|
| Q 1 | 21 | 66 | 32 | 68 |
| Q 2 | 20 | 83 | 24 | 114 |
| Q 3 | 32 | 188 | 17 | 55 |
| Q 4 | 37 | 176 | 21 | 110 |
| **Total** | **110** | 117 | **94** | 72 |

4. *Product strengths and weaknesses*: Discerning attractive market opportunities is valuable only if an organization has the capability of taking advantage of them. Organizations need to evaluate internal strengths and weaknesses in marketing, finance, manufacturing, and other organizational capabilities. Clearly, the organization does not have to correct all of its weaknesses or be complacent concerning its strengths. The key question is whether the organization should limit itself to those opportunities in which it possesses the required strengths or consider opportunities that might mean acquiring or developing other strengths.

Sometimes an organization does poorly because its departments do not work together well as a team. It is therefore critically important to assess interdepartmental working relationships as part of an internal audit. Larger, more bureaucratic organizations tend to have problems with communication between departmental "silos" that are not incentivized to collaborate. Unfortunately, this cultural norm can prevent these organizations from effectively meeting changing market needs.

It is important that an organization understand its strengths and weaknesses from the customer perspective. Typically, routine customer survey information is collected through a convenience sample. Customers have the opportunity to respond to a satisfaction survey for example, but the vast majority of customers do not actually respond. It is a mistake to assume that information from these surveys can be extrapolated to all an organization's customers. Using a random sample of customers, where each customer has an equal chance of responding, generally provides responses that can be generalized and used to make decisions.

## SHOULDER SHOP—PRODUCT STRENGTHS AND WEAKNESSES

*Strengths*

- Niche practice with special expertise and focus on shoulder surgery only. This focus should lead to increased expertise, better patient outcomes, and lower unit costs.
- Physician director leads the organization. He has over 15 years of experience in orthopedic and shoulder surgery, sports injuries, academic medicine, and private practice.
- All physicians have expertise in minimally-invasive arthroscopic shoulder surgery.
- Newly-constructed ambulatory surgery center has state-of-the-art medical technology and evidence-based design. These elements will support high levels of clinical outcomes.
- The pain management clinic is directed by a full-time anesthesiologist, and it uses indwelling regional anesthesia infusion catheters that provide continuous local anesthetic infusion.
- The organization is customer-centric. Referral sources have real-time access to Shoulder Shop patient records. Consumers are supported through concierge-style customer service.

*Weaknesses*
- Competitive orthopedic practices are well-funded and growing aggressively.
- The organization has assumed a high level of financial debt to fund development.
- Continuous surgeon and administrative recruitment efforts must be conducted and funded to ensure that growth targets are reached.
- An alliance needs to be developed immediately with an innovative radiology practice to collaborate on comprehensive care.

*C. Primary Marketing Challenges*   The purpose of this section of the plan is to draw conclusions from your analysis of the preceding market summary and product summary. What are the most pressing market and product issues? For example, what product changes may be necessary to better align your product offering with market trends? How can you further differentiate it from competitors? Is there evidence to support a new product that will offer value? Is there an opportunity to benefit from establishing a new channel partnership? Overcoming these marketing challenges will be your focus in the strategies sections of the plan.

## SHOULDER SHOP—PRIMARY MARKETING CHALLENGES

- Brand differentiation of Shoulder Shop is a major challenge. Targeted referral sources and consumers need to believe that the offering delivers a more meaningful benefit than competitors.
- Employee engagement and loyalty are critical. The company cannot build relationships with customers if employees are not customer-centric and empowered to serve customers.
- Adequate investment capital for the first 24 months is an important priority. We need to raise twice as much capital than we project we will need. This challenge and solution is common in start-up development.

### III. Marketing Goals and Objectives

Marketing goals are developed based on the situation analysis. Goals are used to direct resource allocation for managing the product. Effective goals are realistic and based on data and evidence. Goals represent the two or three most important marketing achievements that are expected to be reached in the next

12 months, and one of them is usually financial. The different goals need to be coordinated. For example, many believe that goals of maximizing sales and simultaneously maximizing profits is not possible. Each goal calls for a different marketing strategy. Objectives are quantified goals that measure progress. Objectives are specific and can be measured daily, weekly, monthly, and quarterly. Measuring objectives carefully will allow the organization to monitor performance and change strategies if necessary.

## SHOULDER SHOP—GOALS AND OBJECTIVES

*A. Goal*—Breakeven in the fourth quarter of year 1.

Objective—Year 1 revenue is projected to be $2.147 million. Breakeven will occur in month 10.

*B. Goal*—Establish Shoulder Shop as the orthopedic customer loyalty leader.

Objective—Referral source and consumer NPS will be in the 90th percentile or higher.

*C. Goal*—Become the market leader for orthopedic value-based purchasing contracting.

Objective—Contract with four payers and a pool of value partners for capitation contracts.

### IV. Overall Strategies—Concepts and Examples

Overall strategies are used to achieve plan goals and objectives and explain the target market strategy, marketing research strategy, and positioning strategy. These three overall strategies also direct the four marketing mix strategies: product, price, place, and promotion.

*A. Target Market Strategy* The *target market* is the subset of the qualified available market. In evaluating different market segments, the organization must look at two factors: the segment's overall attractiveness and the organization's objectives and resources. An ideal segment selected for targeting is generally attractive, sufficiently large, rapidly growing, highly profitability, has substantial scale economies, and is low risk. Some attractive segments may not mesh with the organization's long-run objectives, or the organization may lack one or more necessary competencies to offer superior value. There are five approaches to selecting segments to target:

1. *Single-segment concentration*: Quorum Health Resources concentrates on the small hospital market for consulting and management services, unlike the EY consultancy that focuses on larger hospitals. Concentrated marketing gives an organization deep knowledge of its target segment's needs and behaviors and it

achieves a strong segment presence. It also achieves operating economies by specializing in the segment's product needs, channels, and promotion. The risks are that a particular market segment can decrease buying patterns or a competitor may invade the segment with a higher value offering. Many organizations prefer to operate in more than one segment.

2. *Selective specialization*: The organization selects a number of segments, each objectively attractive and appropriate. There may be little or no synergy among the segments but each promises to be profitable. This multi-segment strategy has the advantage of diversifying risk. When Procter & Gamble launched Crest Whitestrips, initial target segments included newly engaged women, bridal parties, as well as gay men.

3. *Product specialization*: Another approach is to specialize in designing a product for several different segments. The microscope marketplace is roughly divided into the bio-med, industrial, and geology segments. Although the frames may be the same across markets, the optics and accessory modules are segment-specific. Each segment has its defining uses and sales requirements. The organization makes different microscopes for the different customer groups and builds a strong reputation in the specific product area. The downside risk is that the product may be supplanted by an entirely new technology.

4. *Market specialization*: The firm concentrates on serving the many needs of a particular customer group. An example is a health care company that sells an assortment of products solely to university research laboratories. The company gains a strong reputation in serving this customer group and becomes a channel for additional products that the customer group can use. The downside risk is that the overall customer group may suffer budget cuts or shrink in size.

5. *Full market coverage*: Some organizations attempt to serve all customer groups with all the products they might need. In *undifferentiated marketing*, the organization ignores segment differences and goes after the whole market with one offer. Many community hospitals try to serve all segments in their service areas and profitability is a secondary concern. In *differentiated marketing*, the organization creates several different divisions, operates in several market segments, and designs different products for each segment. Differentiated marketing typically creates more total sales and more costs than undifferentiated marketing. This lack of centralization can also be a problem. Baxter, a leading supplier of sterile solutions, had several divisions selling different products and services to hospitals with each division sending out its own invoices. Receiving as many as seven different Baxter monthly invoices confused some hospitals. Baxter's marketers convinced the divisions to consolidate their billing through a single, comprehensive invoice.

Market targeting can also generate public controversy.[7] The public is concerned when marketers are perceived to take unfair advantage of vulnerable or disadvantaged groups. Turing Pharmaceuticals was widely criticized for purchasing the rights to a drug used by AIDS and cancer patients and raising prices from less than $17 to $750 per pill.[8] Socially responsible marketing calls for targeting that serves not only the organization's interests but also the interests of those targeted.

## SHOULDER SHOP—TARGET MARKET STRATEGY

Shoulder Shop is using a selective specialization targeting strategy. The primary target market is referral sources. The majority of orthopedic consumers are referred to orthopedic specialists by a trusted physician, health club, and Workers' Compensation insurance coordinators, based on our marketing research with 50 prospective customers.

A secondary target is consumers likely to experience shoulder disorders in our primary market area. The consumers are athletes typically between 15 and 25 years old as well as exercise conscious males and females over 45 years old. We will also target manual laborers between 20 and 40 years old.

**B. Marketing Research Strategy** Marketing research is routinely used to make informed marketing decisions. Research data and information are analyzed during preparation of the plan situation analysis. It is also used to select particular strategies. The purpose of this section of the plan is to describe the marketing research that is needed in the next 12 months.

Secondary marketing research includes information and data that have been previously collected and is easily accessible. Sources include directories, databases, population demographics, health disease statistics, company information, hospital and physician utilization data, and other information that is often available online (Table 2.2).

*Primary marketing* research is conducted when specific decisions need data and information that are not available through secondary research. Primary data can be collected in five main ways: through observation, focus groups, surveys, behavioral data, and experiments. Examples include ethnographic studies, in-depth individual interviews, brand awareness surveys, and psychographic studies. A hospital needed to know how to react to a highly publicized death caused by medical error. The potential damage to the hospital's reputation could cost millions of dollars in lost research funding and patient revenue.

TABLE 2.2 **Sample of Secondary Research Sources**

- FierceHealthCare: www.fiercehealthcare.com
- HealthLeaders Media: www.healthleadersmedia.com
- Healthcare Finance News: www.healthfinancenews.com
- Kaiser Family Foundation: www.kff.org
- AdvaMed for medical technology innovations: www.advamed.org
- Bioworld Today daily biopharmaceutical news: www.bioworld.com
- American Medical Association data: www.ama-assn.org/
- Centers for Medicare & Medicaid Services data: www.cms.gov

A quantitative telephone survey of 1,000 consumers was quickly conducted to measure awareness and attitudes toward the error. Consumers understood that accidents happen, the hospital needed to solve the problem immediately, and it was very important that the hospital be more clear about the circumstances. The hospital then used the research to respond to these points through media relations and advertising.

## SHOULDER SHOP—MARKETING RESEARCH STRATEGY

Shoulder Shop will focus on customer loyalty in the next year and will survey referral sources and consumers using the Net Promoter Score (NPS). NPS respondents use a 0 to 10 scale to answer a single question: How likely are you to recommend Shoulder Shop to a colleague or patient? We will calculate baselines for referral sources and consumers, and we will also measure competitor NPS. This information will be used to develop strategies that increase the number of Promoters (ratings of 9 or 10) and decrease the number of Detractors (ratings of 0 to 6).

*C. Positioning Strategy*   The concept of strategic positioning was popularized in the 1980s by two advertising executives, Al Ries and Jack Trout. They were concerned with increasing advertising clutter and how consumers were coping with message overload. Positioning was their solution to the problem. In their words, "Positioning starts with a product. A piece of merchandise, a service, a company, an institution, or even a person … but positioning is not what you do to a product. Positioning is what you do to the mind of the prospect. That is, you position the product in the mind of the prospect."[9]

Product positioning helps guide marketing strategy by clarifying the brand's essence, what goals it helps the consumer achieve, and how it does so in a unique way. The positioning of many organizations cannot be discerned because they do not have a positioning. Research has shown that most companies do a poor job of positioning or they attempt to be all things to all people.[10] Having a meaningful benefit is a prerequisite. Research is needed to confirm the value of the benefit with the target market. Research is also needed to validate that the benefit is clearly differentiated from competitors. An effective positioning strategy focuses on a single benefit, point of differentiation, and is implemented consistently through all marketing communication.

The standard positioning format is a helpful tool for developing a positioning strategy:

> *To (the target market), the (product) is the brand (frame of reference) that (primary benefit) because (key differentiating attributes).*

While an organization welcomes the purchase of its products by anyone, marketing resources focus on a particular target market. The frame of reference is a product's relationship to a product category. It suggests the points-of-parity it has with other products in the category. The primary benefit should meet a need that is not already being met and communicated by a competitor. The product's differentiating attributes validate the benefit and further separate it from competitors.

## SHOULDER SHOP—POSITIONING STRATEGY

Shoulder Shop will use the following positioning:

> *To referral sources and active consumers, Shoulder Shop is the brand of comprehensive shoulder care that prevents, treats, and rehabilitates shoulder injuries because it has superior clinical expertise and puts the customer first.*

Referral sources and active consumers represent the primary market. Shoulder Shop has created a new frame of reference by offering shoulder injury prevention, diagnosis, treatment, and rehab in one location. Its unique offering focuses on a narrow subspecialty and comprehensive services. Other orthopedic practices in the market are not focused on shoulders or on complete care. Benefit support is that Shoulder Shop orthopedists provide academic medical center clinical quality care in a convenient and customer-centric practice.

### V. Marketing Mix Strategies and Tactics

Strategies are defined as *how* goals and objectives are reached. Tactics are *what* tasks need to be performed to implement the strategy. The marketing mix section of the plan explains the product, price, place (or channels), and promotion strategies. These four strategies are often referred to as the 4Ps of marketing. They work together with the overall targeting and positioning strategies to achieve the goals.

For example, if a cosmetic dermatology practice in Beverly Hills, California, targets high-income females age 35 to 65, their product strategies need to meet customer expectations for superior clinical results, discretion, and luxury. The pricing strategy reflects the high perceived value and clinical results of the cosmetic services. The channels strategy, or value network, is composed of customer inbound and outbound referral sources that are positioned similarly to the cosmetic dermatology practice. The focus of the promotion strategy is based on maintaining loyal customers who generate personal word-of-mouth referrals.

**A. Product Strategy and Tactics**   Branding is the foundation of product strategy, and branding unifies the four marketing mix strategies. A brand is not simply a product name or logo. *A brand is essentially a promise about an experience with a product.* It is a seller's commitment to consistently deliver a specific set of benefits, features, and services. Effective brands strive to engage customers on a deep level by satisfying multiple needs and fostering a relationship with the product. The best brands convey a sense of trust. Brands can also signal a certain level of quality so that satisfied buyers can easily choose the product again.

Branding can be applied virtually anywhere a consumer has a choice. The key to branding is that consumers must not think that all brands in the category are the same.[11] Branding is about creating differences. For branding strategies to be successful and brand value to be created, consumers must be convinced that there are meaningful differences among brands in the product category. To brand a product, it is necessary to teach consumers "who" the product is—by giving it a name and using other brand elements to help identify it—as well as "what" the product does and "why" consumers should care. For example, the Mayo Clinic brand can convey up to five levels of meaning: attributes, benefits, culture, personality, and user (Table 2.3).[12]

The product strategy is the most important element in the marketing mix. Products are developed to meet target customers' needs or wants. The customer will judge the product offering by the criteria of (1) product features and quality, (2) services mix and quality, and (3) price. All three elements must be woven into a competitively attractive offering.[13] Product strategy calls for making coordinated decisions on product mixes, product lines, brands, and packaging and labeling. Many people usually think of a product as a tangible offering, but a product can be much more. A product is anything that can be offered to a market to satisfy a want or need. Health care products that are marketed include physical goods, services, experiences, events, places, properties, organizations, information, and ideas.

TABLE 2.3 **Levels of Brand Meaning**

| Meaning | Description | Example |
|---|---|---|
| 1. Attributes | A brand brings to mind certain attributes. | Mayo Clinic suggests "patients first," treatment of last resort, and collaborative doctors. |
| 2. Benefits | Attributes must be translated into functional and emotional benefits. | The attribute "patients first" could translate into the functional benefit of "I feel less tension and stress as a patient." |
| 3. Culture | The brand may represent a certain culture. | Mayo represents a tradition based on founder William Mayo's 1910 vision that medicine is a "cooperative science." |
| 4. Personality | The brand can project a certain personality. | Mayo may suggest an intelligent, wise, and caring doctor or a peaceful healing oasis (place). |
| 5. User | The brand suggests the kind of customer who buys or uses the product. | Mayo services are purchased by a diverse group ranging from international royalty to people living near one of its more than 60 primary care clinics or 21 owned or managed hospitals. |

The health care organization needs to address five product levels in planning its market offering (Figure 2.1).[14] The fundamental level is the **core benefit** that the customer is really seeking. A patient visiting a hospital to deliver a baby is seeking "a safe, healthy birth." The purchaser of aspirin is buying "headache relief." Marketers must see themselves as benefit providers.

The marketer turns the core benefit into a *basic product* at the second level. Thus, a patient hospital room in a maternity department includes a bed that doubles as a delivery table, a scale, an ultrasound machine, a recliner, and high intensity lights. At the third level, the marketer prepares an *expected product*, a set of attributes and conditions buyers normally expect when they purchase this product. Maternity patients can expect a clean gown, fresh bedding, working lamps, acceptable food, and a relative degree of quiet.

At the fourth level, the marketer may offer an *augmented product* that exceeds customer expectations. *Product differentiation takes place mostly at the augmentation*

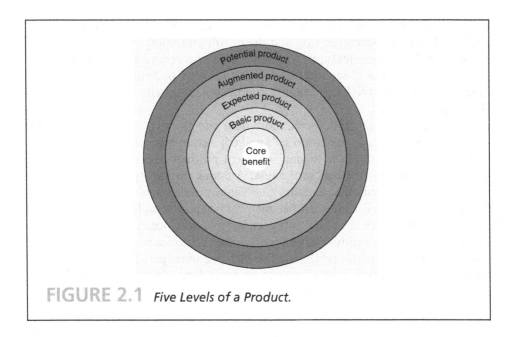

FIGURE 2.1   *Five Levels of a Product.*

*level.* Product augmentation leads the marketer to look at the user's total consumption system, which is the way the user performs the tasks of getting and using products and related services.[15] For hospitals in developed countries, these augmented products often include the following features: access to specialized care, coordination of care, information and education, physical comfort, continuity and transition to home, emotional support, involvement of family and friends, and respect for patient preferences.[16] This augmented offering is triggered by the intense competition for maternity patients in developed countries. In developing countries and emerging markets such as China and India, however, competition takes place mostly at the expected product level.

Each augmentation adds cost. Augmented benefits soon become expected benefits and necessary competitive points-of-parity. Today's hospital customers expect cable TV, Wi-Fi, and a wide range of dining choices. As organizations raise the price of their augmented product, some competitors may offer a stripped-down version at a much lower price. Two medical device examples are companies that manufacture simpler medication administration pumps and those that produce glucose monitors with fewer features.

At the fifth and last level stands the *potential product* which encompasses all the possible augmentations and transformations the product or offering might undergo in the future. Here is where companies search for new ways to delight customers and distinguish their offering. An example is the driving force behind The Birthplace at CaroMont Regional Medical Center. CaroMont wanted to address the many preferences of women's families throughout the birthing process, both inpatient and outpatient. They designed a world-class birthing center dedicated to family-centered care and the health and safety of both mother and baby. The Birthplace features 52 labor, delivery, recovery, and postpartum (LDRP) rooms, three C-section operating suites, a 16-bed single-room Neonatal Intensive Care Unit (NICU), a family dining area, children's play area. and family resource center.[17]

Finally, most organizations sell more than one product. A product mix is the set of all products an organization sells and consists of various product lines. The width of a product mix is how many different product lines are carried, and the depth is the number of items in the mix. A community hospital usually has an outpatient product mix that includes emergency, routine, and diagnostic services. An academic medical center outpatient product mix is wider and deeper with additional services for specialty, subspecialty, and advanced diagnostic lines in a number of locations. Product mix analysis is used to decide which product lines to grow, maintain, harvest, and divest. Product-line managers need to understand the product mix market profile, revenue, costs, and margin to determine the optimal resource and investment allocation for that line.

## SHOULDER SHOP—PRODUCT STRATEGY AND TACTICS

The practice has created an augmented product that exceeds customer expectations and is highly differentiated in the market. Shoulder Shop will offer a comprehensive shoulder health product line. An important underlying differentiator of this product line is that the customer relationship will begin and continue longer than relationships with competing orthopedic practices.

The first product is preventive services to enhance shoulder wellness. The customer relationship will begin before a shoulder injury. The services include exercise evaluations, coaching for avoiding shoulder injuries for specific sports, and educational information briefings on cutting-edge developments in shoulder health and injury.

The second product will be diagnostic and treatment services. These services are clinically state-of-the-art and medically holistic. Exercise, pharmaceutical, myofascial trigger point dry needling, and other procedures will be used before surgery is considered. Shoulder Shop orthopedists are former academic medical center physicians who are national key opinion leaders with interests in clinical innovations and medical collaborations with other types of providers. Shoulder Shop also has the latest technology to improve shoulder treatment outcomes and lower costs.

The third product focuses on rehabilitation. Shoulder Shop has physical therapists, a physiatrist, occupational therapists, and nutritionists who tailor services and products that treat as well as prevent shoulder injuries from recurring. This product extends the customer relationship beyond the relationship of a traditional orthopedic practice.

**B. Pricing Strategy and Tactics**  Health care consumers have traditionally been price-takers and accepted prices without question. Consumers are becoming more interested in pricing because they are now responsible for a higher share of their total health care costs. Price is the only marketing mix element that produces revenue. The others produce costs. Health care organizations that use pricing as a strategic tool will profit more than those that simply let shifting market costs determine their pricing. In setting pricing strategy, a health care organization should follow a six-step procedure (Figure 2.2).[18]

*Step 1: Selecting the pricing objective*

An organization first decides where it wants to position its marketing offerings. It can pursue five major objectives through pricing:

1. *Survival*: Organizations pursue survival as their major objective if they are plagued with overcapacity, intense competition, or changing consumer wants. As long as prices cover variable costs and some fixed costs, the organization stays in business. A struggling rural hospital with overcapacity may choose survival as a short-term strategy.

2. *Maximize current profit*: Organizations use this objective, focused on short-term financial results, by estimating the demand and costs associated with alternative prices and choose the price that produces maximum current profit, cash flow, or rate of return on investment. A publicly-traded company like Humana may use this objective to reach or exceed quarterly earnings targets. In the long-term, however, underspending for brand development and ignoring competitor moves may sacrifice long-run performance.

3. *Maximize market share*: Organizations that choose the maximum market share objective believe that higher sales volume will lead to lower unit costs and higher long-term profit. Also known as penetration pricing, a low price in a price sensitive market will lead to lower production and distribution costs in addition to high product volume.

4. *Maximize market skimming*: Organizations unveiling a new product or technology favor setting high prices to maximize market skimming. Pharmaceutical companies that introduce innovative new drugs use market

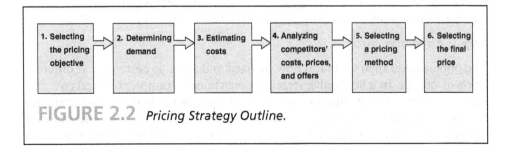

FIGURE 2.2  *Pricing Strategy Outline.*

skimming to gain revenue quickly in a market with high expected demand. Prices are slowly reduced when competitors enter the market or drug patents expire.

5. *Product-quality leadership*: An organization may aim to be the product-quality leader in the market. This pricing objective has become more wide-spread since the enactment of the Affordable Care Act and financial incentives for higher clinical quality and lower prices. Advanced Home Care, a large home health company in the Southeast, has entered a risk-based payment arrangement to treat congestive heart failure, asthma, pneumonia, and other chronic conditions by bundling services and developing stronger relationships with other health care organizations.

### Step 2: Determining demand

The next step is to estimate the demand curve and the probable quantities that it will sell at each possible price. In most industries, the higher the price, the lower the demand. The quantity of health care products and services sold, however, does not necessarily change with price. Prices for newer treatments are often higher for the products they replace.[19] Estimating demand is influenced by what affects price sensitivity. One approach is to conduct a field experiment to observe the effect of different pricing on the same product. A chain of urgent care centers could vary the prices of services offered in different locations and observe changes in customer volume.

The sensitivity of the volume change for different prices is called elasticity of demand. If the price of a product increases, and the change in market demand is minimal, demand for this product is inelastic. Many insurance-reimbursed health products and services are inelastic because, after paying an annual deductible, consumers often pay a low percentage of total costs.

If market demand for a product varies with price, then demand is elastic. Prices for non-reimbursed products like *in vitro* fertilization procedures or LASIK eye surgery are typically elastic. The lower the price the higher the volume. Health care product prices are often decreased in an attempt to increase product volume. This strategy, however, has commonly resulted in a decrease in revenue per customer and no increase in volume. Market research can be used to test price elasticity with customers before decreasing or increasing prices to forecast potential changes in volume. Demand sets the ceiling on the price and internal costs set the floor.

### Step 3: Estimating costs

The organization then estimates how its fixed and variable costs vary at different levels of output. In a hospital emergency department, examples of fixed costs are electricity, beds, the information system, and equipment. Variable cost examples are employee labor costs, supply costs, and maintenance. It is also important to estimate competitors' costs and prices to further understand their strengths and weaknesses. Pharmaceutical companies frequently introduce second-to-market products at prices slightly below competitors in a particular therapeutic category. This practice of setting prices just below competitors is called shadow pricing.

***Step 4:*** *Analyzing competitors' costs, prices, and offers*

Within the range of possible prices determined by market demand and internal costs, the organization must take competitors' costs, prices, and possible public price reactions into account. If the organization's offer contains features not offered by the nearest competitor, it should evaluate their worth to the customer and add that value to the competitor's price. Conversely, if the competitor's offer contains some features not offered by the organization, the firm should subtract their value from its own price. Now the organization can potentially decide whether it can charge more, the same, or less than the competitor. The introduction or change of any price can provoke a response from customers, competitors, distributors, payers, the media, and government. Competitors are most likely to react when the number of firms is few, the products are undifferentiated, and buyers are familiar with product benefits and features. Competitor reactions can be a special problem when these firms have a strong value proposition.

Mylan produces the EpiPen auto-injector that is often used to treat potentially life-threatening allergic reactions in children. Parents became alarmed when Mylan raised prices from $250 in 2013 to over $600 in 2016.[20] Mylan responded to this negative publicity by offering a new generic version of the EpiPen identical to the original product but at half the price. The generic EpiPen now competes with the original product.[21]

***Step 5:*** *Selecting a pricing method*

Four commonly used pricing methods are markup pricing, target-return pricing, perceived value pricing, and going-rate pricing.

1. *Markup pricing*: This method adds a standard revenue amount or percentage of cost to the total price of the product. It focuses on product costs, and its weakness is that it does not consider perceived product value, competitors, or estimated market demand. Prescription drugs often use this method with markups of 100% by manufacturers, wholesalers, and retailers.

2. *Target-return pricing*: The organization determines the price that would yield its target ROI. The organization must consider different prices and estimate their probable impacts on demand, sales volume, and profits. Sony uses this method to sell radiology monitors by carefully forecasting sales and estimating the time required to reach set ROI targets.

3. *Value-based pricing*: Under the Affordable Care Act, value is measured by medical quality scores, outcome measures, and actively managing the overall health of a specified population. A wide range of health care organizations

now have new financial incentives to focus on these three elements. Physicians and health systems enter capitation payment contracts that give them a flat monthly payment per consumer. They are responsible for preventing, diagnosing, and treating health problems as well as providing and coordinating ongoing care management for chronic conditions. These care providers earn a profit if consumers have lower total costs than the capitation amount, and they lose money when consumer costs are higher than the capitation amount.

4.  *Going-rate pricing*: A fourth pricing method is where organizations set prices largely based on competitors' prices. Usually this method is used when costs are difficult to measure and competitive responses are uncertain. An example is pricing for "second-to-market" products that have an innovative technology. When Merck launched Vioxx to treat arthritis in the new Cox-2 inhibitors category, its pricing was similar to the first entrant, Celebrex. Organizations using a going-rate pricing method need to consider their legality. A specialty dental practice scheduled annual meetings with a competing practice to share pricing information and discuss price changes for the next year. This was price collusion, and the Federal Trade Commission would likely determine that the dentists were illegally fixing prices.

### *Step 6: Setting the price*

Setting the price also must consider the influence of other marketing strategies such as positioning. Since Target department stores are positioned as upscale discount stores, their retail medical clinics inside their stores should be consistent with this positioning. The clinics have a modern product design with lower prices than those charged by a competing retail clinic operated by an academic medical center.

Pricing should also be consistent with organization pricing policies. Since the finance department is responsible for setting prices in most health care organizations, the marketing department needs to provide finance with customer and competitor market data and information. The Vanderbilt University Medical Center marketing department worked with the health system finance department to help negotiate higher payer reimbursement. The marketing department supplied market share data and consumer and clinical quality ratings that supported Vanderbilt's competitive clinical advantage and led to higher reimbursement. Marketing departments can also work with a marketing research firm to conduct mystery shopper interviews with competitive organizations. The objective is to understand the competitor customer experience and to learn about competitive pricing.

Pricing needs to take into account the potential risks of gain-sharing and risk-sharing agreements. MedBill, a physician billing company, contracted with physician practices and hospitals to improve their physician reimbursement and billing results. MedBill guaranteed a monthly cash flow projection for the first 12 months of service to reduce client risk. MedBill service pricing needed to take into consideration market conditions, payer collection cycles, and its own billing performance to ensure accurate client reimbursement and payment forecasts.

Pricing decisions will also be affected by competitor and consumer reactions as well as regulations. Organizations must carefully manage perceptions in raising or lowering prices. How will competitors react to a lower price? Will suppliers raise their prices when they see the organization's higher price? If a service is not reimbursable, such as LASIK surgery, customers may shop for the best price. Will the government or the media intervene to prevent higher prices from being charged? Medicare regulations determine the amount paid for a laboratory test or a physician visit.

## SHOULDER SHOP—PRICING STRATEGY AND TACTICS

Shoulder Shop is using the product-quality pricing objective, and it is entering into traditional fee-for-service payment agreements as well as value-based agreements. It has analyzed market demand and estimated its costs. The going-rate pricing strategy is being used for fee-for-service agreements. Prices will be similar to the orthopedic prices of a local academic center because clinical results are expected to be the same or better.

Shoulder Shop offers injury prevention services—in addition to diagnosis, treatment, and rehabilitation services—that competitors do not offer. It will offer allowances to self-pay customers for these services. Self-pay customers, especially targeting those out of network, will receive the same pricing as commercial insurance customers. The prevention-diagnosis-treatment-rehab bundle of services will also be specially priced and targeted toward innovative payers. Value-based pricing will be communicated clearly through positioning, messaging, and personal and non-personal communication.

*C. Channels Strategy and Tactics*  What are marketing channels and why are they needed? *Marketing channels are defined as sets of interdependent organizations that make a product or service available for use or consumption.*[22] Health care organizations often do not distribute or sell their products or services directly to final users. Between them stands a set of intermediaries performing a variety of functions. These intermediaries form a marketing channel system.

The steps in developing an effective channels strategy begin with analyzing customer flow, assessing the value added by each channel member, calculating how each channel member contributes to the plan marketing objectives, and identifying opportunities for channel innovation. Channel strategy innovation often leads to better integration of channels, product, price, and promotion strategies. You should be able to understand the importance and role of channels, how channels function, and how you can use innovative channel strategies and tactics in your marketing plan.

## What are Marketing Channels?

A marketing channel system performs the work of moving goods from producers to consumers. It overcomes the time, place, and possession gaps that separate goods and services from those who need or want them. Each channel member performs a necessary function. For example, a hospital has Valium on its list of available drugs, and physicians can order prescriptions for their hospitalized patients. The Valium follows a channels process beginning with the hospital purchasing tablets from the manufacturer, Roche USA. The drug is sent from the Roche manufacturing plant to a regional warehouse.

A local drug wholesaler, jobber, or hospital group purchasing organization receives shipments of the drug from the warehouse. These intermediaries then ship the Valium to the hospital pharmacy. The physician orders the Valium at the patient bedside, the pharmacy delivers the drug to the hospital floor, and a nurse brings the tablet to the patient. Other channel systems include patient referral sources, key opinion leaders who influence physicians, retailers, brokers, group purchasing organizations, transportation companies, and warehouses.

## Value Networks

The concept of a value network takes an even broader view. *A value network is a system of partnerships and alliances that an organization creates to source, augment, and deliver its offerings.* A hospital focused on increasing cardiac procedures must consider a series of relationships to form a value network. A family medicine physician sees a patient presenting with chest discomfort and decides to refer the patient to a cardiologist for a heart evaluation. The cardiologist determines that the patient needs a heart valve replacement. The cardiologist then refers the patient to a preferred heart surgeon to replace the valve. The surgeon must decide which hospital they will use for the valve surgery.

Once the patient recovers from surgery, the hospital discharge planner needs to decide which outpatient cardiac rehabilitation program to recommend to the patient for diet counseling and exercise therapy. Depending on the hospital's relationships with the primary care physician, the cardiologist, the cardiac surgeon, and the rehabilitation service, it could potentially influence the choices of some or all of these participants in the value network. The increasing number of value-based payment arrangements, based on bundled services and coordination of care, further reinforces the importance of value networks.

### Roles of Marketing Channels

Although producers lose some control, they find it economically advantageous to delegate some marketing functions to intermediaries. Many producers lack the financial resources to carry out every phase of marketing. The two core competencies of the drug company GSK had traditionally been the research and development (R&D) of new compounds and targeting physicians for sales. The cost of pharma R&D began increasing sharply in the 1990s. GSK abandoned internal R&D and moved to "in-licensing" promising new compounds developed by small biotechs and pharma research specialist companies.

Producers also generally earn a higher return on product manufacturing than on product retailing. A generous retail financial margin is close to 10%. Companies in the artificial knee industry have manufacturing margins as high as 70%, and it does not make financial sense to be involved in retailing. Another reason to engage intermediaries is that direct marketing is simply not feasible. Bayer not surprisingly finds it easier and more profitable to distribute aspirin and its other products through wholesalers and retailers rather than have its own retail outlets.

Intermediaries normally achieve superior efficiency in making goods widely available and accessible to target markets. Through their contacts, experience, specialization, and scale of operation, intermediaries usually offer a manufacturing partner more than it can achieve on its own. Market forces are making health care more available and convenient, and new channels are emerging especially in retail distribution. These new channels offer enhanced access, shorter waiting times, and lower prices.

### Channel Functions and Flows

Members of the marketing channel system perform a number of key functions. Some functions like providing physical possession or title to goods constitute a forward flow of activity from the organization to the customer. Other functions such as ordering and payment constitute a backward flow from customers to the organization. Still others occur in both directions including the flow of information, negotiation, finance, and risk taking. Siemens manufactures and sells MRI imaging equipment and requires at least three channels: a sales channel, a delivery channel, and a service channel. Channel flows can be very complex and require a considerable amount of time to organize.

All channel functions have three things in common: they use up scarce resources, they can often be performed better through specialization, and they can be shifted among channel members. When the manufacturer shifts some functions to intermediaries, the producer's costs and prices are lower, but the intermediary must add a charge to cover its work. If the intermediaries are more efficient than the manufacturer, prices to consumers should be lower. If consumers perform some functions themselves, they should enjoy even lower prices. Changes in channel systems often occur when more cost-effective logistics are adopted to move goods to target customers.

### Service Sector Channels

Marketing channels are not limited to the distribution of physical goods. Producers of services and ideas also face the problem of making their output available and accessible to target populations. While most medical appointments and procedures involve customers traveling to a physician office, hospital, or lab, reversing this channel flow by having clinicians making home visits may result in more value. In UnitedHealth Group's HouseCalls program, physicians or mid-level providers perform comprehensive geriatric assessments for seniors in their homes and make referrals to community providers and health plan resources as needed. This program has been available to UnitedHealth's Medicare Advantage plan members in Arkansas, Georgia, Missouri, South Carolina, and Texas since 2008.

Research found that HouseCalls members had lower levels of hospital admissions and nursing home admissions compared to non-HouseCalls Medicare Advantage members and fee-for-service beneficiaries. HouseCalls members had an average of 4% more office visits to specialist physicians. The study concluded that a thorough home-based clinical assessment of a member's health, their home environment, and prompt referrals as needed supported aging in place and averted costly hospital care.[23]

### Channel Design Decisions

Designing a marketing channel system starts with analyzing customer needs. Because the point of a marketing channel is to make a product available to customers, marketers must understand how its target customers prefer to buy the product. An organization supply chain is best designed from the customer's point of view. This process is called demand-chain planning. It is based on how customers prefer to buy a solution rather than how the organization wants to sell their product.

Examples of channel outputs that need to be considered are lot size, waiting time, convenience, product variety, and added services such as delivery and repair. Does the customer want to buy a large lot, like a fleet of ambulances, or does a household want to buy a lot size of one nasal decongestant? Highly perishable products like blood and organs used for transplant will require three or more intermediary channels to purchase, but they must also have a streamlined delivery channel when ordered. Non-standardized products, such as health care information systems, are sold directly by company sales representatives. Products requiring installation or maintenance services, such as lab centrifuges and PET scanners, are usually sold and maintained by the company or by franchised dealers.

Channel design is also important because the channels chosen affect other marketing mix strategies. There are many different options in selecting channels, and most organizations use a variety of channels to cost-effectively reach different market segments. A channel can be analyzed by the types of intermediaries available, the number of intermediaries needed, and the terms and responsibilities of each channel member. An example of a type of channel known as a *facilitator* is IndUShealth, a company that arranges trips to India for U.S. patients interested in complex medical procedures. InUShealth prices are well below those offered at U.S. hospitals. Employers and consumers benefit financially from the IndUShealth bundled medical packages (Table 2.4).[24]

### Channel Strategy Tactics

After a channel system has been designed, individual intermediaries are selected, trained, motivated, and evaluated. Organizations need to select their channel partners carefully because channels are an extension of the organization's brand. Organizations should evaluate the fit of each channel member with its positioning.

## TABLE 2.4  IndUShealth Selected Medical Package Price Ranges ($000s)

| Type of Procedure | Retail Price US | Overseas Package Price India | Overseas Package Price Costa Rica |
|---|---|---|---|
| Laparoscopic Gastric Bypass | 35–50 | 15–25 | 19–22 |
| Hip Replacement—Unilateral | 40–60 | 14–24 | 20–24 |
| Knee Replacement—Bilateral | 65–110 | 20–30 | 32–36 |
| ACL Repair | 25–35 | 9–19 | 10–13 |
| Shoulder Replacement | 35–55 | 15–25 | 17–21 |
| Rotator Cuff Repair | 20–30 | 12–22 | 12–16 |
| Hysterectomy | 20–30 | 12–22 | 14–17 |
| Lumbar Fusion (1-level) | 80–120 | 18–28 | 28–32 |
| Cervical Fusion (2-level) | 100–150 | 22–32 | 28–32 |
| Cervical Disc Replacement (1-level) | 120–220 | 18–28 | 36–40 |
| CABG | 100–170 | 14–24 | – |
| Single Heart Valve Replacement | 140–220 | 19–29 | – |

Blue Cross Blue Shield health plans use independent brokers to represent and sell their plans. The customer experience and the performance of each broker needs to be consistent with the experience and performance of the Blue Cross Blue Shield brand.

Since all channel partners need to be paid, each one will add to the price of the product or service. Marketers need to ensure that the final product price is not too high and is in alignment with its positioning strategy. From a promotion perspective, the marketing communication by each channel partner needs to be consistent with the organization's messaging strategy. Local durable medical equipment dealers contract with a regional home health agency to distribute oxygen, walkers, hospital beds, and other equipment. Dealer advertising, corporate identity, and social media content need to be monitored by the home health agency to safeguard how its brand is being communicated.

## SHOULDER SHOP—CHANNELS STRATEGY AND TACTICS

Shoulder Shop has designed channels strategies to build referral relationships.

The customer service team has a database of area primary care physicians, employers, and payers. It tracks customer referrals by source, and customer service analyzes and reports referral patterns monthly. Additionally, customer service makes sales calls to new referral sources to introduce the practice, and it visits current referral sources to communicate customer results. Customer service is a liaison with referrers collecting feedback, competitive information, and identifying new clinical approaches.

The practice is also using a direct channel to reach targeted consumers. Customer service tracks practice prospects using the Shoulder Shop website to offer information, tips, and eventually convert them to self-referred customers.

***D. Promotion Strategy and Tactics*** Strategic health care marketing calls for more than developing a good product, pricing it attractively, and making it accessible. Organizations must also communicate with their present and potential stakeholders and the general public. The question is not whether to communicate but rather what to say, how and when to say it, to whom, and how often.

### Role of Marketing Communication

Marketing communication is the means by which firms attempt to inform, persuade, and remind consumers—directly or indirectly—about the products and brands that they sell. Marketing communication represents the "voice" of the brand and are one way to establish a dialogue and build relationships with consumers and stakeholders. Marketers need to know what information is needed and wanted by the target market and how the target prefers to receive this information. Marketing communication allows organizations to link their brands to other people, places, events, brands, experiences, feelings, and things. In these ways, marketing communication can contribute to brand equity by forming the brand in memory and establishing a brand image.

### Developing Effective Communication Strategies

Effective marketing communication strategies can be developed by (1) identifying the target audience, (2) determining the communication objectives, (3) designing the communication, (4) selecting the communication channels, (5) estimating the communication budget, (6) deciding on the communication mix, (7) measuring the results, and (8) managing the integrated communication process.

*Step 1: Identify the target audience*

The first step is to identify a clear target audience. The audience could be potential buyers, current customers, deciders, or influencers. Other targets include individuals, groups, particular publics, or the general public. The needs and preferences of a target audience determine message content, tone, and how it should be delivered. A major part of audience analysis is assessing the current image of the organization, its products, and its competitors.

*Step 2: Determine the communication objectives*

The most effective communication often achieves multiple objectives. There are usually four types of communication objectives:

1. *Category need*: Consumers recognize a product or service category in which they have a need. Communicating a new class of health care product, such as when Viagra became available, always begins with a statement that establishes the category need.

2. *Brand awareness*: Consumers identify, recognize, or recall the name of a brand within the category. Brand awareness leads to brand preference and then to brand purchase.

3. *Brand attitude*: Consumers evaluate whether a particular brand might meet a currently relevant need. Relevant brand needs may be *negatively originated*

(problem removal, problem avoidance, incomplete satisfaction, normal depletion) or *positively* oriented (sensory gratification, intellectual stimulation, or social approval).

4. *Brand purchase intention*: Consumers give self-instructions to purchase the brand or to take purchase-related action.

***Step 3: Design the communications***

Designing the communications to achieve the desired response will require both a *message strategy* and a *creative strategy*.

*Message strategy*: Health care message appeals, themes, and ideas need to tie into the brand's positioning, benefits, and points of differentiation. Some of these points may be directly related to product or service performance, such as the quality or the value of the brand. Others may relate to more extrinsic considerations, such as the perception of the brand as safe, respected, or ethical. It is widely believed that government, commercial, and employer buyers are most responsive to performance messages. They are usually knowledgeable about the product, trained to recognize value, and are accountable to others for their choices. Consumers, when they buy high acuity services, like cancer or heart care, also tend to gather information and estimate benefits.

*Creative strategies*: A creative strategy is how marketers translate their messages into a specific communication. Creative strategies can be classified as either informational appeal or transformational appeal.[25] *An informational appeal elaborates on attributes or benefits.* Examples of rational advertising messages are problem-solution ads (Excedrin stops headache pain quickly), product demonstration ads (Effergrip Denture Adhesive Cream can withstand the pressure of biting into an apple), and product comparison ads (Crestor the cholesterol-lowering drug prices all dosages the same, while Lipitor uses higher prices for higher doses). Product testimonials by customers also use informational appeals. The singer Jon Bon Jovi endorsed Pfizer's Advil on television, and basketball player Chris Bosh endorses the Bayer anticoagulant drug Xarelto.

*A transformational appeal elaborates on a non-product-related benefit or image.* Claritin allergy tablet ads show different types of people before and after taking the drug to help them with allergies. Methodist Hospital in Houston advertised to compassionate, mission-driven people to recruit them to work as nurses. The "Leading Medicine" multimedia campaign communicated the type of work experience to expect. Transformational appeals often attempt to stir up negative or positive emotions that will motivate purchase. Examples are communications of the negative results of failing to brush teeth or avoiding regular physical examinations. Showing new mothers with happy, healthy infants is a positive appeal to motivate pregnant women seek prenatal care.

*Step 4:* *Select the communication channels*

Selecting efficient channels to carry the message becomes more difficult as channels of communication become more fragmented and cluttered. Communication channels may be personal or non-personal, and many organizations use both. Pharmaceutical sales people can rarely see busy physicians for more than a few seconds to build brand preference for their drugs. Because personal selling is relatively expensive, the industry also uses non-personal communications including ads in medical journals, online advertising, apps, sampling, and videoconferencing.

Personal communication channels involve two or more persons communicating directly with each other face-to-face, person-to-audience, by telephone, by email, and through websites like Yelp or Amazon with a cross-section of consumer reviews. The strength of personal communication channels is their ability to offer individualized presentation and feedback. Kiehl's has been retailing skin care health products since 1851. Its products are in department stores nationwide, and they are available online. Kiehl's does not advertise or create exciting packaging. Instead it relies on personal word-of-mouth communication. One of the byproducts of Kiehl's well-managed word-of-mouth referral channel is widespread media coverage.[26]

Non-personal channels are communications directed to more than one person. Most non-personal messages come through paid media advertising. Media include print, broadcast, digital, and outdoor such as billboards, signs, and posters. Other non-personal channels are sales promotion, events, and publicity. Consumer promotions include product samples, coupons, and premiums. Common trade promotions are retail advertising and display allowances or discounts, and salesforce promotional contests for sales reps. Events and experiences include sports, arts, entertainment, and nonprofit advocacy events, as well as less formal activities that create novel brand interactions with consumers. Public relations include communication directed internally to employees of the company or externally to consumers, other firms, the government, and media.

*Step 5:* *Estimate the total marketing communication budget*

How do companies decide on the promotion budget? There are four common methods: the affordable method, percentage-of-sales method, competitive-parity method, and objective-and-task method.

1. *Affordable method*: Many companies set the promotion budget at what they think the company can afford. The affordable method completely ignores the role of promotion as an investment and the immediate impact of promotion on sales volume. It leads to an uncertain annual budget and makes long-range planning difficult.

2. *Percentage-of-sales method*: Many companies set promotion expenditures at a specified percentage of sales or of the sales price. Promotion expenditures

will vary with what the company can "afford." It also encourages management to think of the relationship among promotion cost, selling price, and profit per unit. This method has many flaws. One of the most serious is that it does not encourage building the promotion budget by determining what each product and territory deserves.

3. *Competitive-parity method*: Some companies set their promotion budget to achieve share-of-voice parity with competitors. The assumptions are that competitors' expenditures represent the collective wisdom of the industry, and that maintaining competitive parity prevents promotion wars. Neither argument is valid.

4. *Objective-and-task method*: The objective-and-task method calls upon marketers to develop promotion budgets by defining specific objectives, determining the tasks that must be performed to achieve these objectives, and estimating the costs of performing these tasks. The sum of these costs is the proposed promotion spending budget. Examples of objectives and tasks are establishing the market share goal, determining the percentage of the market that should be reached by advertising, and determining the percentage of prospects with brand awareness that should be trying the brand.

A major question is: What is the level of expense that marketing communications should receive in relation to alternatives such as product improvement, lower prices, or better service? The answer depends on where the organization's products are in their life cycles, whether they are commodities or highly differentiable products, whether they are routinely needed or have to be "sold," and other considerations.

***Step 6:** Decide on the marketing communication mix*

Organizations must allocate the marketing communication budget over seven modes of communication. Each communication tool has its own unique characteristics and costs.

a) Advertising

*Definition*: *Any paid form of non-personal presentation and promotion of ideas, goods, or services by an identified sponsor.*

*Examples*: print, broadcast, online, outdoor ads.

*Characteristics*: Advertising can be used to form a long-term image for a product or quick sales. It permits the seller to repeat a message many times. It also allows the buyer to receive and compare the messages of various competitors. Large-scale advertising says something positive about the seller's size, power, and success. Advertising provides opportunities for dramatizing the company and its brands and products through the artful use of print, sound, and color.

b) Sales promotion

*Definition: A variety of short-term incentives to encourage trial or purchase of a product or service.*

*Examples*: sampling, coupons, rebates, contests, trade discounts and allowances.

*Characteristics*: They incorporate some concession, inducement, or contribution that gives value to the consumer. They also include a clear call to action to complete the transaction now.

c) Events and experiences

*Definition: Organization-sponsored activities and program designed to create daily or special brand-related interactions.*

*Examples*: street teams, health fairs, open-house receptions, sports sponsorships, "cause" sponsorships.

*Characteristics*: They can be seen as highly relevant because the consumer is often personally invested in the outcome. Given their live, real-time quality, events and experiences are more actively engaging for consumers. They are typically an indirect "soft sell."

d) Public relations

*Definition: A variety of programs directed internally to employees of the organization or externally to consumers, other firms, the government, and media to promote or protect a company's image or its individual product communications.*

*Examples*: media relations, product publicity, corporate communications, lobbying, counseling.

*Characteristics*: The appeal of public relations is based on three distinctive qualities. News stories and features have higher credibility and are more credible to readers than ads. Public relations can reach prospects who prefer to avoid mass media and targeted promotions. Public relations can use dramatization to tell the story behind a company, brand, or product.

e) Direct and interactive marketing

*Definition: Use of mail, telephone, or online activities to communicate and solicit responses directly with customers or prospects. The objective is to raise awareness, improve image, or elicit sales of products and services.*

*Examples*: catalogues, sales letters, telemarketing, email.

*Characteristics*: A customized message can be prepared to appeal to the addressed individual. The message can be prepared and updated very quickly. The message can be interactive and changed depending on the person's response.

f) Word-of-mouth marketing

*Definition: People-to-people oral, written, or electronic communications that relate to the merits or experiences of purchasing or using products or services.*

*Examples*: managed personal conversations, chat rooms, blogs.

*Characteristics*: Influential because people trust others they know and respect, and so word-of-mouth can be highly influential. Word-of-mouth can be a very intimate dialogue that reflects personal facts, opinions, and experiences. Word-of-mouth occurs when people want it to and are most interested, and it often follows noteworthy or meaningful events or experiences.

g) Personal selling

*Definition: Face-to-face interactions with one or more prospective purchasers for the purpose of making presentations, answering questions, and procuring orders.*

*Examples*: sales presentations, sales meetings, samples, trade shows, incentive programs.

*Characteristics*: Personal selling is the most effective tool at later stages of the buying process, particularly in building up buyer preference, conviction, and action. Personal selling creates an immediate and interactive episode between two or more persons. Each is able to observe the other's reactions. It also permits all kinds of relationships to spring up, ranging from a matter-of-fact selling relationship to a deep personal friendship. The buyer is often given personal choices and encouraged to directly respond.

**Step 7:** *Measure the results*

Marketing results ROI needs to be projected before marketing communication tactics are implemented. Marketing investment spending should have a positive ROI, or the spending cannot be justified financially. After implementing the communication plan, the organization must measure actual impact against projections. Did marketing communication lead to incremental revenue and profit?

Too often, however, marketers supply only outputs and expenses: online views, numbers of ads placed, media costs. Marketers try to translate outputs into intermediate outputs such as reach and frequency, recall and recognition scores, persuasion changes, and cost-per-thousand calculations. Ultimately, behavior change measures capture the real payoff from communications.

Measuring results for health care products and services is particularly challenging. Consumers cannot typically decide to use a health care product or service on a whim, as they would after seeing an ad for a hamburger or a beer. Members of the target audience are asked whether they recognize or recall the message, how many times they saw it, what points they recall, how they felt about the message, and their previous and current attitudes toward the product and company.

The marketer should also collect behavioral measures of audience response, such as how many consumers preferred the product, intended to purchase the product, or talked to others about it. Ultimately, a hospital, for example, would want to know the average cost for each incremental admission resulting from its marketing communication spending. Answering this question is possible with a purposefully programmed health information management system.

***Step 8:*** *Manage the integrated communications process*

Integrated marketing communications can produce stronger message consistency and greater sales impact. It forces management to think about every way the customer comes into contact with the company, how the company communicates its positioning, the relative importance of each vehicle, and timing issues. As defined by the American Association of Advertising Agencies, integrated marketing communications (IMC) is a concept of marketing communication planning that recognizes the added value of a comprehensive plan.

Such a plan evaluates the strategic roles of a variety of communication disciplines like general advertising, direct response, sales promotion, and public relations—and combines these disciplines to provide clarity, consistency, and maximum impact through the seamless integration of discrete messages. The wide range of communication tools, messages, and audiences makes it imperative that companies move toward integrated marketing communications.

## SHOULDER SHOP—PROMOTION STRATEGY AND TACTICS

The primary target audience is referral sources, with an emphasis on physicians since they represent 85% of procedures. The objective is to build awareness with 100% of qualified referring physicians in the geographic market area. A personal selling strategy will be used to establish relationships with primary care physicians and their office staff. The initial tactic will be a lunch presentation meeting with each office. The message will focus on the benefits of referring to Shoulder Shop and how Shoulder Shop is differentiated from other orthopedic practices. Lunch will be catered. A supply of one-page backgrounders will be printed and distributed to each practice. This informational material is designed to be given to prospective patient end-users.

Shoulder Shop's website will be designed to be used by both referral sources and end-users. In addition to orthopedic problem and solution information, online scheduling and messaging will be included. Shoulder Shop will also select several advocacy and charitable organizations for financial support and a tie-in to the practice. Alliances will be formed with two athletic teams to build awareness with potential customers. Additionally, two athletic events will be sponsored annually. Finally, free consultations and clinics will be offered once per month to improve community health and generate awareness. The results of all of these tactics will be measured to determine their ROI.

## VI. Implementation and Controls

How do health care organizations know whether their marketing plans are achieving the marketing and financial objectives that have been set? The last section of the marketing plan includes controls for monitoring activities and adjusting plan implementation.

**A. Plan Performance Tracking**  Effective marketing relies on results. Strategies and tactics to meet goals and objectives may need to be modified. Marketing measures relate to customer-level concerns such as their attitudes and behavior or loyalty. Other measures relate to brand-level concerns such as market share, relative price premium, or profitability. Marketers are increasingly being held accountable for marketing investments and financial return on marketing expenditure investments. When marketers can estimate the dollar contribution of marketing activities, they are better able to justify the value of marketing investments to senior management.

**B. Revenue, Spending, and Market Share Measures**  Three ways to measure key aspects of the marketing plan's performance are revenue analysis, marketing spending analysis, and market share analysis. A fourth plan performance measure is behavioral change, and this is explored in Chapter 9 Social Cause Marketing in Health Care.

*1. Revenue analysis:*  Revenue or sales analysis consists of measuring and evaluating actual revenue compared to forecast revenue. A table is used to compare revenue forecast by month with actual revenue results. If actual revenue performance lags the forecast, a revenue analysis will alert management to identify opportunities to improve performance or revise the forecast.

*2. Marketing spending analysis:*  There are a number of methods for budgeting marketing spending, and the objective-and-task budgeting method is commonly used. At the beginning of the fiscal year, funding is allocated across the various marketing activities scheduled for the year. Your marketing plan should include a budget spreadsheet that is updated monthly with actual and year-to-date spending for each activity. Spending for all marketing activities is tracked and reported monthly.

Data and information used to measure marketing effectiveness—such as brand awareness, preference, sales, market share, trade allowances, and others— are compared to their respective spending allocations. If the performance of marketing programs is below expectations, they should be evaluated to identify the reasons for the variances. Increasing or decreasing allocated spending may result. This analysis of budgeting, performance, and control measurement supports marketing accountability.

*3. Market share analysis:* Market share measures how the organization performs relative to competitors. Market share is the organization's or a product's sales expressed as a percentage of total market sales. IQVIA (iqvia. com) collects and sells health care data to help pharmaceutical companies and payers measure market size, sales activity, and market share. The subscription fees for these services offer a positive ROI for global pharmaceutical companies. Hospitals can also purchase market data from IBM/Truven that will enable them to measure service line market share in their market area. Syndicated market share data, unfortunately, are either not available or are unaffordable for many types of health care organizations.

## SHOULDER SHOP—IMPLEMENTATION AND CONTROLS

Our expenses and marketing spending will be matched as best as possible to ascertain marketing effectiveness. By monitoring sources of customers and referral patterns, we should be able to estimate a return on investment for marketing investments. We will track marketing expenditures monthly, and the marketing budget will be redirected as needed to address changes in our budgetary, cost, and revenue assumptions.

The Shoulder Shop is operating in a market with high gross margins and very low variable costs. Costs relating to revenues per unit are estimated at 8% of sales. Monthly fixed costs are projected to be $76,742, and monthly fixed costs are expected to increase 3% annually based on inflation. We estimate that the Shoulder Shop will breakeven when monthly sales reach $82,435, or 210 units.

| Breakeven Analysis | |
|---|---|
| *Assumptions* | Average per unit revenue $392 |
| | Average per unit variable cost $27 |
| | Estimated monthly fixed cost $76,742 |
| *Breakeven* | Monthly units to breakeven 210 |
| | Monthly revenue to breakeven $82,435 |

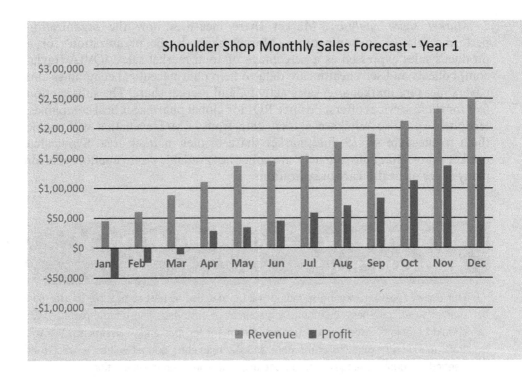

## CHAPTER SUMMARY

A strategic marketing plan can effectively guide a health care organization and help it reach its goals and objectives. The basis of the plan is understanding the environment, customer needs, and competitors. The marketing plan is a collaborative, accessible, and dynamic document based on management consensus. Plan implementation is critical and can be threatened by a range of hurdles. Eight steps, beginning before the plan is written, are recommended to support success: build a cross-functional team, check the long-term direction, clarify the goals and objectives, conduct a comprehensive analysis, recommend the most important strategies and tactics, verify the numbers, sell the plan, and execute and track progress.

A strategic marketing plan is essentially a battle plan. It focuses and communicates an organization's attack and defense plans for its market. It is different from a strategic plan and a business plan because it is chiefly influenced by environmental trends and competitors, and it is centered on customer needs. The typical time horizon is 12 months while other types of plans often have a three- to five-year horizon.

The chapter focuses on explaining each concept of a comprehensive strategic marketing plan. The situation analysis sets the stage. Marketing goals and objectives reflect the three most important areas of organizational emphasis. Overall targeting, marketing research, and positioning strategies take advantage of market opportunities, prepare for market threats, and tackle primary marketing challenges. The marketing mix strategies—product, price, channels, and promotion—develop and implement the overall strategies. All marketing strategies and tactics are measured, evaluated, and modified to achieve the organization's goals.`

## DISCUSSION QUESTIONS

1. How could strategic marketing contribute to developing an effective health care pricing strategy?

2. The number of retail store-based basic primary care clinics is currently increasing. This health care distribution innovation is straightforward with low barriers of entry into this market. Why was this distribution strategy not implemented earlier? What other types of new health care distribution strategies could be successful?

3. Health organization managers struggling with increasing customer volume and revenue often think that the solution is educating prospective buyers and "getting the word out." As a strategic marketer, how would you respond to this assumption? What steps would you recommend to increase customer volume and revenue?

## CASE: A MARKETING PLAN FOR DR. AGATSTON

Dr. Arthur Agatston, MD, is a cardiologist in Miami, the author of the book *The South Beach Diet*, and he does not take a conventional approach to practicing medicine. Convinced of the benefits of smoking cessation, exercise, and diet, he claims that only 3 of his 2,800 patients had a heart attack this past year. Cardiologists estimate that the right preventive care can reduce heart attacks by 80%.

The U.S. health care system, however, has traditionally focused on treating acute illness. Doctors and hospitals were rewarded for performing expensive tests and procedures when cheaper preventive measures might actually produce better results. Consider heart care: nuclear scans and invasive procedures such as bypass surgery have high levels of reimbursement. Medicare paid almost $15 billion, or about 5% of its total budget, for bypasses, stents, and other invasive cardiology, according to Jonathan Skinner of Dartmouth University. Yet the appropriateness of such measures for many patients remains unproven.

According to Dr. Gregg W. Stone, director of cardiovascular research at Columbia University, the three keys to effective disease prevention are (1) frequent patient visits to a physician, (2) a close relationship between the physician and the patient, and (3) a very committed patient. These characteristics represent the value proposition of Dr. Agatston's practice. Nurses give patients specific cholesterol goals to meet and help them deal with drug side-effects. Physical therapists offer exercises that improve joint mobility. A nutritionist explains strategies for sticking to a high-fiber Mediterranean diet, even on a cruise or a business trip.

Unfortunately, while stressing this preventive approach to medicine, Dr. Agatston's practice is actually losing money. He is able to make up for this short-fall through his best-selling book sales, but other physicians who practice prevention and who are not celebrities often suffer financially.[27]

## CASE QUESTIONS

You are a strategic health care marketing consultant, and Dr. Agatston has hired you to grow his practice and improve its financial performance. Answer the three questions that follow to outline a strategic marketing plan for Dr. Agatston's practice.

1.  Identify three marketing goals and corresponding objectives for the Agatston marketing plan. Describe how you would develop these goals.

2.  Develop three overall marketing strategies including targeting, marketing research, and positioning to guide the marketing mix strategies. Use the standard format for the positioning strategy. Explain your reasoning for each strategy.

3.  What product, pricing, channels, and promotion marketing mix strategies do you recommend? Include at least one to two tactics for each strategy.

# CHAPTER

# RESEARCHING THE HEALTH CARE ENVIRONMENT

## LEARNING OBJECTIVES

In this chapter we will address the following questions:

1. Why is it important to understand the health care environment?
2. What are the three components of a marketing information system?
3. What constitutes good marketing research?
4. How do six environmental forces effect nine health care market participants?

Making marketing decisions in a fast-changing world is both an art and a science. To provide context, insight, and inspiration for marketing decision-making, health care organizations need up-to-date information about environmental macro trends and the micro effects particular to their business. Virtually every health care organization has been touched by dramatic shifts in the demographic, economic, technological, social-cultural, natural, and political-legal environments.

This chapter will explain how to use marketing information, market intelligence, and marketing research systems to make decisions. It will also cover how to identify and use secondary marketing research, describe the six steps for conducting primary research, and demonstrate how an analysis of environmental forces and market participants will reveal market opportunities and threats.

## THE NEED FOR MARKET INFORMATION

Organizations with timely and accurate market information are better at selecting target markets, developing offerings that meet market needs, and executing effective marketing plans. Medical technology is creating radical shifts in treatment outcomes, locations, costs, and prices. Federal and state reimbursement regulations and payments change frequently. Consumers are becoming increasingly savvy in how they select health care providers and treatments. Marketing managers need a continuous flow of accurate data and information to understand and track changes in customer needs, wants, preferences, and consumption patterns. Public health data are often collected by governments and associations, and they can be two years old, inconsistent, or incomplete. During the Covid-19 pandemic, the collection of accurate morbidity, mortality, and utilization data has been a problem for effective public health decision-making and policy. Most state health departments rely on hospital-reported data, but if 73% of hospitals report on some days and 93% report on other days then public health decisions will suffer.

At one end of the spectrum, market-driven health plans and pharmaceutical firms have developed marketing information systems that rapidly provide detailed data about customer wants, preferences, and behavior. These data are used to measure and forecast disease patterns, price products against competitor brands, and make corporate acquisitions. At the other end of the spectrum are physician practices that lack any data compiling capability, rely on paper medical charts and faxing, and outsource all of their billing. Many other health care organizations fall in between and have marketing departments focused primarily on promotion or collecting HIPAA-mandated patient satisfaction surveys.

## USING MARKETING INFORMATION, INTELLIGENCE, AND RESEARCH SYSTEMS

The purpose of a marketing information system is to make decisions. A marketing information system consists of people, equipment, and procedures to gather, sort, analyze, evaluate, and distribute needed, timely, and accurate information to marketing decision-makers. Such a system is developed from (1) internal company records, (2) marketing intelligence activities, and (3) marketing research.

### *Internal Records System*

Marketers need internal operations and financial data to understand organization trends related to volume, revenue, prices, costs, capacity, expenses, margins, and other activities. Analyzing internal records helps identify product strengths and weaknesses. For example, organizations are increasingly using databases to store information on prospects, customers, clinical activity, and financial activity. A customer database can contain not only names, addresses, and past transactions, but also demographic and psychographic data like activities, interests, opinions, and attitudes. Table 3.1 offers five examples of how internal records can support marketing analysis.

The use of "big data" in health care can offer insights into areas such as neglected customer segments, new customer trends, and predicting outbreaks of contagious diseases. Although the widespread use of electronic health records (EHR) is improving data management, there continue to be problems with integrating data from diverse sources. The Argonaut Project, a consortium of health providers and IT vendors, was launched in 2014 to simplify and standardize the exchange of basic clinical data. Their long-term goal is to make health data-sharing easier by using internet-based open source messaging and document standards in place of more complex health care specific standards.[1]

### *Marketing Intelligence System*

The internal records system supplies results data, but the marketing intelligence system supplies happenings data. A marketing intelligence system is a set of procedures and sources that managers use to obtain everyday information about developments in the marketing environment. Marketers collect marketing intelligence through reading digital and print newsletters, books, newspapers, journals, social media, trade and professional publications, discussion groups, ratings and reviews. They also speak with managers in their organization, customers, competitors, suppliers, and distributors.

Large pharmaceutical companies can buy syndicated research data from IQVIA, an international contract research organization and clinical data company, to estimate product market share by physician, by drug, and by market. The organization's employees can be given incentives and special communication

TABLE 3.1   **Using Internal Records to Support Health Care Marketing.**

| Marketing Application | Internal data and information | Locations of data |
|---|---|---|
| Heart center marketing plan | Primary care physician referral data over the past three years, current baseline use, and capacity of the facility. | Physician call center, billing department, personnel staffing records. |
| Service-line profitability analysis | Admissions data sorted by ICD-10 CM diagnosis code, charge master pricing data, gross and net revenue by payer. | Admissions department, health information management department, patient accounting department. |
| Physician billing service company market share analysis | Number of physician clients, medical specialty, current and potential reimbursement by CPT code, collection rate by payer by state. | Client service department, finance department, coding department, remittance and collections department. |
| Health plan member profitability forecast | New member volume trends, premium revenue trends by market segment, medical cost trends, administrative cost data. | Sales department, finance department, actuarial department. |
| Hospital information system company sales performance analysis | Number of leads and referrals, number of sales calls and product demonstrations, sales closed to sales proposals ratios. | Marketing call center, field sales database, finance department. |

channels to convey new market information. Although salespeople often are best positioned to discover intelligence, anyone in the organization can contribute to a better understanding of customers, including nurses, patient registration employees, telephone operators, maintenance workers, and other employees. A range of actions that can improve the quality marketing intelligence are shown in Table 3.2.

## Marketing Research System

Marketing research is defined as *the systematic design, collection, analysis, and reporting of data and findings relevant to a specific marketing situation facing the*

TABLE 3.2  **Improving the Quality of Marketing Intelligence.**

| Action | Example |
| --- | --- |
| Train and motivate the sales force to spot and report new developments that may be missed by other means. | Have sales reps observe how customers use the organization's products and services in innovative ways, which can lead to new product ideas. |
| Motivate distributors, retailers, and other intermediaries to pass along important intelligence. | Use mystery shoppers to identify service problems that can be addressed by revamping processes and retraining employees. |
| Network externally to gather data in legal and ethical ways. | Offer rewards to employees who submit new information about what competitors are doing. |
| Establish a customer advisory panel. | Invite the largest or the most representative, outspoken, or sophisticated customers to provide feedback on products and services. |
| Take advantage of government data resources. | Check CMS and U.S. Census data to learn more about Medicare payment patterns, physician practice patterns, demographic shifts, and changing family structure. |
| Buy information from outside suppliers at a lower cost than gathering it directly. | Obtain competitive medical service line data from Truven/IBM, analysis of new health care regulations from Advisory Board Company, or competitive advertising spending data from Nielsen Media Research. |
| Use online customer feedback to collect competitive intelligence. | Check consumer ratings on websites like RateMDs, Healthgrades, and Consumer Reports to learn more about competitors' strengths and weaknesses. |

*organization.* It is the job of the marketing researcher to produce insight into the customer's attitudes and buying behavior. The marketing research system includes both secondary research that has been previously collected as well as newly acquired primary research.

***What is Secondary Health Care Marketing Research?*** Secondary research data are data that were collected for another purpose and already exist. Secondary data provide a starting point and offer the advantages of low cost and ready availability. For instance, physician practice managers can join the Medical Group Management Association to receive low-cost physician compensation data, practice operations data, and practice cost and revenue data to benchmark their practice against national norms.

Most secondary marketing research starts with "Googling it." The websites shown next offer a wide range of available data and information.

1. FierceHealthcare, www.fiercehealthcare.com
   FierceHealthcare is the leading source of health care management news for health care industry executives. News summaries and links to complete articles are provided. The FierceMarkets Network includes nine total health care sites that cover electronic medical records, finance, information technology, payers, mobile health care, practice management, and hospitals. It also has 13 life science sites that report on biotechnology, contract research organizations, diagnostics, pharmaceuticals, medical devices, and animal health.

2. HealthLeaders Media, www.healthleadersmedia.com
   HealthLeaders Media provides staff reports and links to news sources related to health care leadership, business strategy, finance, billing, information technology, managed care, Medicare reimbursement, quality of care and patient safety, marketing, nursing management, and hospitals.

3. Becker's Hospital Review, www.beckershospitalreview.com
   Becker's website publishes daily online newsletters covering hospitals, spine, ambulatory surgery centers, clinical, health IT, health CFO, dental, and payer markets.

4. MedCity, https://medcitynews.com
   MedCity News is an online news source for the business of innovation in health care. The focus is on startups, industry leaders, personalities, policies, and M&A.

5. HIMSS Media, www.himssmedia.com
   HIMSS Media primarily offers information for health and health care technology marketers. Electronic newsletters cover health care finance, mobile health, government health information technology, medical practice management technology, payers, and European health information technology.

6. Kaiser Family Foundation, www.kff.org
   The Foundation analyzes domestic and global health policy, conducts public opinion and survey research, provides an information clearinghouse, and offers the Kaiser Health News e-newsletter. The Foundation is not associated with Kaiser Permanente or Kaiser Industries.

7. Mathematica Policy Research, www.mathematica-mpr.com/our-focus-areas/health

    Mathematica conducts research and publishes data on care delivery and financing, quality measures, health systems change, controlling health care costs, and designing delivery systems to meet diverse needs. Center for Studying Health System Change was a Mathematica affiliate until December 2014.

8. Commonwealth Fund, www.commonwealthfund.org

    The Commonwealth Fund is a private foundation that promotes a high value and innovative global health care system. The focus is on publications and data related to better access, improved quality, greater efficiency, and helping society's most vulnerable populations. The Fund supports independent research on health care issues and makes grants to improve health care practice and policy.

9. PwC Health Research Institute (HRI), www.pwc.com/us/en/health-industries/health-research-institute.html

    PwC's HRI provides intelligence, perspectives, and analysis on trends affecting health care industries. The site specializes in health services, health technology, the Affordable Care Act, pharma and life sciences, and regulation. The "HRI Annual Top Ten Health Industry Issues" is particularly insightful.

10. Deloitte Center for Health Solutions (DCHS), www.deloitte.com/centerforhealthsolutions

    DCHS is the research division of Deloitte's Life Sciences and Health Care practice. The goal of DCHS is to inform stakeholders across the health care system about emerging trends, challenges, and opportunities.

11. SmartBrief, www.smartbrief.com/industry/health-care

    SmartBrief publishes more than 40 e-newsletters in health care, serving medical professionals such as family physicians, specialists, and nurses, and exploring diverse topics such as medical devices, pharmaceuticals, insurance, and health IT.

12. Hospitals & Health Networks (H&HN), www.hhnmag.com

    H&HN is published by the American Hospital Association. It focuses on topics concerning hospital managers such as operations, finance, governance, patient care, nursing, physicians, and delivery system transformation.

13. Medscape, www.medscape.com

    Medscape is a web resource for physicians and health professionals. It features peer-reviewed original medical journal articles, CME, and a customized version of the National Library of Medicine's MEDLINE.

14. RAND Health, www.rand.org/health

RAND Health is one of the largest independent health research groups in the world. This site includes access to free research briefs, surveys, policy papers, publications, and other tools that address a wide range of health care issues.

***What is Primary Marketing Research?*** There are situations when secondary research is dated, inaccurate, incomplete, or unreliable. Primary research can be customized to collect information that meets a particular need. Primary data are data freshly gathered for a specific purpose or for specific research projects. Marketers design, collect, analyze, and report findings relevant to specific problems and opportunities facing the organization. The purpose of research is to identify evidence that will support effective decisions. It is too easy to dismiss research findings as simply "interesting" or "we know that already" if research is not connected to specific management decisions.

Marketing research may be used to explore attitudes and behavior by market segment, compare product preferences, test market demand and price elasticity to support a sales forecast, evaluate advertising effectiveness, and other uses. An organization can obtain this marketing research in a number of ways. Most large companies have their own marketing research departments, which often play crucial roles within the organization. At smaller organizations, marketing research is often carried out by everyone in the organization—and by customers too. Organizations normally budget marketing research at 1 to 2% of sales. A large portion of that is spent on the services of outside research firms. Marketing research firms fall into three categories:

1. *Syndicated-service research firms*: These firms gather consumer and trade information, which they sell for a fee. Examples include the Nielsen Company, Kantar Group, Westat, and IRI.

2. *Custom marketing research firms*: These firms are hired to carry out specific projects. They design the study and report the findings.

3. *Specialty-line marketing research firms*: These firms provide specialized research services. The best example is the field-service firm, which sells field interviewing services to other firms.

***The Primary Marketing Research Process.*** To take advantage of all these different resources and practices, good marketers adopt a formal marketing research process. Effective marketing research involves the six steps shown in Figure 3.1.

***Case Example: Regional Radiology.***   The six-step primary research process will be illustrated based on a study completed for Regional Radiology, a 20-physician radiology group practice in the Southeast. Preceding this study, Regional Radiology used secondary marketing research to identify a potential location for a new satellite office. The research showed that there may be an opportunity to meet the needs of referring physicians and consumers in a North Carolina beach community.

The group also prepared a pro forma financial forecast for its four-slice computed tomography (CT) imaging service. The new office would break even financially if 800 scans, approximately 3.5 scans per day, were completed annually. Regional Radiology then contracted with a custom health care marketing research firm to complete a primary research study to understand market needs and test the decision to expand.

***Step 1:*** *Define the problem, decision alternatives, and research objectives*

Problem analysis leads to decision options which are followed by research objectives. Marketing management must be careful not to define the problem too

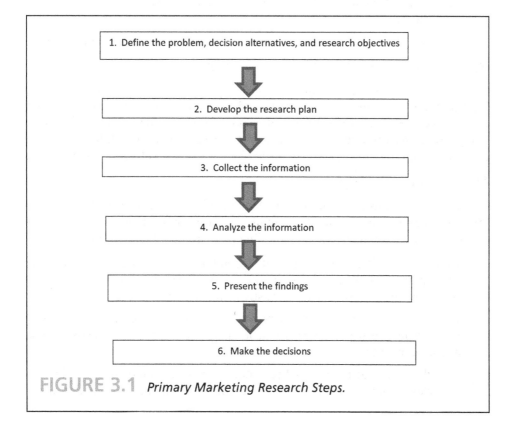

FIGURE 3.1   *Primary Marketing Research Steps.*

broadly or too narrowly for the marketing researcher. Regional Radiology defined the problem this way: "Will opening a new satellite office, with four-slice CT imaging services in this new market, have a higher long-term return-on-investment compared to other potential investments?"

Decision alternatives can be a critical element of research or they can be inconsequential. Alan Andreasen believes that marketers should take a "backwards" approach to research and first identify the most important management decisions.[2] Once the decisions are defined, then the research can be narrowly focused on collecting only the information needed to make the decisions. This approach avoids common criticisms of research such as "since we already knew that information, the research was not valuable." The decision facing Regional Radiology was either to enter a new geographic market or not. This decision led to the following research objectives:

a) Estimate the size of the total available market for CT imaging referrals by area physicians.

b) Identify the specific physicians likely to refer patients to the new imaging office.

c) Rank the factors most important for referral decisions and in changing referral patterns.

d) Measure physician satisfaction and loyalty with competing imaging centers.

e) Estimate CT imaging market share by competitor.

Exploratory research is not decision-focused by design. Its goal is to shed light on the real nature of the problem and to suggest possible solutions or new ideas. Other research is descriptive, it seeks to quantify demand, such as how many physicians would refer CT scan patients on weekends and holidays. Research can also be causal with the purpose of testing a cause-and-effect relationship.

***Step 2:*** *Develop the research plan*

The second step calls for designing an efficient, affordable research plan for gathering the needed information. This entails decisions about data sources, research approaches, research instruments, sampling plan, and contact methods.

1. *Data sources*: The plan can include secondary data, primary data, or both. Most plans first examine secondary data to see whether the problem can be partly or wholly solved without costly primary data.

2. *Research approaches*: Researchers can collect primary data for marketing research in five ways: observation, focus groups, surveys, behavioral data, and experiments.

   a) Observational research—Fresh data can be gathered by observing the relevant actors and settings. *Ethnographic research* is a particular observational research approach that uses concepts and tools from anthropology and other social science disciplines to provide deep cultural understanding of how people live and work. The goal is to immerse the researcher into consumers' lives to uncover unarticulated desires that might not surface in any other form of research. For example, an ethnographic researcher working for Regional Radiology may shadow a primary care or specialist physician for several days. The purpose of the research could be to find opportunities to improve the imaging referral process and to better understand the role of the end-user.

b)  Focus group research—A focus group is a gathering of 6 to 10 people carefully selected by researchers based on certain demographic, psychographic, or other considerations. They are brought together, either in a room or online, to discuss various topics of interest at length and have a "focused" discussion. A professional research moderator guides the conversation through questions and probes based on the marketing managers' discussion guide or agenda. The objective is to identify insights through having participants discuss, listen, and react to each other's perspectives.

Focus group research is a useful exploratory step, but researchers must avoid generalizing from focus group participants to the whole market because the sample size is small and not random. Focus group findings are most valuable if they are objective, consistent, and confirmed through quantitative research. Pitfalls include conducting only a single focus group, using an untrained moderator or one without health industry knowledge, and biasing participant responses by disclosing the name of the study sponsor.

If Regional Radiology used focus group research, the moderator in a referring physician focus group might start with a broad question, such as "How do you feel about imaging services?" Questions then move to how physicians view the different types of imaging, different existing imaging services, and different proposed services.

c)  Survey research—Surveys are best suited for descriptive research. Organizations undertake surveys to learn about people's knowledge, beliefs, preferences, and satisfaction, and to measure these magnitudes in the general population. A physician survey was used by Regional Radiology to understand the 20 referring practices in the target market. A telephone survey was planned, but Regional Radiology could also have used an online survey or scheduled personal interviews with respondents.

d)  Behavioral data—Customers leave traces of their purchasing behavior in store scanning data, catalogue purchases, and customer databases. Much can be learned by analyzing these data. Customers' actual purchases reflect revealed preferences and often are more reliable than statements they offer to market researchers. Definitive Healthcare is a company that sells national imaging center database information. It has detailed profiles and analytics on over 16,700 imaging centers across the nation, and it collects volume and cost data for all types of radiology procedures including CT Scans, MRIs, X-rays, and others. These data and information may have helped Regional Radiology if it were considering national instead of regional expansion.

e) Experimental research—The most scientifically valid research is experimental research. The purpose of experimental research is to capture cause-and-effect relationships by eliminating competing explanations of the observed findings. Regional Radiology might experiment by temporarily staffing a CT imaging service by subletting office space for several months at or near their proposed practice location. If this test market was successful, then Regional Radiology could purchase office space and further invest in developing patient volume.

3. *Research instruments*: Marketing researchers have a choice of three main research instruments in collecting primary data: questionnaires, qualitative measures, and technological devices.

a) Questionnaires—A questionnaire consists of a set of questions presented to respondents. Because of its flexibility, the questionnaire is the most common instrument used to collect primary data. Questionnaires need to be carefully developed, tested, and debugged before they are administered on a large scale.

Marketing researchers distinguish between closed-end and open-end questions. Closed-end questions specify all the possible answers and provide answers that are easier to interpret and tabulate. Open-end questions allow respondents to answer in their own words and often reveal more about how people think. They are especially useful in exploratory research, where the researcher is looking for insight into how people think rather than in measuring how many people think a certain way.

In-depth interviews are one-on-one personal or telephone interviews that are designed to probe more wide-ranging attitudes and behavior. The interviewer uses open-ended questions to get participants to offer detailed insights and to learn what motivates behavior. Conducting 20 to 25 in-depth interviews can often lead to valuable insights. The study limitations of extrapolating focus group findings to the overall market also apply to in-depth interviews.

b) Qualitative measures—Some marketers prefer more qualitative methods for gauging consumer opinion because consumer behavior does not always match their responses to survey questions. Qualitative research is indirect by nature, so consumers may be less guarded and reveal more about themselves in the process. Unstructured measurement approaches permit a range of possible responses. Because of the freedom it affords both researchers in their probes and consumers in their responses, qualitative research can often be an especially useful first step in exploring consumers' brand and product perceptions. Qualitative approaches are limited only by the creativity of the marketing researcher.

Different qualitative researchers examining the same results may draw very different conclusions due to personal bias. Another drawback of qualitative research is that marketers must temper the in-depth insights that emerge with the fact that the samples are often very small and may not necessarily reflect the overall market. Quantitative research often follows and is used to test qualitative conclusions.

c) Electronic devices—Galvanometers can measure the interest or emotions aroused by exposure to a specific ad or picture. The tachistoscope flashes an ad to a subject with an exposure interval that may range from less than one hundredth of a second to several seconds. After each exposure, the respondent describes everything he or she recalls. Eye cameras study respondents' eye movements to see where their eyes land first, how long they linger on a given item, and so on.

Digital technology has now advanced to such a degree that marketers can use devices such as skin sensors, brain wave scanners, and full body scanners to get consumer responses. Some researchers study eye movements and brain activity to see which online ads grab their attention. Technology has replaced the diaries that participants in media surveys used to keep. Audiometers attached to television sets in participating homes now record when the set is on and to which channel it is tuned. Electronic devices can record the number of radio programs a person is exposed to during the day, or, using Global Positioning System (GPS) technology, how many billboards a person may walk or drive by during a day.

4. *Sampling plan*: After deciding on the research approach and instruments, the marketing researcher must design a sampling plan based on three decisions:

a) Sampling unit—*Who is to be surveyed?* The researcher must define the target population that will be sampled. In the Regional Radiology survey, should the sampling unit be only primary care physicians, specialty physicians, or both? The sampling unit is determined and a sampling frame must be developed so that everyone in the target population has an equal or known chance of being sampled. A sampling plan is needed to define the target population for the research. Those involved in the product buying decision process need to be outlined. The gatekeepers, influencers, economic buyers, and approvers need to be considered. Purchase of Regional Radiology imaging services could involve referring physicians, consumers, health plans, and employers.

b)   Sample size—*How many people should be surveyed?* Large samples give more reliable results than small samples. It is not necessary to sample the entire target population or even a substantial portion to achieve reliable results. Samples of less than 1% of a population can be reliable with a credible sampling procedure.

c)   Sampling procedure—*How should the respondents be chosen?* To obtain a representative sample, a probability sample of the population should be drawn. Probability sampling allows the calculation of confidence limits for sampling error. When the cost or time involved in probability sampling is too high, marketing researchers will take nonprobability samples, even though they do not allow sampling error to be measured. Regional Radiology used a nonprobability sample of local physicians and referral coordinators who were judged to be important sources of information.

5.   *Contact methods*: Once the sampling plan has been determined, the marketing researcher must decide how to contact subjects. Choices include mail, telephone, personal, or online interviews. The advantages and disadvantages of these methods are summarized in Table 3.3.

### *Step 3*: *Collect the information*

The data collection phase of marketing research is generally the most expensive and the most prone to error. Marketers may conduct surveys in homes, over the phone, online, or at a central interviewing location like a shopping mall. Four major problems arise in surveys. Some respondents will be away from home or otherwise inaccessible and must be contacted again or replaced. Other respondents will refuse to cooperate. Still others will give biased or dishonest answers. Finally, some interviewers will be biased or dishonest.

Although it was not initially planned, Regional Radiology used a qualitative written research survey. This method was used to target 20 prospective referring physicians and physician extenders in four ZIP codes. These survey respondents were contacted by telephone to schedule phone interviews, but most of them declined to schedule an interview. Instead, they asked to complete a written questionnaire at their convenience. The study sampling plan was modified, written questionnaires were faxed to the practices, and the completed surveys were returned by fax. Each respondent received an incentive of $50 for participating in the survey.

Internationally, one of the biggest obstacles to collecting information is the need to achieve consistency.[3] Latin American respondents may be uncomfortable with the impersonal nature of online interviewing and need interactive elements

TABLE 3.3  **Marketing Research Contact Methods.**

| Contact Method | Advantages | Disadvantages |
|---|---|---|
| **Mail or email questionnaire** | Ability to reach people who would not give personal interviews or whose responses might be biased or distorted by the interviews. | Response rate is usually low and slow. |
| **Telephone interview** | Ability to gather information quickly and clarify questions respondents do not understand; higher response rate than mail questionnaires. | Interviews must be short and not too personal, contacting is more difficult because of consumers' growing antipathy toward being called at home, and the Federal "Do Not Call" registry, e.g. mobile phones must be manually dialed. |
| **Personal interview** | Ability to ask more questions and record additional observations about respondents, such as dress and body language. | Most expensive contact method; requires more planning and supervision; is subject to interviewer bias or distortion. |
| **Online interview** | Ability to post questions online using a moderated focus group "bulletin board"; or a narrowly defined panel of consumers, employees, physicians, and others who meet specific targeting criteria. Online product testing, in which companies float trial balloons for new products, is also growing and providing information much faster than traditional new product marketing research techniques. Less expensive compared to telephone or personal interviews. Respondents tend to be more candid online. | Samples can be small and skewed. These convenience samples do not have statistical validity and reliability. |

in a survey so they feel they're talking to a real person. Respondents in Asia, on the other hand, may feel more pressure to conform and may therefore not be as forthcoming in focus groups as online. Sometimes the solution may be as simple as ensuring the right language is used.

***Step 4****: Analyze the information*

The next-to-last step in the process is to extract findings by tabulating the data and developing summary measures. The researchers now compute averages and measures of dispersion for the major variables and apply some advanced statistical techniques and decision models in the hope of discovering additional findings. They may test different hypotheses and theories, applying sensitivity analysis to test assumptions and the strength of the conclusions. The analysis of the Regional Radiology study used tabulations, mean and median analysis, market share calculations, and interpretations of numerous verbatim comments made by respondents.

***Step 5****: Present the findings*

In this step, the researcher should present findings that are relevant to the major marketing decisions facing management. The conclusions presented to Regional Radiology were:

1. *Regional Radiology will need to capture a 32% share of the CT market to breakeven*—Research estimated that the total available CT scan market was 11 scans per day. Management projected breakeven volume at 3.5 scans per day, covering fixed and variable costs (3.5 ÷ 11 = 32%).

2. *There is a market opportunity for Regional Radiology to offer a differentiated service product*—Effective communication and speed in obtaining an appointment were the two most important benefits in referring patients for imaging services. The benefit of convenient hours and days available for appointments was ranked third. Fortunately for Regional Radiology, these three factors were also rated as the primary weaknesses of their competition.

3. *The respondents indicated that they were likely to send referrals to a new imaging service that met their needs*—The physicians were also asked how they would like to receive information about a new imaging service. Surprisingly, there was no interest in electronic communications. The physicians had a clear preference for direct mail and fax communication.

***Step 6****: Make the decision*

Managers who commission primary marketing research need to weigh the evidence. For example, if Regional Radiology has little confidence in the findings, they may decide against investing in the new satellite office. If they are predisposed to launching the service, the findings support their inclination. They may even decide to do additional research to confirm their decision.

The Regional Radiology board weighed the evidence and decided to invest in the new imaging service. The decision was theirs, but marketing research provided them with insight into the problem. Aside from the research, an additional factor supported the decision to enter the new market. It was a pledge from a nearby ENT specialty physician practice for an average of two patient referrals per week to the new imaging office.

Adhering to the following seven-step primary marketing research guidelines will lead to the effective design of primary marketing research studies:[4]

(1) *Scientific method*: Effective marketing research uses the principles of the scientific method: careful observation, formulation of hypotheses, prediction, and testing.

(2) *Research creativity*: Innovation and collaboration in research is important. For example, a hospital targeting heart patients built relationships using its website to collect demographic data, cardiac care information preferences, and consent to send consumers information on heart disease prevention. This database was the basis of a new hospital heart affinity "club" with regular meetings at the hospital and member discounts on heart healthy products and services.

(3) *Multiple methods*: Marketing researchers shy away from overreliance on any one method. They also recognize the value of using two or three methods to increase confidence in the results.

(4) *Interdependence of models and data*: Marketing researchers recognize that data are interpreted from underlying models that guide the type of information sought.

(5) *Value and cost of information*: Marketing researchers show concern for estimating the value of information against its cost. Costs are typically easy to determine, but the value of research is harder to quantify. It depends on the reliability and validity of the findings and management's willingness to accept and act on those findings.

(6) *Healthy skepticism*: Marketing researchers show a healthy skepticism toward glib assumptions made by managers about how a market works. They are alert to the problems caused by "marketing myths."

(7) *Ethical marketing*: Marketing research benefits both the sponsoring company and its customers. The misuse of marketing research can harm or annoy consumers, increasing resentment at what consumers regard as an invasion of their privacy or a disguised sales pitch.

## DEVELOPING AN ENVIRONMENTAL ANALYSIS

An environmental analysis uses secondary data to understand how participants are affected by forces and trends in the macroenvironment (Table 3.4). An environmental analysis informs a marketing plan but is not part of the plan.

## MAJOR PARTICIPANTS IN THE HEALTH CARE MARKET

The nine types of participants in the health care environment are consumers, care providers, payers, employers, government, medical and trade associations, health care advocacy groups, health care suppliers, and competitors.

1. *Consumers*: The U.S. had a population of 330 million people in 2019, with a net gain of one person every 18 seconds.[5] Consumption of health care varies widely with 1% of consumers accounting for 23% of health care spending in a given year. An estimated 5% of the population account for 50% of health spending. The healthier 50% of the population has little or no health care spending (3%).[6]

2. *Providers*: Health care providers include physicians, nurses, physical therapists, nurse practitioners, physician assistants, psychologists, pharmacists, podiatrists, dentists, and others that provide clinical care. There were 479,856 primary care physicians and 525,439 specialty physicians for a total of 1,005,295 U.S. physicians in 2019.[7] The most physicians were in California, New York, and Texas. Physicians are employed in group practices, hospitals, governments, health plans, pharmaceutical companies, and public clinics.

3. *Payers*: The Centers for Medicare & Medicaid Services (CMS) track health care spending by sponsor. A sponsor is defined as the entity that is ultimately responsible for financing the health care bill. The three primary sponsors or payers are businesses, government, and consumer households. These sponsors pay health insurance premiums, out-of-pocket expenses, or finance health care through taxes or other revenues.

    Federal government spending increased based on faster growth in Medicare and Medicaid. Consumer household spending increased in out-of-pocket expenditures and decreased in employer-sponsored health insurance premiums. Private business costs increased due to higher health insurance premiums, and state and local government had slower growth in Medicaid spending versus 2017 (Table 3.5).[8]

4. *Employers*: Employers started offering health insurance during World War II to compete for scarce employees. Health benefits have grown to represent 8% of employee costs.[9] Employers are concentrating on four strategies. First, they are focusing on managing costs of benefits, modeling and projecting health insurance costs, using a high-performance drug formulary restricting brand name drugs for some conditions, and benchmarking costs against

TABLE 3.4  **Health Care Environmental Analysis Framework.**

| NINE MARKET PARTICIPANTS | Six Environmental Forces | | | | | |
|---|---|---|---|---|---|---|
| | Demographics | Economic | Social-Cultural | Natural | Technological | Political-Legal |
| CONSUMERS | | | | | | |
| CARE PROVIDERS | | | | | | |
| PAYERS | | | | | | |
| EMPLOYERS | | | | | | |
| GOVERNMENT | | | | | | |
| PROFESSIONAL ASSOCIATIONS | | | | | | |
| HEALTH CARE ADVOCACY GROUPS | | | | | | |
| HEALTH CARE SUPPLIERS | | | | | | |
| COMPETITORS | | | | | | |

TABLE 3.5  **2018 Health Payers.**

| Payer | 2018 Percentage | Percentage increase vs. 2017 |
|-------|-----------------|------------------------------|
| Federal government | 28% | 5.6% |
| Consumer households | 28% | 4.4% |
| Private businesses | 20% | 6.2% |
| State & local government | 17% | 2.5% |

peers. Second, employers are adding value to benefits. Examples include using data to evaluate the performance of physicians and hospitals, adding telemedicine services, and adopting narrow provider networks and centers of excellence. A center of excellence uses a universal certification or set of standards established by a medical specialty's professional society, a government entity such as the National Cancer Institute, or a consumer group organized in response to a disease.[10]

Third, employers want employees to become more engaged in managing their health. Employees are being given health care pricing and quality information, health and wellness messages through apps, and employers are changing organization culture to better support healthy behaviors. Employees can win prizes for improving health scores, and lululemon will reimburse employees for two fitness classes per week. Finally, employers are experimenting with innovative channels. These include contracting directly with physicians, hospitals, accountable care organizations, and medical homes. Employers have also found that using private health insurance exchanges, for active employees and retired employees, has reduced costs and simplified administration.[11]

5.  *Governments*: Federal, state, and local governments are active health care participants primarily through regulation, licensing, and reimbursement. For example, the federal government responded to problems with access to health insurance by passing the Affordable Care Act (ACA) in 2010. The controversial ACA offers subsidies to consumers without health insurance, created online health insurance exchanges to enroll consumers in health plans, and prohibits insurers from denying coverage for pre-existing health problems. The percentage uninsured at the time of interview decreased from 16.0% in 2010 to 8.5% in 2018.[12] As of January 2020, 33 states plus the District of Columbia had expanded Medicaid coverage, three were in the process of expanding, and 14 states had decided against expanding Medicaid coverage.

6. *Medical and trade associations*: Health care special interest groups are often represented by nonprofit professional associations. These organizations monitor market changes, publish research, lobby legislators to influence government policy, solicit funds, and sponsor educational programs. One of the most widely recognized organizations is the American Medical Association (AMA). Its membership includes a diverse group of physicians, but the AMA represents only about one-third of all U.S. physicians.

   The Pharmaceutical Research and Manufacturers of America (PhRMA) represents pharmaceutical and biotechnology companies. Pharma and biotech companies are strongly regulated to ensure patient safety. A major function of PhRMA is to act as a self-regulating entity to preempt additional government regulation. For example, the intent and effects of direct-to-consumer (DTC) advertising has been contentious. The PhRMA published its "Guiding Principles on Direct to Consumer Advertising about Prescription Medicines" on the PhRMA website to demonstrate the industry's commitment to improving the educational value of DTC.

7. *Health care advocacy organizations*: A health care advocacy organization is also usually a nonprofit entity that is devoted to a particular disease, medical condition, or health care problem. Advocacy organizations focus on increasing awareness, raising funds, providing information, developing support groups, and lobbying legislators to affect policy.

   The American Legacy Foundation launched its "truth" campaign in 2000 to target the 5.6 million teens at risk for premature death from tobacco use. American Legacy has prevented millions of young people from becoming smokers including 2.5 million between 2015 and 2018 alone. The Legacy Foundations uses marketing research-driven anti-smoking awareness advertising, "street teams" that meet and speak with teens on their own territory, a web-based smoking cessation program, and other tactics.

8. *Health care product and service suppliers*: There is a large number of diverse companies that market products and services to physicians, hospitals, health plans, employers, consumers, and other participants in the health care environment. Examples of these supplier categories are pharmaceutical companies, biotechnology companies, medical technology companies, medical supply and equipment companies, health plans, health information management companies, diagnostics companies, pharmacies, and many others.

   Most supplier product categories are made up of a few large companies with high market share along with hundreds of smaller companies. For example, it is estimated that the top 20 "Big Pharma" companies represent 60% of the world pharmaceutical market. There are more than 6,500 medical device companies in the U.S., but over 80% have fewer than 50 employees. The majority of U.S. metropolitan areas have a dominant health plan with a concentrated 50% or higher market share.[13]

9. *Competitors*: An organization's competitors can be identified from both an industry and a market point of view.[14] An industry is defined as a group of organizations that offer a product or class of products that are close substitutes for each other. Using the market approach, competitors are organizations that satisfy the same customer need.

   The market approach to competition reveals a broader set of actual and potential competitors. For example, a customer who buys a flu vaccine really wants the benefit of avoiding the flu. A vaccine can be purchased at a physician practice, a pharmacy, an employee health clinic, or an urgent care center. To identify a company's direct and indirect competitors, they map the buyer's steps taken to obtain and use a product.[15] Once competitors are identified through mapping, their strengths, weaknesses, market share, positioning, and apparent strategy can be evaluated.

## MACROENVIRONMENTAL FORCES

Marketers find many opportunities by identifying trends in the macroenvironment. A trend is a direction or sequence of events that has some momentum and durability. A fad is unpredictable, short-lived, and without social, economic, and political significance.[16] Trends are more predictable and durable than fads. A new product or marketing program is likely to be more successful if it is in line with strong trends rather than opposed to them.

For example, the percentage of people who value physical fitness and well-being has risen steadily over the years, especially in the under-30 group, the young women and upscale group, and people living in the West. Marketers of health foods and exercise equipment cater to this trend with appropriate products and communications. Marketers benefit from trendspotting skills, but detecting a new market opportunity does not guarantee its success even if it is technically feasible.

Companies and their suppliers, marketing intermediaries, customers, competitors, and publics all operate in a macroenvironment of forces and trends that shape opportunities and pose threats. Within the rapidly changing global picture, six major forces represent "noncontrollables" which the organization must monitor and to which it must respond. These forces are demographic, economic, social-cultural, natural, technological, and political-legal.

Marketers must also pay attention to the interactions among forces to identify new opportunities and threats. For example, explosive population growth (demographic) leads to more infectious diseases (natural), which lead governments to call for more regulations (political-legal), which stimulate new health care technological solutions and products (technological), which, if they are affordable (economic), may actually change attitudes and behavior (social-cultural).

### Demographic Environment

The main demographic force that marketers monitor is population because people make up markets. Marketers are interested in the size and growth rate of the population in different cities, regions, and nations. Marketers also pay attention to age distribution. Health status has been found to be affected by demographics such as the geographical distribution of people, birth and death rates, age, ethnic mix, educational levels, household patterns, and regional characteristics and movements.

Marketers can use demographic data to help understand market behavior and identify health care needs and wants. The Agency for Healthcare Research and Quality (AHRQ) analyzes demographic data to understand health care utilization. The AHRQ periodically segments health care cost data by demographics that include the number of chronic conditions, age, race, sex, insurance status, and income. Those consumers in the top decile of spenders are more likely to be in fair or poor health, elderly, female, non-Hispanic whites, and those with public-only coverage. Those in the bottom half of spenders are more likely to be in excellent health, children and young adults, men, Hispanics, and the uninsured.[17]

***Worldwide Population Growth.***    The world population is undergoing explosive growth, standing at over 7.8 billion and expected to exceed 8 billion by the year 2023.[18] Population growth is a source of concern for two reasons. First, resources needed to support this much human life—such as food, health care, and land—are limited and may be depleted at some point. Second, population growth is highest in areas that can least afford it. Africa has the highest rate of population growth, and it is expected to have more than half of world growth between 2015 and 2050 due to high birth rates and young populations. In comparison, births barely exceed deaths in developed countries, and deaths are expected to exceed births in developed countries for the first time in 2025.[19]

Although worldwide population growth has major implications for health care, these growing markets may not have sufficient purchasing power. Nonetheless, organizations that carefully analyze their markets can find major opportunities. With the growth of senior markets, for example, there is greater demand for long-term care and nursing home services. Not all seniors have the same wants and needs, however, and segmenting the senior market will help marketers serve specific populations.

***Population Age Mix.***    National populations vary in their age mix. At one extreme is Mexico, a country with a very young population and rapid population growth. At the other extreme is Japan, a country with one of the world's oldest populations. Milk, diapers, school supplies, and toys would be important products in Mexico. Japan's population would consume many more adult products. A population can be subdivided into six age groups: preschool, school-age children, teens, young adults age 25 to 40, middle-aged adults age 40 to 65, and older adults age 65 and up. For marketers, the most populous age groups are most influential in the marketing environment.

In the U.S., the 77 million baby boomers born between 1946 and 1964 are a powerful force shaping the health care marketplace. Boomers are fixated on their youth, not their age. According to one survey, half of all boomers were depressed that they were no longer young and nearly 1 in 5 were actively resisting the aging process. In fact, obesity afflicts 40% of 65- to 74-year-olds. Searching for the "fountain of youth," new diets, sales of health club memberships, home gym equipment, skin-tightening creams, nutritional supplements, and organic foods have all soared.

Boomers are becoming more involved with health care decisions not only for themselves, but also for their aging parents who require long-term care services. An estimated 75% of boomers and their parents, 2.3 million people, are projected to require nursing home care by 2030, up from 1.3 million in 2010. Those living with Alzheimer's disease are expected to nearly triple from 5 million in 2013 to 14 million in 2050.[20] Understanding these trends is important for hospital facility planning, drug development, medical school enrollment, and a wide range of other health care services and products.

*Ethnic Health Care Markets.*   Countries also vary in ethnic and racial makeup. The U.S. was originally called a "melting pot," but there are increasing signs that the melting didn't occur. Now people call the U.S. a "salad bowl" society with ethnic groups maintaining their ethnic differences, neighborhoods, and cultures. The U.S. is increasingly becoming more racially and ethnically diverse.

The population of the U.S. in 2020 was 330.2 million people, which ranked it the third most populous country. The population by race and ethnicity in 2018 was 60% white, 18% Hispanic, 12% black, 6% Asian, 3% two or more races, and 1% American Indian.[21] According to the Pew Research Center, the U.S. will not have a single racial or ethnic majority by 2055. Much of this change is because of immigration. Most of the 59 million immigrants to the U.S. since 1965 have come from Latin America and Asia. In 1965, 5% of the U.S. population was foreign-born compared to 14% in 2019.[22]

Each group has specific needs, wants, and buying habits that marketers need to understand. After PacifiCare Health Systems (now part of United Health Group) learned that 20% of its 3 million health plan customers were Latino, it set up a new unit, Latino Health Solutions department. This department created an innovative health benefits program named PlanBien to better reach this market segment. PlanBien offers bilingual health information and services for Hispanic and Latino families, employers, and its affiliated brokers and consultants. PlanBien also refers Hispanic and Latino members to Spanish-speaking doctors.[23]

Market segmentation and targeting is also important for health plans interested in the Medicare/Medicaid dual-eligible market. This group is made up of

9 million lower-income people over age 65 who are also eligible for Medicaid. The size of this segment is 40 million people, and 21 million are in various ethnic groups. Many health plans simply target the 65 and over segment and rely on one message to communicate their dual-eligible product.

Marketing communications would be more cost-effective, and sales would be higher, if communications were more targeted. Research has found that on average African-American seniors view seven hours of television a day, more than any other ethnic group. Asian-Americans and Hispanic seniors have a tendency to prefer online sources for information. Bilingual Asian-American seniors have higher levels of trust in media and services that are communicated in their native language, while 43% of Hispanic seniors use Spanish-only media. Overgeneralizing ethnic group preferences, however, can be risky because individuals within groups have a range of preferences.

Senior purchasing decisions are also influenced by their caregivers and influencers. Adult children and other caregivers want communications that help them better understand the health of their loved ones, support their role as caregiver, and help reduce caregiver stress. Influencers such as doctors and friends have a wide range of communication needs and preferences. These needs should be analyzed to ensure that communication is effective.

### *Economic Environment*

Markets, as well as people, require purchasing power. The available purchasing power in an economy depends on current income, prices, savings, debt, and credit availability. Marketers must pay careful attention to trends affecting purchasing power because they can have a strong impact on revenue, especially for health care organizations with high-priced products and services and price-sensitive consumers. For example, people with lower incomes are not good prospects for expensive concierge physician services with high monthly fees or high-deductible health plans.

*Income Distribution.*   Nations vary greatly in level and distribution of income and industrial structure. The four types of industrial structures are subsistence economies (few opportunities for marketers), raw-material exporting economies such as Zaire (copper) and Saudi Arabia (oil), industrializing economies such as India, Egypt, and the Philippines, and industrial economies that are rich markets for all sorts of goods and services like the U.S. and Western Europe.

Marketers often distinguish countries with five different income-distribution patterns: (1) very low incomes, (2) mostly low incomes, (3) very low and very high incomes, (4) low, medium, high incomes, and (5) mostly medium incomes. In the U.S., recent trends in health care costs, insurance coverage, and household income have increased disparities between different income groups.

Improvements in life expectancy have been highly unequal, with low-income consumers having smaller gains in life expectancy compared with higher-income consumers. For example, the average life expectancy of a 66-year-old man who was in the top 10% career income segment is expected to live 79.3 years. A man of the same age in the lowest 10% income segment is likely to live five years less.[24]

***Health Care Costs.***    An estimated $3.6 trillion was spent on national health expenditure in 2018. The majority of spending (53%) was for hospital (33%) and physician (20%) care. Overall expenditure increased 4.6% compared to 2017. U.S. health expenditure represented 17.7% of gross national product, and average expenditure per person was $11,172 (Table 3.6 and Figure 3.2).[25]

The primary sources of spending for national health expenditures came from private health insurance, Medicare, Medicaid, and consumer out-of-pocket. Private health insurance—such as Blue Cross/Blue Shield, United Healthcare, and Kaiser Permanente—represented 34% of total health spending. It increased by 5.8% in 2018 to $1,243.0 billion. Medicare spending represented 21% at $750.2 billion and grew 6.4% in 2018. Overall Medicaid spending was 16% of the total, and Medicaid grew 3.0% to $597.4 billion in 2018. Consumers paid 10% of total health care spending out-of-pocket. Consumer spending increased 2.8% to $375.6 billion (Figure 3.3).[26]

**TABLE 3.6**  **2018 National Health Expenditures.**

| Type of Health Care | Percentage of Total Expenditures | 2018 Cost (billions) | Percentage Increase vs. 2017 |
|---|---|---|---|
| Hospital | 33% | $1,200.0 | 4.5% |
| Physician | 20% | $725.6 | 4.1% |
| Prescription drugs | 9% | $335.0 | 2.5% |
| Non-traditional settings | 5% | $191.6 | 4.6% |
| Nursing & continuing care | 5% | $168.5 | 1.4% |
| Dental | 4% | $135.6 | 4.6% |
| Home health | 3% | $102.2 | 5.2% |

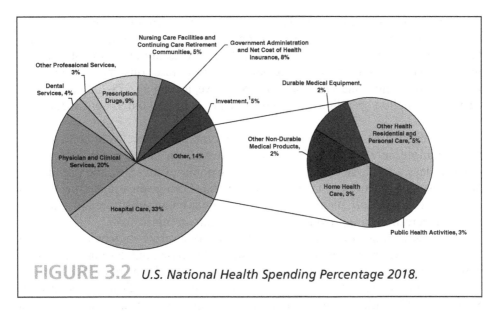

FIGURE 3.2  *U.S. National Health Spending Percentage 2018.*

*National Health Expenditure Data, CMS, December 5, 2019, www.cms.gov/Research-Statistics-Data-and-Systems/Statistics-Trends-and-Reports/NationalHealthExpendData/NHE-Fact-Sheet, accessed 12/13/19.*

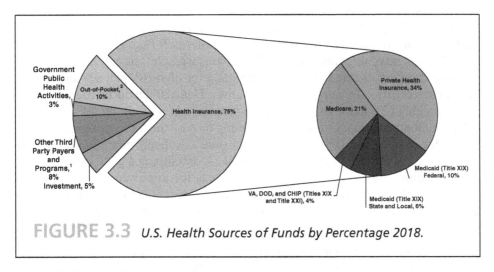

FIGURE 3.3  *U.S. Health Sources of Funds by Percentage 2018.*

*National Health Expenditure Data 2018 Fact Sheet, CMS, www.cms.gov/files/document/nations-health-dollar-where-it-came-where-it-went.pdf, accessed 1/1/20.*

Health care spending by consumer ranges widely. About 5% of the population accounts for nearly half the spending in a given year. Meanwhile, the other half of the population has little or no health care costs, about 3% of total spending.[27] AHRQ analyzed consumer segment costs and those consumers with four or more chronic conditions were the most expensive, averaging $78,200 per person. The second highest spending group, consumers age 65 and older, were $63,800 on average.

Starting in 2014, the ACA began the economic shift from "volume to value." CMS changed care provider financial incentives from billing more procedures, hospital days, and physician visits to achieving quality, outcomes, and population health results. For example, health promotion has been given a higher priority to avoid acute illness, outpatient care and home care is being substituted for hospital inpatient care, and care provider collaboration has strengthened.

CMS is testing new clinical care models to improve outcomes, investing resources to advance community health, using value-based purchasing, supporting patient-centered medical homes, and mandating the development of Accountable Care Organizations (ACOs). For example, the Heartland Medical Center ACO in St. Joseph, Missouri, was one of 114 ACOs to join the Medicare Shared Savings Program in 2012, and it now oversees care for 12,600 Medicare beneficiaries. The ACO focused its first-year strategy on enhancing quality reporting at the point of care. It adapted the medical center's electronic health record (EHR) system to enable physicians to identify consumers' unmet medical needs. The EHR data dashboard flags how clinical treatment diverges from evidence-based standards. The dashboard also gives members of the care team a quick synopsis of diagnoses, medication history, and health care utilization patterns. It flags gaps in care such as missed cancer screenings and lab tests for patients with chronic conditions.

By expanding its care management program for high-risk patients and engaging employees in quality improvement initiatives, Heartland reduced overall spending by roughly 15% in the first year of the program. As a result, the ACO received a $2.9 million performance bonus representing 60% of the total savings. The most important reasons for Heartland's success were effectively communicating and educating providers about the goals of the ACO, developing a good care management program, and using data to monitor areas for improvement.[28] Heartland engaged employees by restructuring their financial incentives to support the new quality measures. Physicians, nurses, and traditional hourly-wage workers—such as medical assistants—were able to increase their compensation by 12%.

***Savings, Debt, and Credit Availability.***   Consumer savings, debt, and credit availability affect health consumer expenditures. Physicians and hospitals are now working with financial services companies to market credit cards to patients. The purpose of these joint ventures is to help physicians and hospitals reduce their mounting collection efforts, which are due to patients bearing more responsibility for out-of-pocket spending on health care.

CareCredit, CapitalOne Healthcare Finance, GE Money CareCredit, and other health care credit cards offer consumers credit for elective procedures like LASIK eye surgery or cosmetic Botox treatments as well as for services like cancer treatment. The cards often have no-interest promotional periods, but if the balance is not paid in full, interest charges as high as 27.99% are assessed retroactively for the entire paid and unpaid balances. These credit offerings are controversial. Consumers have reported that medical providers have pressured them to sign credit applications. When hospitals encourage patients to tap unused credit from these cards, consumers have lost bargaining leverage for discounts as well as the opportunity for charity care.[29]

## Social-Cultural Environment

Society shapes our beliefs, values, and norms that largely define consumer preferences. People almost unconsciously absorb a world view that defines their relationship to themselves, others, organizations, society, and the universe. Other cultural characteristics of interest to marketers include the persistence of core cultural values, the existence of subcultures, and shifts of values through time.

1. *Views of themselves*: Consumers are becoming increasingly involved in their health care. Nine out of 10 consumers prefer to be in control of medical decisions or participate in shared decision-making with their doctors. Only 7% of consumers want their doctor to take the lead role. These findings support an ongoing trend toward a health care model in which the consumer plays a central role in making choices that meet their needs.[30] A primary reason for this trend is that consumers are being given more responsibility for paying for their health care.

2. *Views of others*: People are concerned about health care for the homeless, for their aging parents, and for residents of developing countries. At the same time, 56% of consumers have concerns about the privacy and security of their medical information that would prevent them from telling their doctors "everything" about their personal health.

3. *Views of organizations*: The requirement that all consumers have health insurance and the growth of high-deductible health plans have resulted in consumers wanting more price transparency, affordability, the ability to compare prices, and get speedy service. Retail health care organizations have taken advantage of this market opportunity. For example, CVS opened its first MinuteClinics in 2006 staffed with nurse practitioners that offered a range of primary care from flu shots to physicals. Now there are more than 960 MinuteClinics nationwide that post their prices, allow consumers to choose which services they want, and do not require appointments.[31]

4. *Views of society*: Those who want to change society do not always act in its best interest. Many refuse to get their children immunized because of fears

about side effects and their distrust of policymakers and pharmaceutical companies. Not all of these concerns are unfounded. Merck, the manufacturer of the MMR vaccine, is currently embroiled in two lawsuits for allegedly falsifying data on the effectiveness of the mumps vaccine.[32]

5. *Views of nature*: People vary in their attitudes toward nature. To treat minor illnesses, 17% of consumers said they prefer to use natural homeopathic remedies like herbal medicines over mainstream or allopathic medicines. The use of natural remedies may increase in coming years since they are more preferred by millennials (22%), and generation X (19%) consumers, compared to baby boomers (14%) and seniors (11%).[33]

**High Persistence of Core Values.**    Most people in the U.S. still believe in working, getting married, giving to charity, and being honest. *Core beliefs* and values are passed from parents to children and are reinforced by social institutions—schools, religious institutions, businesses, and governments. *Secondary beliefs* and values are more open to change. Believing in the institution of marriage is a core belief. Believing people should marry early is a secondary belief.

Marketers have some chance of changing secondary values but little chance of changing core values. For instance, the nonprofit organization Mothers Against Drunk Drivers (MADD) does not try to stop the sale of alcohol, but it does promote the idea of appointing a designated driver who will not drink. MADD also lobbies against drugged driving, underage drinking, and lowering the legal drinking age to 18.

Although core values are fairly persistent, cultural swings do take place. In the 1960s, hippies, the Beatles, Elvis Presley, and other cultural phenomena had a major impact on hairstyles, clothing, sexual norms, and life goals. Young boys are now being influenced by the superhero culture and video games while young girls are influenced by the Disney princess culture. Sports figures like tennis player Serena Williams and footballer Ronaldo, as well as pop singers like Taylor Swift, are also influencing the culture.

Additionally, each society contains subcultures, groups with shared values, beliefs, preferences, and behaviors emerging from their special life experiences or circumstances. Many brands target young people to develop them as lifetime customers. Marketers at community hospitals like Timpanogos Regional Hospital in Orem, Utah, and the Department of Pediatric Newborn Medicine at the Brigham and Women's Hospital academic medical center in Boston, promote maternity services to meet the needs of two very different markets. The underlying shared goal, however, is to attract younger consumers who will have positive customer experiences and who will then return for other hospital services as they age.

### Natural Environment

Natural environmental forces can take several forms. The deterioration of the natural environment is a major global concern. In many world cities, air and water pollution have reached dangerous levels and have triggered or worsened such health problems as asthma and certain types of cancer. Experts have documented the ecological damage and the global warming phenomenon. Watchdog groups such as the Sierra Club and Friends of the Earth carry these concerns into the political and social action.

Pollutants can trigger and exacerbate asthma, COPD, and cancers. Opportunities await those who can reconcile prosperity with environmental protection. Due to millions of rural cooking fires, parts of Southern Asia suffer extremely poor air quality. A person cooking over an open wood or kerosene fire inhales the equivalent of two packs of cigarettes a day. Illinois-based Sun Ovens International (sunoven.com/around-the-world) makes family-sized and institutional solar ovens that use mirrors to redirect the sun's rays into an insulated box. Used in more than 100 countries, the oven improves health, saves money, and reduces greenhouse gas emissions.

Diseases are natural forces that have been classified into three types by the Centers for Disease Control and Prevention (CDC). A disease *outbreak* is characterized by its inability to be controlled.[34] Sometimes a single case of a contagious disease is considered an outbreak. This may be true if it is an unknown disease, is new to a community, or has been absent from a population for a long time. CDC considered the 2014 cases of the Ebola virus in West Africa to be an outbreak.[35]

An *epidemic* is a disease that affects many people at the same time. In 2003, the severe acute respiratory syndrome (SARS) epidemic took the lives of nearly 800 people worldwide.[36] A *pandemic* is a very extensive epidemic, like a plague, that is prevalent in a country, continent, or the world. HIV/AIDS is an example of a major pandemic that is being better controlled through public health management. In 2020, Covid-19 was classified as a global respiratory pandemic that caught countries unaware of virtually every aspect of the disease. The CDC has developed a Pandemic Severity Index, with categories of increasing severity (Level 1 to Level 5). It uses a ratio to estimate the number of expected deaths. Similar to preparing for a hurricane, this index can help communities with pandemic preparedness and planning.[37] Covid-19 was classified a Level 3 Warning Avoid Nonessential Travel—Widespread Ongoing Transmission on March 27, 2020.[38]

Natural environmental trends can lead to market opportunities for health care companies. One-third of nosocomial or hospital-acquired infections are considered preventable. The CDC estimates that 2 million people in the U.S. are infected annually by hospital-acquired infections, resulting in 20,000 deaths.[39] The most common nosocomial infections are of the urinary tract, surgical site, and various pneumonias. Roche Molecular Diagnostics developed the cobas® MRSA/SA Test to detect Staphylococcus aureus (SA) and methicillin-resistant Staphylococcus aureus (MRSA) infections. This test is used by hospitals to screen for both organisms using a single nasal swab specimen with results in a matter of hours.[40]

### Technological Environment

One of the most dramatic forces shaping health care is technology. New health care technology has led to such breakthroughs as penicillin, open-heart surgery, and the birth control pill. Every new technology can also be a force for "creative destruction." Christensen defined both sustainable and destructive technologies.[41] A sustainable technology adds an incremental improvement to an established technology. Xanax is a sedative prescribed for anxiety, and time- released Xanax was introduced to reduce the number of daily doses needed.

A destructive technology displaces an established technology and creates a new industry. For example, cholesterol-lowering statin drugs like Lipitor and heart stents have substantially reduced the demand for coronary bypass surgery. Software "robots" can be used to automate manual workflows for processing complicated medical claims and consequently eliminate administrative jobs. Disruptive technologies may have performance problems or low market demand. Examples are a new health information technology that may have a negative impact on the consumer or physician experience, or a virtual reality application designed to distract pain patients that may not have clinical support.

New health care technology also creates major long-term social consequences that are not always foreseeable. The contraceptive pill led to smaller families, more working wives, and larger discretionary incomes—resulting in higher expenditures on vacation travel, durable goods, and luxury items. Marketers should monitor such technology trends as the pace of change, the opportunities for innovation, varying R&D budgets, and increased regulation.

**Accelerating Pace of Technological Change.**   Many health care technology products such as MRI scanners were not available 30 years ago. The lag between new ideas and their successful implementation is all but disappearing, as is the time between introduction and peak production. These technologies are changing markets and needs. For example, technologies enabling physicians to treat patients in remote geographic locations using telehealth can save time, increase access to care, and reduce costs.

The Mayo Clinic has been expanding its brand through its adoption of innovative technology. It uses telemedicine services to assess, diagnose, and treat consumers for stroke, neonatology, and emergency medicine. Through its Center for Connected Care, Mayo is using video communications to help its specialty physicians expand the brand to 45 participating hospitals across nine states.

**Unlimited Opportunities for Innovation.**   Scientists today are working on a startling range of new technologies that will revolutionize products and production processes. Some of the most exciting work is being done in biotechnology, computers, microelectronics, telecommunications, robotics, and designer materials. Researchers are working on AIDS vaccines, safer contraceptives, more potent and less addicting painkillers, and tastier nonfattening foods. They are developing new classes of antibiotics to fight ultra-resistant infections, designing robots for heart surgery and home nursing. The challenge in innovation is not only technical but commercial—to develop affordable new versions of products.

Companies are already harnessing the power of genome sequencing. This trend began with the Human Genome Project (HGP) that sequenced the first human genome to better understand, prevent, diagnose, and treat diseases and conditions. The HGP has spawned a $20 billion DNA technology industry. The UK Biobank has plans to decipher the genomes of 500,000 individuals, while Iceland is studying the genomes of its entire human population. Complete Genomics, a company based in California and owned by BGI-Shenzhen in China, claims to be on the verge of roughly sequencing genomes for whole species for about $100 by using rapidly improving sequencing technology.[42]

***Increased Regulation of Technological Change.*** As products become more complex, the public needs to be reassured about their safety. Consequently, government agencies' powers to investigate and ban potentially unsafe products have been expanded. In the U.S., the Federal Food and Drug Administration must approve all drugs before they can be sold. Safety and health regulations have also increased in the areas of food, automobiles, clothing, electrical appliances, and construction. Marketers must be aware of these regulations when proposing, developing, and launching new products.

### *Political-Legal Environment*

Marketing decisions are strongly affected by developments in the political and legal environment. This environment comprises laws, government agencies, and pressure groups that influence and limit various organizations and individuals. An example of an innovative state government initiative that effectively improves population health outcomes is the Health Access at the Right Time program (HeART) started by the South Carolina Department of Health and Human Services (SCDHHS) in February 2014.

HeART is a collaborative program involving 50 state agencies, providers, and community stakeholders. HeART targets 75,000 residents in the sickest Medicaid geographical "hotspots." It improves care coordination through retail clinics, telemedicine, school-based health clinics, and the use of community health workers. Community health workers effectively increase access to health care services through better patient communications with primary care practices. South Carolina estimates that its fiscal year 2014 spending would have been 64% higher without HeART.[43]

Sometimes new laws lead to new opportunities for businesses. Regulations related to the licensing and training of emergency medical technicians (EMTs) and paramedics have created dozens of new companies dedicated to meeting the increased demand for mandatory training.

Four major trends in the health care political-legal environment are the implementation of the ACA, access to clinical and financial health care data, increased business legislation, and the growth of special-interest groups.

***Implementation of the Affordable Care Act.*** The ACA has affected health care economics, as described earlier in this chapter, and it also has had a far-reaching impact on politics and society. Two key goals of the ACA were to increase the number of consumers with health insurance and to expand coverage of the Medicaid program.

In 2010, the uninsured rate was an all-time high of 18.2%. ACA implementation began in January 2014, and the uninsured rate for those under age 65 plummeted to 10.3% by the first nine months of 2016, according to data from CDC. This was the lowest percentage of uninsured consumers since the CDC began tracking in 1971.[44]

Unfortunately, the uninsured rate has reversed and climbed to 13.7% in 2018. Women, younger adults, the lower-income group have the greatest increases, and all regions except for the East reported increases.[45] One reason may be the increase in the rates of insurance premiums in many states, and another is may be that insurers have increasingly withdrawn from the ACA exchanges resulting in fewer choices and less premium price competition.

Having health insurance affects health care because it determines how and when people seek medical care, where they can get their care, and how healthy they are overall. Uninsured adults are more likely to delay medical diagnosis or treatment when they are acutely sick or injured because of cost. Additionally, consumers without health insurance are less likely to receive preventive care or screenings for early detection of chronic diseases.[46] The states that expanded Medicaid under the ACA had a 7.3% uninsured rate in 2016, and the states that did not expand Medicaid had a 14.1% uninsured rate. An estimated 9 to 10 million mostly low-income consumers gained Medicaid coverage. Over half of the national uninsured population lived in those states.

***Access to Financial and Clinical Health Care Data.***   CMS proposed in its 2014 Inpatient Prospective Payment System rule that hospitals "undertake efforts to engage in consumer-friendly communication of their charges."[47] This purpose is to help patients understand specific costs before treatment and allow them to compare hospital prices. Pricing data is becoming more accessible to the public through resources such as CMS's physician payment data as well as through private companies. Consumers facing high-deductible health plans are also requesting cash prices for procedures from physicians and hospitals.

Another example of the trend toward pricing transparency is health plan reference pricing. Plans set the amount they will pay for procedures and the different fees providers charge. Consumers can select the provider and decide if they will pay a higher price if it is higher than what the plan will pay. After the California Public Employees' Retirement System (CalPERS) began using reference pricing for hip and knee replacements, consumer choices for those procedures resulted in a 26% decrease in costs for CalPERS from 2010 to 2011.

Clinical data access is also becoming more common. The U.S. Department of Health and Human Services proposed new rules that would require clinical trial sponsors to report the summary results of all clinical trials, not just trials for products that receive FDA approval. The OpenFDA initiative provides a public database for analyzing drug and medical device adverse events, recalls, side effects, and labeling information. The FDA is also interested in having patients share their experiences using mobile health apps.[48]

*Increase of Business Legislation.*    Business legislation has three main purposes: to protect businesses from unfair competition, to protect consumers from unfair business practices, and to protect the interests of society from unfair business behavior. A major purpose of business legislation and enforcement is to charge businesses with the social costs created by their products or production processes.

At what point do the costs of regulation exceed the benefits? Although each new law may have a legitimate rationale, it may have the unintended effect of sapping initiative and impeding economic growth. Regulators and enforcers may be lax or overzealous. For example, there are 35 states that require certificate of need (CON) approval before hospitals can begin new construction or remodeling of hospital facilities. These CON laws are designed to control supply of what could be unneeded health services and extra costs to the system. An alternative approach would be to let market forces influence changes in capacity to make hospitals accountable and at risk for their initiatives so as to protect taxpayers. Marketers need a good working knowledge of relevant business legislation, legal review procedures, major laws protecting competition, consumers, and society, and ethical standards.

While increased hospital financial accountability may reduce the need for CON regulation, there are increased needs for health care business legislation. Most assume that the FDA can require prescription and over-the-counter companies to stop marketing products that are unsafe, but the FDA does not currently have that ability. Pending legislation, the Recall Unsafe Drugs Act bill, was introduced to Congress in February 2017, and it would give the FDA recall authority. Under current legislation, the FDA can only request that companies voluntarily recall products, but companies are not legally required to comply. The agency can only mandatorily recall infant formula, medical devices, human tissue products, biologics, and tobacco.[49]

The New England Compounding Center produced contaminated drugs in 2012, and there were no regulations for compounding pharmacies at the time. The drugs led to a fatal fungal meningitis outbreak affecting 778 patients and causing 64 deaths nationwide. Regulations for these pharmacies have subsequently been approved. Standard Homeopathic Company, the manufacturer of the Hyland's brand of homeopathic products, marketed teething tablets with inconsistent levels of belladonna. Belladonna is an herb that has toxic side effects if taken orally. Hyland's teething tablets have been linked to over 400 adverse events including death, seizures, shortness of breath, and tremors. Neither New England Compounding Center or Standard Homeopathic complied with the voluntary recall requested by the FDA.

*Growth of Special-Interest Groups.*    The number and power of special-interest groups have increased since the early 1990s. Political action committees (PACs) lobby government officials and pressure businesses to pay more attention to the rights of consumers, women, senior citizens, minorities, the disabled, and the LGBTQ community.

An important force affecting health care organizations is consumerism—an effort of citizens and government to strengthen the rights and powers of buyers in relation to sellers. The National Association of Healthcare Advocacy Consultants uses education, national standards of practice, and policy change to support better consumer health. They help consumers understand their diagnoses and procedures, assist in considering second opinions and alternate treatment options, clarify their personal values as they relate to medical treatments, coordinate case management and discharge planning, and arrange home community-based services.[50]

Yet new laws and growing pressure from special-interest groups continue to add more restraints on marketers, moving many private marketing transactions into the public domain. Marketing managers in the pharmaceutical sector feel particularly constrained by their legal departments. Pharma legal staff is increasingly focused on fraud and abuse laws, especially in the international market, as well as ensuring that advertising claims fall within the law.

## CHAPTER SUMMARY

Understanding the health care environment is the basis of effective strategic marketing. Marketing information and data are necessary to know what target markets want and need. A marketing information system consists of the people, equipment, and procedures used to collect, analyze, and distribute information to decision-makers. It includes an internal records system, a marketing intelligence system, and a marketing research system.

Marketing research is broadly divided between secondary research that is already collected and primary marketing research that has not been collected. The secondary research sources described represent a cross-section of health care research options. An important element of primary research is to begin the research process with marketing decisions. Once the decisions have been identified, the research can be designed to collect the specific information needed to make the decisions.

An environmental analysis analyzes how health care market participants are affected by market forces. The nine groups of health care participants affected by environmental forces are consumers, care providers, payers, employers, government, professional associations, health care advocacy groups, health care product and service suppliers, and health care competitors. The six environmental forces affecting the participants are demographic, economic, social-cultural, natural, technological, and political-legal forces. The primary purpose of an environmental analysis for health care organizations is to identify market opportunities and market threats.

## DISCUSSION QUESTIONS

1. Online marketing research surveys are becoming more common based on their lower costs. What are the pros and cons of using web-based series of focus group versus a traditional in-person focus group?

2. Physicians and other scientists are often concerned with survey data validity and reliability because they make decisions based on statistical significance. Statistical significance requires random selection of survey respondents. Quantitative telephone surveys randomly select survey respondents, and online surveys rely on respondent panels that are not random samples. Telephone surveys have a higher cost than online surveys. Your marketing research client is a group of academic medical center faculty researchers. What questions would you ask this client before you proposed either a phone survey or an online survey?

3. Your company just received marketing approval in the European Union (EU) for an implantable orthopedic device, and you have been transferred to Frankfurt, Germany, to manage the rollout. Unfortunately, you know very little about European health care systems. Pick one EU country and use the environmental analysis framework in this chapter to help you understand that country's health care system with respect to your product.

4. You are working for a U.S. Senator who is very concerned about rising health care costs. In order to address this problem, she and her colleagues are proposing a single, national fee schedule that would apply to all providers and suppliers. What do you tell her are the three most important marketing issues facing this approach to reduce costs?

## EXERCISE: ENVIRONMENTAL ANALYSIS

Conduct an environmental analysis for a health care product or service of your choice. Download a copy of the "Health Care Environmental Analysis Framework" (Table 3.4) from the Book Companion site to organize your analysis.

1. Use the secondary marketing research sources to research the six health care environmental forces and the nine participants for your selected product, service, or organization. You can also use other secondary research sources.

2. Use the Health Care Environmental Analysis Framework to organize the impact of each environmental force on the nine participants. Analyze how the environmental forces affect the different health care participants in your market. (Note: Not all of the forces will have an effect on all of the participants.)

3. Write a health care environmental analysis that identifies the most important forces, the participants most affected, and then analyze the market opportunities and threats for your product or organization.

# CHAPTER

# CONSUMER HEALTH CARE MARKETING

## LEARNING OBJECTIVES

In this chapter we will address the following questions:

1. Why do consumers buy health care?
2. What determines health care behavior?
3. How do consumers make health care buying decisions?
4. How have market-driven organizations used innovative strategies to leverage market opportunities?

Everyone is a health care consumer, but consumer demand for different health care services and products varies widely. Consumer marketing behavior plays an important role in understanding how consumers make different health care buying decisions. Marketers need to know the answers to the following "who, what, when, where, how, and why" questions:[1]

a) Who buys our product or service?

b) Who makes the decision to buy the product?

c) Who influences the decision to buy the product?

d) How is the purchase decision made? Who assumes what role?

e) What does the customer buy? What needs must be satisfied?

f) Why do customers buy a particular brand?

g) Where do they buy the product or service?

h) When do they buy? Any seasonality factors?

i) How is our product perceived by customers?

j) What are customers' attitudes toward our product?

k) What social factors might influence the purchase decision?

l) Does the customer's lifestyle influence their decisions?

m) How do personal or demographic factors influence the purchase decision?

Marketers will get the answers to these questions and leverage market opportunities if they can estimate consumer health care demand, understand consumer health care behavior and psychology, and apply a five-stage buying decision model.

## CONSUMER DEMAND FOR HEALTH CARE

Analyzing consumer life span, morbidity, mortality data, health care spending patterns, and changes in health status can help explain why health care is needed, who uses it, and how the U.S. compares to other countries.

### Life Expectancy Fell

Life expectancy is the most basic measure of the health of a society, and it is strongly influenced by infant mortality. The overall U.S. life expectancy in 2018 was 78.7 years at birth. Female life expectancy was 81.2 years, and male life expectancy was five years less at 76.2 years. That same year, overall life expectancy increased for the first time in four years, rising from 78.6 years in 2017. Life expectancy had peaked at 78.9 in 2014, and then dropped by 0.1 annually from 2015 to 2017. Although these 0.1 differences are small, life expectancy declines in developed countries are extremely unusual. The previous decline occurred in 1993 during the

AIDS epidemic. The recent decline is associated with the opioid epidemic or the "deaths of despair" of younger people who died from overdoses, suicide, and alcoholism. Using another measure, expected additional lifespan for consumers at age 65 in 2018 was 20.7 years for females and 18.1 years for males (Figure 4.1).[2]

According to the Organization for Economic Cooperation and Development (OECD), an intergovernmental economic organization with 37 member countries with market economies, a person born in 2019 can expect to live almost 81 years. Global gains in life expectancy, however, are stalling and chronic diseases (including mental illness) have replaced such acute conditions as infectious diseases as the major causes of morbidity and mortality. Life expectancy in 2015 decreased in 19 countries especially in the United States, France, and the Netherlands.

U.S. life expectancy ranked 28th among the 36 OECD countries reporting in 2018 (Figure 4.2).[3] The reasons for this change include rising rates of obesity and diabetes in OECD countries, with 56% of adults overweight or obese and almost one-third of children aged 5 to 9 overweight. Other reasons for this include: slower progress in reducing deaths from heart disease and stroke, respiratory diseases such as influenza and pneumonia that have claimed more lives in recent years, and opioid-related deaths that have increased by about 20% since 2011. Almost one-third of adults live with two or more chronic conditions. Mental illness has also taken its toll, with an estimated one in two people experiencing a mental health problem in their lifetime.

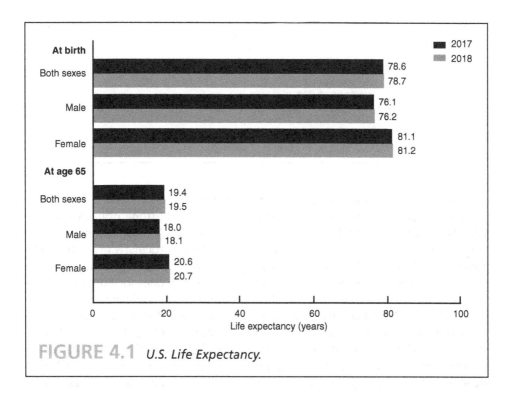

**FIGURE 4.1** *U.S. Life Expectancy.*

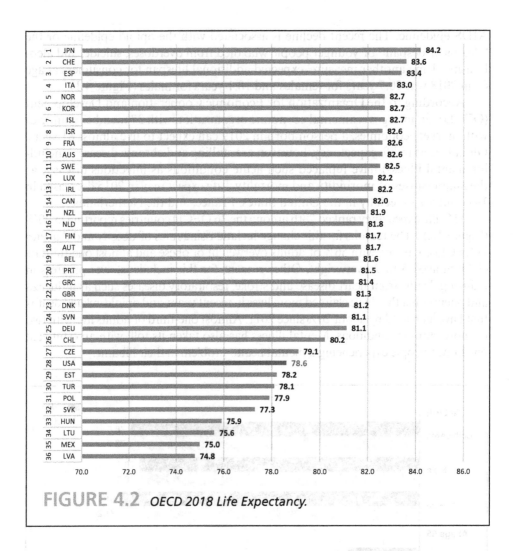

**FIGURE 4.2** *OECD 2018 Life Expectancy.*

Quality of care is improving in terms of safety and effectiveness, but patient-reported outcomes and experiences need more attention. Strong primary care systems keep people well and relieve pressure on hospitals. Avoidable admissions for chronic conditions have fallen in most OECD countries, particularly in South Korea, Lithuania, Mexico, and Sweden. Fewer people are dying following a heart attack or stroke, with Norway and Iceland having low case-fatality rates for both conditions. Survival rates for a range of cancers reflect better preventive and curative care.

Across all OECD countries, women diagnosed early for breast cancer have a 90% or higher probability of surviving their cancer for at least five years. A more thorough understanding of quality of care requires measuring what matters to people. Yet few health systems routinely ask patients about the outcomes and experiences of their care to get a complete understanding of the customer experience.[4]

## Morbidity Data

Virtually everyone is a health care consumer at birth. Nearly all U.S. infants (99%) are born in a hospital.[5] The demand for health care then begins to change for different consumer segments. Morbidity includes both prevalence and incidence of disease. Incidence is the number of new cases of illnesses over a time period, and prevalence is the total number of cases at a particular time.[6] The prevalence of obesity was 93.3 million of U.S. adults in 2015–2016, which represented 39.8% of the population. Obesity-related conditions include heart disease, stroke, type 2 diabetes, and certain types of cancer, which are some of the leading causes of preventable, premature death. Hispanics and non-Hispanic blacks had the highest age-adjusted prevalence of obesity, followed by non-Hispanic whites and non-Hispanic Asians (Figure 4.3).[7]

Another approach to inferring illness and injury morbidity is to analyze physician visits. Visits can take place in physician practices, hospital emergency departments and clinics, in-home, urgent care centers, and other locations. While 85% of consumers have at least one physician visit in a typical year, those with higher morbidity generally have more visits.[8] There were 278 visits per 100 people in 2016, and consumer visits can be segmented by age and gender. Women had significantly higher visit rate of 315 compared to men with a rate of 239. Infants under age 1 had the highest rate of visits with 736 followed by 498 for those age 65 and older (Figure 4.4).[9]

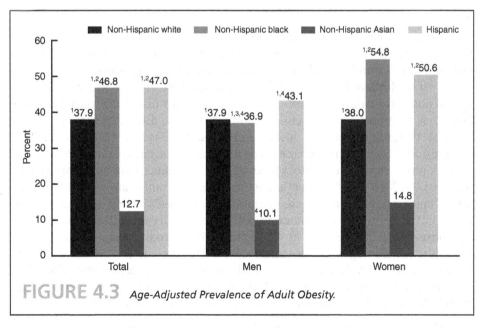

FIGURE 4.3    *Age-Adjusted Prevalence of Adult Obesity.*

*Source:* "Comorbidity and the Use of Primary Care and Specialist Care in the Elderly," Annals of Family Medicine, American Academy of Family Physicians, www.ncbi.nlm.nih.gov/pmc/articles/ PMC1466877/#!po=7.14286, accessed 1/13/20.

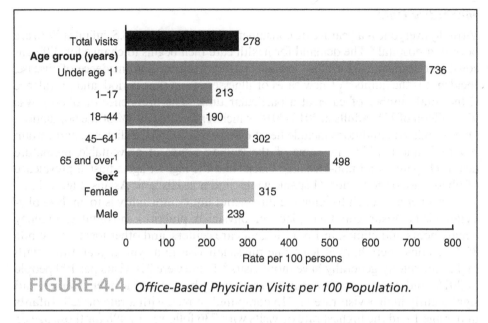

**FIGURE 4.4** *Office-Based Physician Visits per 100 Population.*

*Source:* "Characteristics of Office-based Physician Visits, 2016," NCHS Data Brief, No. 331, January 2019, CDC, www.cdc.gov/nchs/data/databriefs/db331-h.pdf, accessed 1/13/20.

### Mortality Data

One of the fundamental ways the well-being of a nation is measured is through tracking the rate at which its citizens die and how long they can be expected to live. Importantly, understanding how people die helps us to understand important consumer health problems. Determining who has these diseases and how they are spread not only guides the investment and research for discovering more effective diagnosis, treatment, and prevention efforts, but it also directs marketing.

The 10 leading causes of death accounted for 74% of all deaths in 2018 (Figure 4.5).[10] Significant decreases in deaths due to heart disease, cancer, unintentional injuries, chronic respiratory illnesses, and Alzheimer's disease were reported from 2017 to 2018. A 30% reduction in the cancer mortality rate and a 25% reduction in unintentional injury rates—mainly drug overdoses—were the main reasons for improved overall life expectancy in 2018. The overall cancer death rate dropped significantly by 2.2% from 2017 to 2018 primarily due to the decline in lung cancer mortality, the leading cause of cancer death. The reasons for the decrease were reduced smoking levels and treatment advances such as precise tumor classification and better surgical techniques. There were significant increases in death rates from influenza and pneumonia and from suicide from 2017 to 2018.

1. *Heart disease*: Heart diseases, also called cardiovascular disease, concern blood vessels, structural problems, and blood clots. Seven types are described

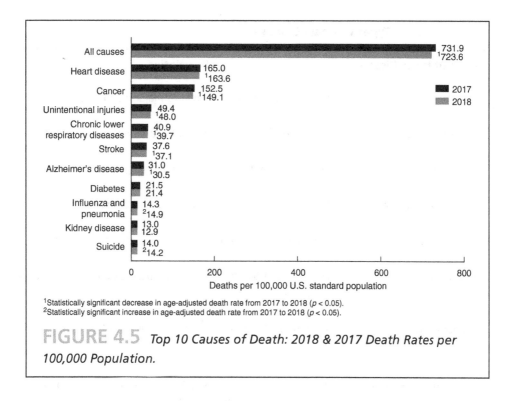

<sup>1</sup>Statistically significant decrease in age-adjusted death rate from 2017 to 2018 ($p < 0.05$).
<sup>2</sup>Statistically significant increase in age-adjusted death rate from 2017 to 2018 ($p < 0.05$).

FIGURE 4.5 *Top 10 Causes of Death: 2018 & 2017 Death Rates per 100,000 Population.*

in Table 4.1. Stroke is also considered a cardiovascular disease, but CDC has listed stroke in a separate category.

The rate of heart disease increased steadily from the beginning of the twentieth century to 1950 and then it began to decline. This trend follows the rise and fall of smoking rates and the proliferation of new smoking cessation programs. Heart disease death rate decreased by 8.3% from 2017 to 2018.

2. *Cancer*: Cancer deaths typically take place at a later age than heart disease deaths. Cancer deaths also reflect the long-term effects of poor health habits, particularly smoking, as well as the aging of the population. About 25% of cancer deaths are caused by lung cancer. The number of lung cancer deaths is higher than breast, prostate, and colon cancers combined. The average age for a lung cancer diagnosis is 70, and 2% are younger than 45.[11]

3. *Accidents*: Motor vehicle accidents, unintentional drug overdoses, and accidental falls and other injuries make up the majority of this category. For consumers age 1 to 44, the leading cause of death is violence and injuries, outpacing cancer, HIV, and the flu. Nearly 200,000 people die from injury each year, one person every three minutes, while millions are injured and survive. Survivors often struggle with mental health, physical health, and

TABLE 4.1 **Types of Heart Disease**

| Types of Heart Disease | Description |
|---|---|
| Coronary artery disease | Damage or disease in the heart's major blood vessels |
| High blood pressure | The force of the blood against the artery walls is too high |
| Cardiac arrest | Sudden loss of heart function, breathing, and consciousness |
| Congestive heart failure | Heart gradually loses its ability to pump blood |
| Arrhythmia | Improper beating of the heart, irregular, too fast, or too slow |
| Peripheral artery disease | Narrowing of blood vessels and reduced blood circulation to the limbs |
| Congenital heart disease | An abnormality in the heart that develops before birth |

financial problems the rest of their lives. Each year, 2.7 million older people are treated in emergency departments for fall injuries.[12]

4. *Chronic lower respiratory diseases*: Chronic obstructive pulmonary disease, also known as COPD, is a progressive disease that makes breathing difficult. Chronic bronchitis, emphysema, and asthma are illnesses in this category. Smoking or secondhand smoke are typically the causes of these diseases and result in the majority of deaths. Up to 25% of people with COPD, however, never smoked. Long-term exposure to lung irritants like air pollution, chemical fumes, or dust may contribute to COPD.

5. *Stroke*: Cerebrovascular disease, or stroke, involves a blood vessel blockage or hemorrhage in the brain that reduces the supply of oxygen or nutrients. Within four minutes without blood and oxygen, brain cells become damaged and may die. Stroke, a leading cause of disability requiring a range of rehabilitation services, has dropped from the third leading cause of death to the fifth. Preventive health behavior—such as smoking cessation, healthy eating, and screening for high blood pressure and cholesterol—along with improved diagnostic imaging and rapid treatments, have increased stroke survival.

6. *Alzheimer's disease*: In this disease, brain cells and the connections among cells degenerate and die. Over time memory and other important mental functions are reduced. The main symptoms are memory loss and confusion. There is no cure, but medications and management strategies may temporarily

improve symptoms. Diagnostic criteria and reporting have improved, and Alzheimer's has risen in this list of causes of death. In the past, cases of Alzheimer's were likely reported erroneously as dementia, a different disease category. Since incidence of Alzheimer's increases with age, and heart disease and stroke have been either averted or survived, more consumers are aging into Alzheimer's.

7. *Diabetes*: Diabetes is a chronic condition that has changed positions on the top 10 list in the 2010s. Diabetics have high levels of blood glucose and complications result directly or indirectly from that imbalance. Type 1 diabetes is inherited, usually diagnosed in children, and is caused by the pancreas's inability to make insulin. Type 2 diabetes is more common, often associated with obesity, and is caused by the body's resistance to the action of insulin. Diabetes affects approximately 29.1 million people, or 9.3% of the U.S. population. An additional 8.1 million people have diabetes but are not aware of it. There are about 76,000 deaths caused by diabetes each year, but it is also listed as a contributing factor on 245,000 death certificates annually. Diabetes can also lead to hardening and narrowing of the arteries as well as to strokes, coronary heart disease, and other large blood vessel diseases.[13]

8. *Influenza and pneumonia*: The CDC combines influenza and pneumonia deaths and estimates that 20% of deaths in this category are associated with the flu and 80% with pneumonia. The flu is an infection of the nose, throat, airways, and lungs caused by a virus. Death certificates with flu as the cause of death are only 3,000 to 5,000 a year, and the CDC does not know exactly how many consumers die annually from the flu. Pneumonia is a common illness affecting approximately 450 million people a year worldwide, and it is most likely to cause death in children less than 5 and adults older than age 75. The viral flu can lead to bacterial pneumonia and approximately one-third of all pneumonia cases are caused by the flu. Flu may also worsen chronic diseases and lead to death from other causes such as congestive heart failure or COPD.

9. *Kidney disease*: This category includes chronic kidney disease (CKD) and kidney failure or end-stage renal disease. There are 200,000 new cases of CKD annually, and 31 million consumers (10% of the population) have CKD. The kidneys filter waste and excess fluid from the blood, and waste builds up when disease causes kidneys to fail. Symptoms develop slowly, and some people have no symptoms at all. In later stages, those with kidney disease need to have their blood filtered using dialysis or a transplant may be needed. More than 661,000 consumers have kidney failure. Of these, 468,000 individuals are on dialysis, and roughly 193,000 have had a kidney transplant. Kidney disease can be caused by diabetes, atherosclerosis, and high blood pressure.[14]

10. *Suicide*: Suicide is the nation's 10th leading cause of death, and the number of cases has been on the rise since 1999. Approximately 44,200 people die by suicide annually, and for every suicide there are 25 attempts. While

males are four times more likely than females to die by suicide, females attempt suicide three times as often as males. Firearms were used for almost 50% of all suicides. No complete count is kept of suicide attempts. The CDC collects data on non-fatal injuries from self-harm and these data suggest that approximately 12 people harm themselves for every reported death by suicide. Suicide attempts often go unreported or untreated, and surveys suggest that at least 1 million people in the U.S. engage in intentionally inflicted self-harm.[15] It is estimated that suicide costs the U.S. $51 billion annually.

Blood poisoning, chronic liver disease, and Parkinson's disease did not make the top 10 mortality list, but they are all increasing. HIV/AIDS has been declining since 1995, but the disease continues to have a significant effect. An estimated 1.1 million people in the U.S. were living with HIV in 2016, and 14% or 1 in 7 do not know it. Medical errors—including wrong diagnoses, botched surgeries, and medication mistakes—kill 250,000 consumers annually, according to a Johns Hopkins study. Medical errors could be considered the third leading cause of death in the U.S. based on this number, but medical errors are not recognized as a major cause of death.[16] Major diseases causing mortality are measured by the CDC using medical billing codes, but there are no billing codes for deaths due to medical errors.

### Health Care Spending

While mortality is increasing and life expectancy is decreasing, the U.S. spends more on health care than other nations. In 2018, the U.S. spent $3.6 trillion on health care, and this represented 17.7% of U.S. gross domestic product (GDP).[17] The OECD analyzed health spending for similarly large and wealthy countries based on GDP and GDP per capita. The U.S. spent more on health care than any other country with $10,586, 45% higher than the second-highest per capita spender Switzerland (Figure 4.6).[18]

The chief reason for higher U.S. per capita spending than other developed countries is not greater health care utilization but higher prices for drugs, medical services, and salaries—physician, nurse, and hospital administrator compensation. According to research published in *Health Affairs*, although U.S. health spending is higher than other countries, its public spending is in line with these countries. Private spending, however, by commercial insurers and self-insured employers was significantly higher than private spending in any comparable country. While the U.S. outspent other countries, overall access to health care was lower.

The U.S. is also experiencing diminishing health care value as costs increase and health status decreases. One cause, identified by the Institute of Medicine (IOM), is that 30% of every dollar spent on health care was wasted due to management inefficiency and resistance to adopting innovation. The study urged

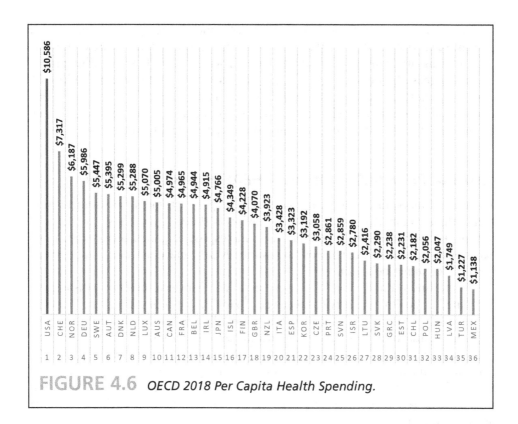

FIGURE 4.6   *OECD 2018 Per Capita Health Spending.*

physicians to more readily accept proven best clinical practices and medical technology, advised scientists to use stricter standards to evaluate clinical research, and recommended that hospitals streamline management processes and increase implementation of advanced health information technology.

An example of the value of improving a management process was when Cincinnati Children's Hospital made the decision to systematically stagger their surgeons' operating schedules. The result was that the hospital was able to decrease physician overtime pay, increase the efficient use of current hospital beds, and eliminate the planned purchase of additional beds that would have cost $100 million.[19] These types of changes need to be accompanied by organizational culture change and a realignment of employee incentives.

The costliest 1% of people account for 23% of total health care expenses, while the costliest 5% are responsible for half of all U.S. health care spending.[20] Demographically, these consumers are typically age 65 and over with multiple chronic conditions. Seniors with multiple chronic conditions can often take as many as 19 medication doses daily, and the average senior sees seven physicians across four different practices annually.

Another study found that less than 50% of seniors were up to date on clinical preventive services, and fewer than half of all non-surgical patients are compliant by following up with their primary care provider after hospital discharge.[21] Changing these trends requires that consumers have a better understanding of how the health system works and how to make more informed decisions. Understanding consumer behavior and how consumers make health care decisions will lead to effective marketing strategies that improve health and increase value.

## WHAT DETERMINES CONSUMER HEALTH CARE BEHAVIOR?

The aim of marketing is to meet and satisfy target customers' needs and wants better than competitors. Consumer behavior is the study of how individuals, groups, and organizations select, buy, use, and dispose of goods, services, ideas, or experiences to satisfy their needs and wants. Marketers must understand every facet of consumer behavior.

Interestingly, only 10 to 15% of an individual's overall health status can be attributed to health care services received.[22] Health status is strongly determined by behavior, genetics, and social determinants like living conditions, access to food, and education.[23] According to health economist Victor Fuchs, changing health care consumer behavior is the essential precondition for improving health. Consumers must first make having good health a priority over other goals, and then make informed lifestyle choices concerning diet, exercise, sleep, and smoking to achieve better health.[24] Behavior that leads to improved health will also reduce health care costs.

The starting point for understanding consumer buying behavior is the stimulus-response model shown in Figure 4.7. Both marketing and environmental stimuli

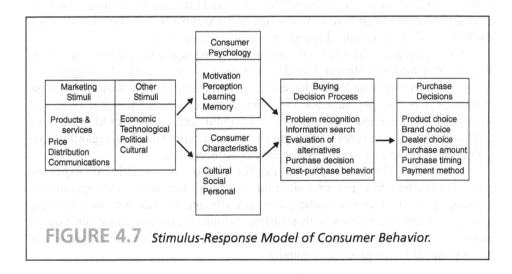

FIGURE 4.7 *Stimulus-Response Model of Consumer Behavior.*

enter the buyer's consciousness. In turn, the combination of consumer character-istics and psychological processes results in decision processes and a purchase. The marketer's task is to understand what happens in the consumer's conscious-ness between the arrival of external marketing stimuli and the ultimate purchase decision. A consumer's health care behavior and purchasing are influenced by their cultural, social, and personal characteristics. Cultural factors have the broad-est and deepest influences.

### *Cultural Factors*

Culture, subculture, and social class are particularly important influences on consumer health care buying behavior. Culture is the shared characteristics, val-ues, and beliefs of particular groups of people. Culture is also the fundamental determinant of a person's wants and behavior. Children acquire values, percep-tions, preferences, and behaviors through their family and other cultural entities. Each culture also consists of smaller *subcultures* that provide more explicit iden-tification and socialization for their members. Subcultures can include nationali-ties, religions, racial groups, and geographic regions. Social class is more than just how much money you have; it is also about your health and how you interact with others.

Multicultural marketing grew out of careful marketing research showing that ethnic and demographic niches did not always respond favorably to mass market advertising. Asians often believe that the number four is unlucky because when pronounced in Japanese or Chinese it sounds very similar to the word for "death." Pictures of pills or syringes in groups of four can symbolize bad luck for those people who believe in numerology. In another example, immigrants may be extremely private about medical, financial, and other personal data. They may also be distrustful of health care organizations based on experiences in their home country. Asking about the ability to pay for medical services may create an uncom-fortable situation. In some countries banks are avoided and cash is kept at home. By discussing their resources, they may believe that thieves will target them. Nearly half of all working-age Latinos may lack health insurance, but this does not mean they cannot pay for their health care.[25]

*Social classes* are relatively homogenous and enduring divisions in a society. They are hierarchically ordered and their members share similar values, interests, and behavior. A classic depiction of social classes in the U.S. defined seven ascend-ing levels: (1) lower lowers, (2) upper lowers, (3) working class, (4) middle class, (5) upper middles, (6) lower uppers, and (7) upper uppers.[26] Social classes differ in dress, speech patterns, recreational preferences, and many other characteristics. Social class is indicated by clusters of variables such as occupation, income, and education rather than by any single variable.

Health studies have found that lower class people have more anxiety and depression and are less physically healthy. People with fewer resources and educa-tion also need to depend more on other people. Psychologists have found that they have a physiological response that is missing in people with more resources. Those with lower class backgrounds are generally better at reading other people's emotions, have greater empathy, and more altruism. Wealthier people do not have to rely on each other as much because wealth, education, and a higher station in life give them the freedom to focus on the self. In psychology experiments, wealthier people do not read other people's emotions as well, and they hoard resources and are less generous than they could be.[27]

Consumers can move up and down the social ladder during their lifetime. Studies have found that as people rise in the classes they become less empathetic, and they become happier—but not as much as may be expected. Marketers need to be aware that social classes show distinct product and brand preferences in many areas. They also need to understand how these preferences affect a target market's health status, proactive attitudes toward health care, and its approach to buying health care resources.

CVS Health decided to remove tobacco products from its stores because it believes that community health is more important than tobacco revenue. At the same time, CVS Health took steps to mirror local communities to further engage customers in preventive care. After reviewing the cultural and social context of their diverse local populations, they replaced their unattended Minute Clinic store kiosks with live interactions with human beings in many locations.

Having employees who understand the local language, the culture, and social contexts improves preventive health through stronger relationships. CVS Health also reevaluated its corporate policies and procedures to recruit, train, and retain employees representative of the community. For example, Hispanics are often very family-oriented, and CVS Health wanted to support the personal time commitments employees may have to their large and extended families.[28]

### Social Factors

In addition to cultural factors, a consumer's health care behavior is influenced by social factors. Research of lower-income minority consumers in the Boston market, conducted by Dana-Farber and the Harvard School of Public Health, found both benefits and downsides of social ties. Consumers with close friends ate more fruits and vegetables than those with fewer friends. The research also showed that consumers with strong family relationships ate more sugary drinks and fast food than those without these relationships.[29] Marketers need to evaluate these types of findings by analyzing social factors related to reference groups, family, and roles and statuses.

Social determinants such as employment status, income level, educational attainment, pollution levels, and neighborhood crime affect personal choices and health behavior. Health behavior is responsible for 80 to 90% of personal health while clinical care accounts for 10 to 20%.[30] Examples of these resources include safe and affordable housing, access to education, public safety, availability of healthy foods, local emergency health services, and environments free of life-threatening toxins. A "place-based" framework reflecting five key areas of social determinants of health was developed by Healthy People 2020, a division of the Office for Disease Prevention and Health Promotion (Figure 4.8).[31]

Market-driven health care organizations are now using delivery models to target the low-cost market segment through reduced fixed costs, rethinking how clinicians deliver care, and addressing the social determinants of health. Since 2012, Ardás Family Medicine (ardasclinic.com) in Denver has provided health services to 60,000 patients who are primarily refugees. Nearly one-third (31%) are age 18 or under and represent a range of ethnicities: Nepalese (26%), Burmese (21%), Somalian (13%), Iraqi (13%), DRC/Rwandan (9%), Eritrean (3%), Eastern European (3%). The payer mix is 90% Medicaid, 7% uninsured, and 3% commercial insurance—and the clinic is profitable.

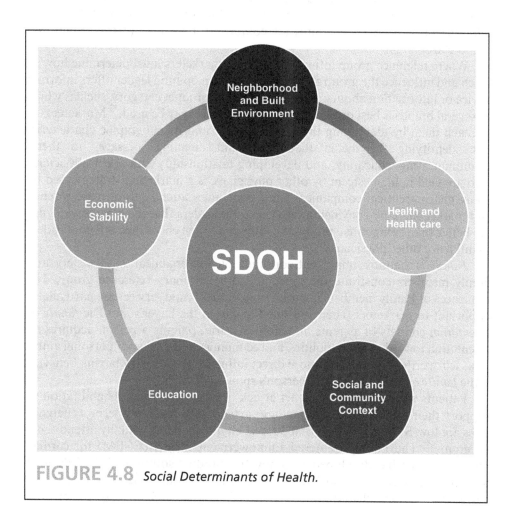

FIGURE 4.8  *Social Determinants of Health.*

Ardás founder Dr. P. J. Parmar designed the clinic around customer needs by addressing local social determinants of health. The clinic offers office visits, labs, vaccines, and travel shots, wound care, EKGs, orthopedic injections, and dental services among others. All services are detailed by CPT code and price on the clinic website for patients who do not have insurance. Patients are seen on a walk-in basis rather than by appointment, and the office is designed to move people in and out quickly. There are evening and weekend hours, and over-the-counter medications are available in the office.[32]

*Reference groups* consist of all the groups that have a direct face to-face or indirect influence on a consumer's attitudes or behavior. Primary groups are family, friends, neighbors, and co-workers with whom individuals interact fairly continuously and informally. Secondary groups, such as professional and trade-union groups, tend to be more formal and require less continuous interaction. Reference groups expose consumers to new behaviors and lifestyles, influence attitudes and self-concept, and create pressures for conformity that may affect product and brand choices.

Where reference group influence is strong, marketers must determine how to reach and influence the group's opinion leaders. An opinion leader offers informal advice or information about a specific product or product category, such as which of several brands is best or how a particular product may be used.[33] Marketers try to reach them by identifying their demographic and psychographic characteristics, identifying the media they read, and directing messages to them. Communicating, educating, and developing relationships with select physicians, who are held in high esteem by other physicians, is a marketing strategy used by many pharmaceutical companies. These companies attempt to increase revenue and market share by convincing select opinion leaders that the company's drugs are better than competitive products. Companies then encourage opinion leaders to influence other physicians.

*Family* is the most important consumer buying organization in society, and family members constitute the most influential primary reference group. The influences of family members in purchasing products and services are particularly important to marketers. There are two families in the buyer's life. The *family of orientation* consists of parents and siblings. From parents a person acquires an orientation toward religion, politics, and economics and a sense of personal ambition, self-worth, and love.[34] A more direct influence on everyday buying behavior is the *family of procreation*, or a person's spouse and children.

Patients who experience a heart attack often need cardiac rehabilitation to support their recovery. Cardiac rehab participation and long-term adherence rates are low. Studies estimate that 30% of eligible patients actually attend these programs.[35] The Family-Centered Empowerment Model (FCEM) for cardiac rehab, however, has developed an innovative product solution. FCEM decided to recruit and coach a cardiac rehab consumer family member to actively participate in the rehabilitation process. Family members bring patients to appointments, support them in practicing rehab exercises, and help them fill, refill, and take their prescription medicines. Research has validated that this family mentoring improves physical health, mental health, and the quality of life of FCEM patients.[36]

*Roles and statuses* in groups—such as families, clubs, places of worship, and other community organizations—often define norms of behavior and offer important sources of information. A role consists of the activities a person is expected to perform and each role in turn connotes a status. People choose products that reflect and communicate their role and their actual or desired status in society. Marketers must be aware of the status-symbol potential of health care products and brands. A woman in Southern California seeking cosmetic surgery may choose a surgeon in Beverly Hills because the practice reputation includes a celebrity clientele. A new cancer patient in Tennessee may decide to visit the renowned M.D. Anderson Cancer Center in Houston for an oncology treatment second opinion. A lower-income consumer in rural Wyoming may choose to seek medical care from the local county health department or a nearby medical school.

### Personal Factors

Personal factors take into account individual differences in patterns of thinking, feeling, and behaving. Personal characteristics that have a strong influence on health care buyers include age and stage in the life cycle, occupation and economic circumstances, personality and self-concept, and lifestyle and values.

*Age and stage in the life cycle* are important because only 20% of lifetime health care expenses occur during the first half of life. Health care needs accelerate between ages 65 and 85, and about half of all health care expenses in a person's lifetime occur after age 65.[37] Family life cycle and the number, age, and gender of people in the household also influence health care. U.S. households are increasingly fragmented with 27% living alone. The growth in the number of men living alone rose from 6% in 1970 to 12% in 2012. The number of women living alone was higher at 15%, but men are more vulnerable to the side effects of the single life.[38] Men in social isolation have been found to have more health risks and a higher mortality rate.[39]

*Occupational and economic circumstance* analysis helps marketers identify above-average interest in their products and services. A blue-collar worker who does physical labor is more likely to need occupational therapy. A Fortune 500 corporate executive may need preventive health services aimed at reducing cardiovascular and other stress-related health problems. Economic circumstances can also impact consumer health care spending. A survey found that 31% of consumers or their family members delayed needed medical care because of costs.[40]

*Personality and self-concept* also affect health care buying behavior. Consumers have individual personality characteristics that influence their buying behavior. Personality is made up of the set of distinguishing human psychological traits that lead to consistent and enduring responses to environmental stimuli. It is often described in terms of such traits as self-confidence, dominance, autonomy, deference, sociability, defensiveness, and adaptability. Personality can be useful in analyzing consumer behavior because brands also have personalities. Consumers are likely to choose brands whose personalities match their own.

Brand personality is the mix of human traits that are attributed to a particular brand. The American Association of Retired People (AARP) has a trustworthy brand personality supported by decades of experience and the characteristics of maturity and trust. A compassionate brand is St. Jude's Research Center because it demonstrates sincerity, heart, love, and devotion. St. Jude's fundraising is based on doing the right thing and making the world a better place. The personality of the Susan G. Komen breast cancer foundation, however, is based on getting things done. There is a sense of duty, action, and excitement that is evident in their messaging, graphics, and racing and walking events.[41]

Marketers often try to develop brand personalities that will attract consumers with the same self-concept because consumers often choose and use brands with a brand personality consistent with how they view themselves.[42] Yet it is possible that a person's *actual self-concept* differs from their *ideal self-concept*. Another variation of self-concept is how a consumer thinks others see them. A consumer who is sensitive about how others see them may purchase branded prescription drugs instead of generic drugs, or they may travel a long distance from home to a residential weight loss or a substance abuse rehabilitation program rather than purchase these health services locally.

*Lifestyle and values* differentiate consumers from the same subculture, social class, and occupation. A *lifestyle* is a person's pattern of living in the world as expressed in activities, interests, and opinions. Lifestyle portrays the "whole person" interacting with their environment. Marketers search for relationships between their products and lifestyle groups. Lifestyles are shaped partly by whether consumers are money constrained or time constrained. Companies aiming to serve money-constrained consumers will create lower-cost products and services. By appealing to thrifty consumers, Teva Pharmaceuticals, the leading generic pharmaceutical manufacturer in the world, makes safe and quality medicines more affordable and accessible.

Consumers who have time pressures are willing to pay others to perform tasks because time is more important to them than money. Duke Signature Care is a concierge medicine service offered by Duke Health (Durham, NC). Subscribers pay a $2,500 annual fee for convenience-related services such as more attention during physician appointments, immediate or next day appointments, 24/7 telephone access to a doctor, and free parking.

Consumer decisions are also influenced by core *values*, the belief systems that underlie attitudes and behaviors. Core values go much deeper than behavior or attitude and determine, at a basic level, people's choices and desires over the long term. Marketers who target consumers on the basis of their values believe that with appeals to people's inner selves, it is possible to influence their outer selves and their purchasing behavior. The National League for Nursing is an organization for nurse faculty and leaders in nursing education, and they recruit new members by accentuating the core values of caring, integrity, diversity, and excellence.

### Marketing Tool—PATH Behavioral Attractors

After understanding consumer cultural, social, and personal factors, marketers need tools to use this information to inform marketing strategies. Patterns of Adapting to Health (PATH) is a psychographic tool that can be used to understand individual health priorities that shape health behavior. Consumers complete a 20-question PATH Inventory that measures indicators of actions or habits in response to health-related situations ("I often play in active or competitive sports") and beliefs ("Doctors often try new drugs on their patients without knowing all the side effects"). A Likert scale is used to measure the level of agreement or disagreement with each statement, and an algorithm analyzes consumer responses in the context of 11 health care behavioral dimensions (Table 4.2).[43]

TABLE 4.2  **PATH Health Care Dimensions**

1. Involvement in family health

2. Trust in medical professionals

3. Propensity to experiment with health care alternatives

4. Propensity to avoid health care

5. Level of health care information seeking

6. Involvement in health care decision-making

7. Level of being health reactive versus health proactive

8. Receptivity to health care advertising

9. Price concern

10. Quality concern

11. Health emphasis and involvement

This consumer health analysis reveals individual patterns of attitudes and behavior that fit nine PATH consumer profiles (Table 4.3).[44] PATH assumes that social context immediately affects a person's expression of health-related behaviors. Marketers understanding these consumer profiles can predict levels of health, risk of illness or disease, health behavior, and demand for particular health care services.

**TABLE 4.3 PATH Consumer Profiles**

| PATH | Profile | Example: Exercise Pattern |
|---|---|---|
| 1. | Critically Discerning | Ambivalent about engaging in regular vigorous exercise and working to maintain an optimum level of fitness. |
| 2. | Health Contented | Extremely low levels of commitment to fitness characterized by avoidance of regular physical activity and habitual avoidance of fitness-related issues. |
| 3. | Wisely Frugal | Show some involvement in regular vigorous activity and a modest commitment to maintaining a high level of physical fitness. |
| 4. | Traditionalist | Avoid regular vigorous physical activity although trying to maintain an optimal level of fitness is something they approach. |
| 5. | Family Centered | Neither engage nor refrain from participation in regular vigorous physical activity. This is consistent with their slightly lower level of commitment to work toward the condition of top physical shape. |
| 6. | Family Driven | Show some involvement in regular vigorous exercise although they are not as engaged in keeping themselves in top physical shape. |
| 7. | Health Care Driven | Report very low involvement in regular vigorous physical activity, although they show a small tendency to be involved in maintaining a top level of physical shape. |
| 8. | Independently Healthy | Adults are associated with a very strong attraction to regular vigorous physical activity. They have a strong commitment to keeping their bodies in top physical shape. |
| 9. | Naturalist | Strongly avoid engaging in regular vigorous physical activity, although they work towards trying to keep themselves in top physical shape. |

Insights provided by the PATH have been used by health systems, medical groups, and health insurance plans. For example, health plans validated the predictive relationship between a member's dominant PATH and medical claims levels for hospital care, physician demand, and prescription demand. Within disease management, the PATH were shown to improve consumer engagement and behavior change following a disease management intervention. Clinicians trained to apply tailored communications to consumers based on their dominant PATH resulted in an 18% improvement in engagement and an 11% improvement in health behavior compared to a control group. The PATH have also been used to support health coaching to increase coaching engagement and improve health behavior.[45]

## CONSUMER MARKETING PSYCHOLOGY

Four key psychological processes—motivation, perception, learning, and memory—fundamentally influence consumer responses to various marketing stimuli.

### Motivation

A person has many needs at any given time. Some needs are biogenic, and they arise from physiological states of tension such as hunger, thirst, or discomfort. Health care needs can also come from a *psychological state* such as the need for recognition, esteem, or belonging. A *motive* is a need that is sufficiently pressing to drive a person to act. Abraham Maslow, a U.S. psychologist who sought to explain why people are driven by particular needs at particular times, hypothesized that human needs are arranged in a hierarchy from the most pressing to the least pressing. In order of importance these needs and examples are physiological (food), safety (security), social (sense of belonging), esteem (status), and self-actualization (altruism).

Marketers can use Maslow's hierarchy of needs to understand how various health care offerings can satisfy different types of needs. For example, a consumer with an infected finger is motivated by a physiological need to visit a retail clinic to relieve pain. Buying health insurance satisfies a need for safety and security. Psychiatric counseling services can meet social needs. Self-esteem could be increased through plastic surgery. Becoming an organ donor can contribute to self-actualization. It is important to note that higher level needs cannot be met before basic needs. Motivating a consumer to exercise to improve health will likely be unsuccessful if the consumer is most concerned with trying to feed and protect their family.

### Perception

A motivated person is ready to act, but how that motivated person actually acts is influenced by their view or perception of the situation. Perception is the process that enables a consumer to select, organize, and interpret information to create a meaningful picture of the world. Perceptions can vary widely among individuals exposed to the same stimuli. One consumer may view an ad for a physician practice as helpful, and another person may perceive that the doctors are desperate for business. Consumers can have different perceptions of the same product or service because of three perceptual processes: selective attention, selective distortion, and selective retention.

The average consumer is exposed to over 1,500 marketing communications every day, and consumers use *selective attention* to avoid sensory overload and screen out most of these communications. The result is that marketers must work hard to attract consumers' attention. Through research, marketers have learned that consumers are more likely to notice a message that meets a current need. For example, smokers who want to stop smoking may notice magazine ads for a product like Nicorette gum that will help them quit. Furthermore, smokers are more likely to notice stimuli that they anticipate, such as Nicorette gum on sale at a drug store. Smokers are also more likely to notice stimuli whose deviations are large in relation to the normal size of the stimuli, such as an ad offering "buy one, get one free" for Nicorette gum over a coupon for 50 cents-off. Likewise, if consumers are not suffering from heart disease, they may not notice digital advertising for cardiac surgery.

Even noticed stimuli do not always come across in the way the senders intended. *Selective distortion* is the tendency to twist information into personal meanings and interpret information that fits our preconceptions. Consumers will often distort information to be consistent with prior product and brand beliefs. The smoker may have a friend who failed to quit smoking using Nicorette gum, and therefore the smoker does not believe that the gum will help him.

People forget much information to which they are exposed but will tend to retain information that supports their attitudes and beliefs. Consumers are also more likely to remember good points about a product they like and to overlook the good points of competing products. This *selective retention* works to the advantage of strong brands, and it also explains why marketers repeat messages to ensure that the information is not overlooked.

### Marketing Tool—The Health Belief Model

The actions taken by consumers are determined by their perceptions of the benefits and barriers of health behavior. The Health Belief Model (HBM) states that the perception of a personal health behavior threat is influenced by at least three factors: general health values including interest and concern about health, specific health beliefs about vulnerability to a particular health threat, and beliefs about the consequences of the health problem.

The HBM was developed in the 1950s by social psychologists working in the U.S. Public Health Services.[46] It has been used extensively to promote health through diet and exercise programs and to reduce health risk through smoking cessation, vaccination, and contraceptive practices. It has also been used to increase compliance with medical recommendations following diagnosis of chronic illnesses. In the example of promoting condom use to avoid HIV, the HBM found that consumers will take health-related actions if they perceive that:

1. A negative health condition, such as contracting HIV, should and can be avoided.

2. A positive expectation that by *taking* a recommended action, like using a condom, HIV can be prevented.

3. They can successfully take a recommended action and can actually use condoms comfortably and with confidence.

The first step for marketers is to conduct marketing research to identify and understand the five HBM concepts shown in Table 4.4 before developing marketing communications strategies.[47]

TABLE 4.4 **Health Belief Model Concepts**

| Concept | Definition | Application |
|---|---|---|
| **1. Perceived susceptibility** | Beliefs about the chances of getting a condition. | ▪ Define what populations(s) are at risk and their levels of risk<br>▪ Tailor risk information based on an individual's characteristics or behaviors<br>▪ Help individuals develop an accurate perception of their own risk. |
| **2. Perceived severity** | Beliefs about the seriousness of a condition and its consequences. | Specify the consequences of a condition and recommended action. |
| **3. Perceived benefits** | Beliefs about the effectiveness of taking action to reduce risk or seriousness. | Explain how, where, and when to take action and what the potential positive results will be. |
| **4. Perceived barriers** | Beliefs about the material and psychological costs of taking action. | Offer reassurance, incentives, and assistance; correct misinformation. |
| **5. Cues to action** | Factors that activate "readiness to change." | Provide "how to" information, promote awareness, and employ reminder systems. |
| **6. Self-efficacy** | Confidence in one's ability to take action. | ▪ Provide training and guidance in performing action<br>▪ Use progressive goal setting<br>▪ Give verbal reinforcement<br>▪ Demonstrate desired behaviors. |

High blood pressure, or hypertension, is a risk factor for heart disease and stroke. It is also a health problem for one in three adults, or 77.9 million of the population. Screening campaigns often identify people with elevated blood pressure but have no symptoms. Consumers who feel normal are unlikely to follow instructions to take prescribed medicine or lose weight.

The National High Blood Pressure Education program (NHBPE), an initiative of the National Heart, Lung, and Blood Institute, has used the HBM to influence desired behaviors like increasing blood pressure monitoring, adhering to healthy lifestyles and medication plans, and noncompliance. The NHBPE used marketing research to understand consumer perceptions of the six HBM concepts among consumers with high blood pressure. The NHBPE was interested in influencing desired behaviors by increasing blood pressure monitoring and compliance with recommended lifestyle and medication plans. Research respondents perceived susceptibility, seriousness, and efficacy barriers such as:

> *"It is hard for me to change my diet and to find the time to exercise."*
> *"My blood pressure is difficult to control."*
> *"My blood pressure varies so much, it's probably not accurate."*
> *"Medications can have undesirable side effects."*
> *"It's too expensive to go to the doctor just to get my blood pressure checked."*
> *"It may be the result of living a full and active life. Not everybody dies from it."*

The marketing research found that asymptomatic people may follow a prescribed treatment regimen, but they must first accept that they do in fact have hypertension (perceived susceptibility). They must also acknowledge that hypertension can lead to heart attacks and strokes (perceived severity). Taking medication or following a recommended weight loss program will reduce the risks (perceived benefits) without negative side effects or excessive difficulty (perceived barriers).

Using the research, along with the HBM, the National Heart Lung and Blood Institute developed social marketing strategies that projected the following concepts:

1. You don't have to make all the changes immediately.
   - *The key is to focus on one or two at a time.*
   - *Sometimes, one change leads naturally to another. For example, increasing physical activity will help you lose weight.*

2. You can keep track of your blood pressure outside of your doctor's office by taking it at home.

3. You don't have to run marathons to benefit from physical activity.
   - *Any activity, if done at least 30 minutes a day over the course of most days, can help.*

These research findings were used in printed materials, reminder letters, and pill calendars to encourage consumers to consistently follow their doctors' recommendations (cues to action). For those who have had difficulty losing weight or maintaining weight loss, research showed that a behavioral contract would help to establish achievable, short-term goals to build confidence (self-efficacy).[48]

The results of the NHBPE social marketing program was increased awareness of the relationship between hypertension, stroke, and heart disease from less than one-quarter of consumers to more than three-quarters of the population. Virtually all consumers have had their blood pressure measured at least once, and a substantial percent of the population has it measured yearly.

### Learning

When people act, they learn. Learning involves changes in an individual's behavior arising from experience. Most human behavior is learned. Theorists believe that learning is produced through the interplay of drives, stimuli, cues, responses, and reinforcement. A *drive* is a strong, internal stimulus that impels action. *Cues* are minor stimuli that determine when, where, and how a person responds.

Suppose you buy a membership at the Duke Health and Fitness Center. If your experience is rewarding, your response to exercise and Duke will be positively reinforced. Later, when you want to see a concierge physician, you may assume that since Duke helped you become more fit, you will have another positive experience with Duke. You *generalize* your response to similar stimuli. A countertendency to generalization is *discrimination* in which the person learns to recognize differences in sets of similar stimuli and can adjust responses accordingly. Applying learning theory, marketers can build up demand for a product by associating it with strong drives, using motivating cues, and providing positive reinforcement.

### Memory

All the information and experiences that individuals encounter as they go through life can end up in their long-term memory. Cognitive psychologists distinguish between short-term memory (STM)—a temporary repository of information—and long-term memory (LTM)—a more permanent repository.

Most widely accepted views of long-term memory structure involve some kind of associative model formation.[49] For example, the *associative network memory model* views LTM as consisting of a set of nodes and links. *Nodes* are stored information connected by *links* that vary in strength. Any type of information can be stored in the memory network, including information that is verbal, visual, abstract, or contextual. A spreading activation process from node to node determines the extent of retrieval and what information can actually be recalled in any given situation. When a node becomes activated because external information is being encoded (e.g., when a person reads or hears a word or phrase) or internal information is retrieved from LTM (e.g., when a person thinks about some concept), other nodes are also activated if they are sufficiently strongly associated with that node.

Following this model, consumer brand knowledge in memory can be conceptualized as consisting of a brand node in memory with a variety of linked associations. The strength and organization of these associations will be important determinants of the information that can be recalled about the brand. *Brand associations* consist of all brand-related thoughts, feelings, perceptions, images, experiences, beliefs, attitudes, and so on that become linked to the brand node.

Some organizations create mental maps that depict consumers' knowledge of a particular brand in terms of the key associations. These associations are likely triggered by marketing and by their relative strength, favorability, and uniqueness. A brand map begins with elicitation of brand associations using a survey with open-ended responses. Responses are added to a card if 50% or more respondents name the specific association. In the second stage, consumers select the cards that are most important to the brand in their opinion. Respondents then connect the associations by making a map using either one, two, or three parallel lines depending on their perceived strength of the connection.

Figure 4.9 displays an individual consumer's hypothetical brand map highlighting beliefs for a large medical practice in the Midwest. According to this

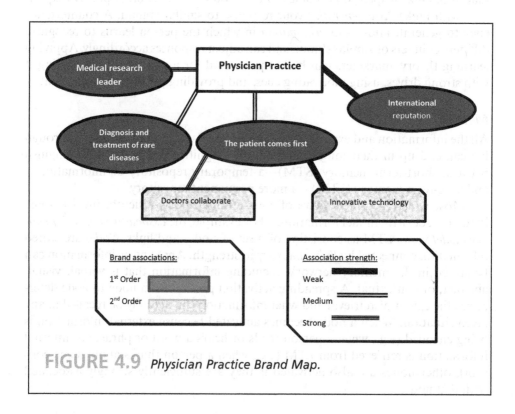

FIGURE 4.9  *Physician Practice Brand Map.*

brand concept map, the practice has first order brand associations with "medical research leadership," "diagnosis and treatment of rare diseases," "the patient comes first," and "international reputation." Second order brand associations are "doctors collaborate" and "innovative technology." Individual consumer brand maps are then aggregated to form consensus maps. Brand maps reveal a brand's strengths and weaknesses and can also be segmented by type of consumer.[50]

*Memory encoding* refers to how and where information gets into memory. Memory encoding can be characterized according to the amount or quantity of processing that information receives at encoding (i.e., how much a person thinks about it) and the nature or quality of processing that information receives at encoding (i.e., the manner in which a person thinks about it). The quantity and quality of processing will be an important determinant of the strength of an association.

In general, the more attention placed on the meaning of information during encoding, the stronger the resulting associations in memory will be.[51] Also, the ease with which new information can be integrated into established knowledge structures clearly depends on the nature of that information, in terms of characteristics such as its inherent simplicity, vividness, and concreteness. Repeated exposures provide greater opportunity for processing and potential for stronger associations. High levels of repetition, however, for an uninvolved, unpersuasive ad are unlikely to have as much sales impact as lower levels of repetition for an involving, persuasive ad.

*Memory retrieval* refers to how information gets out of memory. According to the associative network memory model, the strength of a brand association increases both the likelihood that that information will be accessible and the ease with which it can be recalled by "spreading activation." Successful recall of brand information by consumers relies on more than the initial strength of that information in memory. Three factors are particularly important. First, *other* product information in memory can produce interference effects causing one brand's information to be either overlooked or confused. One challenge facing crowded categories with many competitors—like hospitals, physician or dental practices, or health insurance plans—is that consumers may mix up brands.

Second, the time between exposure to information and encoding affects the strength of a new association—the longer the time delay the weaker is the association. Finally, information may be "available" in memory (i.e., potentially recallable) but may not be "accessible" from memory (i.e., able to be recalled) without the proper retrieval cues or reminders. The particular associations for a brand that "come to mind" depend on the context in which the brand is considered. The more cues linked to a piece of information the better the likelihood that the information can be recalled. For example, a consumer telephone survey of health system brand ad recall, conducted during a holiday weekend, may be hampered by a low level of consumer health interest at the time of the survey.

## THE BUYING DECISION PROCESS: THE FIVE-STAGE MODEL

Marketers must understand every facet of the consumer buying process, from learning about a product to making a brand choice, to using the product, and even disposing of it.[52] Starting with problem recognition, the consumer passes through the stages of information search, evaluation of alternatives, purchase decision, and post-purchase behavior (Figure 4.10). Clearly, the buying process starts long before the actual purchase and has consequences long afterward.[53] Although this model implies that consumers pass sequentially through all five stages in buying, consumers sometimes skip or reverse some stages. The model provides a good frame of reference, however, because it captures the full range of considerations that arise when a consumer faces a highly involving new purchase.[54]

1. *Problem recognition*: The buying process begins when a consumer recognizes a problem or need that is triggered by an internal stimulus (such as feeling pain or discomfort) or an external stimulus (such as seeing an ad for breast cancer awareness month), that then becomes a drive. By gathering information from a number of consumers, marketers can identify the circumstances that trigger a particular need. They can then develop marketing strategies that trigger consumer interest and lead to the second stage in the buying process.

2. *Information search*: An aroused consumer will be inclined to search for more information. We can distinguish between two levels of arousal. At the milder search state of *heightened* attention, a person simply becomes more receptive to information about a product. At the *active information s*earch level, a person talks with friends, searches online, and visits facilities to learn about the product.

   Information sources fall into four groups: personal sources (family, friends, neighbors, acquaintances), commercial sources (advertising, websites, salespersons, dealers, packaging, displays), public sources (mass media, consumer-rating organizations), and experiential sources (handling, examining, using the product). The consumer usually receives the most information from commercial sources, although the most influential information comes from personal sources or public sources that are independent authorities. Information from personal experience or recommendations from trusted sources are typically more valuable to consumers recognizing a problem.

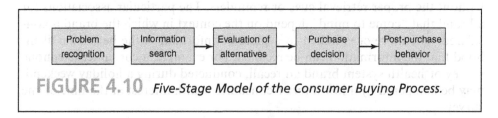

FIGURE 4.10 *Five-Stage Model of the Consumer Buying Process.*

Through gathering information, the consumer learns about competing brands and their features. The first box in Figure 4.11 lists the total set of brands available to the consumer. The individual consumer will come to know only a subset of these brands (*awareness set*). Some brands will meet initial buying criteria (*consideration set*). As the consumer gathers more information, only a few will remain as strong contenders (*choice set*). The consumer makes a final choice from this set.[55]

A health care organization must strategize to get its brand into the awareness set, consideration set, and choice set. Other brands in the consumer's choice set need to be analyzed to develop appropriate competitive appeals. Marketers need to research the type of information consumers want, how they prefer to receive it, and its relative influence to develop targeted communications. A low-involvement purchase like getting a flu shot requires less information than a high-involvement decision like deciding where to go for heart surgery. Figure 4.11 illustrates the heart surgery options that a national employer could consider for its employees.

3. *Evaluation of alternatives*: How do consumers process competitive brand information and make a final value judgment? No single process is used by all consumers or by one consumer in all health care buying situations. Most marketing models view consumers as forming judgments largely on a conscious and rational basis, but circumstance and emotion can also be important for decisions. Consumers initially try to satisfy a need and then begin the search for specific benefits and a product solution. Third, consumers perceive each product as a bundle of attributes with varying capabilities for delivering the benefits sought to satisfy a need.

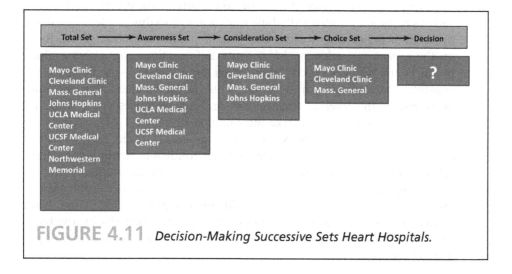

**FIGURE 4.11**  *Decision-Making Successive Sets Heart Hospitals.*

The attributes of interest to buyers vary by product. The attributes sought in a travel medicine clinic might be up-to-date knowledge of disease incidence in foreign countries, web access to information, 24/7 access to a physician in the country being visited, and an affordable service subscription price. The same consumer will be interested in different attributes when selecting an urgent care clinic such as time to next appointment, cost, whether the provider is a physician or a nurse practitioner or physician assistant, and location convenience.

In addition, consumers vary as to which product attributes they see as most relevant and important. Knowing that consumers pay the most attention to attributes that deliver the benefits that they want, marketers can segment their markets according the attributes that are most important to different consumer groups. Conjoint analysis is a marketing research tool used to measure attribute preferences. In conjoint analysis, respondents are shown different paired comparisons of attributes and are asked to rank the various offers. Consumers are then assigned to the market segment with the matching cluster of attributes.

Evaluations often reflect beliefs and attitudes that consumers acquire through experience and learning. These in turn influence buying behavior. A *belief* is a descriptive thought that a person holds about something. People's beliefs about the attributes and benefits of a product or brand influence their buying decisions. Just as important as beliefs are attitudes. An *attitude* is a person's enduring favorable or unfavorable evaluation, emotional feeling, and action tendencies toward some object or idea. Because attitudes economize on energy and thought, they can be very difficult to change. An organization is well-advised to fit its product into existing attitudes, if possible, rather than to try to change attitudes. Segments of consumers with strong attitudes that do not align with a product are likely not good targets.

The consumer arrives at attitudes (i.e., judgments, preferences) toward various brands through an attribute evaluation procedure.[56] He or she develops a set of beliefs about where each brand stands on each attribute. Based on the *expectancy-value model* of attitude formation, consumers evaluate products and services by combining their brand beliefs—the positives and negatives—according to importance. This model assumes high consumer involvement, the level of engagement and active processing a consumer undertakes in response to marketing stimulus.

Anne, a mother of three young children, has narrowed her pediatrician choice set to four practices based on the following attributes: location, office hours, network affiliation with specialists at an academic medical center, physician empathy, and cost. If one pediatric practice dominated the others on all five attributes, we could reliably predict that Anne would choose it. Since not all the practices have the same benefits or attributes, knowing how Anne weighted each of the five attributes would help to predict her choice.

The marketer's task is to identify how target consumers weigh the value of each of the five attributes for the four pediatric practices. The marketer can then segment potential customers into groups with the same or similar preferences and enhance the attractiveness of a practice by one or several of the following steps[57]:

- Expand office hours to include nights and weekends: real positioning
- Alter consumer beliefs about the brand: psychological repositioning
- Alter consumer beliefs about competitors' brands: competitive repositioning
- Alter the importance of weights: persuade buyers to attach more importance to the attributes in which the brand excels
- Call attention to neglected attributes: such as bilingual services
- Shift the buyer's ideals: persuade buyers to change their ideal levels for one or more attributes

4. *Purchase decisions*: In the fourth stage, the consumer forms preferences among brands in the choice set and may also form an intention to buy the most preferred brand. Two factors can intervene between the purchase intention and decision.[58] The first is the *attitudes of others*. The extent to which another person's attitude reduces the preference for an alternative depends on two things: the intensity of the other person's negative or positive attitude toward the consumer's preferred alternative, and the consumer's motivation to comply with the other person's wishes.[59] If Anne prefers pediatric practice A, and her sister Elizabeth strongly recommends practice B, Anne's purchase probability for practice A will be somewhat reduced. Related to the attitudes of others is the role played by information intermediaries who publish their evaluations or recommendations. Online resources like Consumer Reports, Healthgrades, RateMDs, the Leap Frog Group, and others review physician and hospital performance and offer consumer opinions.

The second factor is *unanticipated situational factors* that may erupt to change the purchase intention. Anne could lose her job, some other purchase might become more urgent, or a physician may disappoint her, which is why preferences and purchase intentions are not completely reliable predictors of purchase behavior. A consumer's decision to modify, postpone, or avoid a purchase decision is also heavily influenced by *perceived risk*, such as the amount of money at stake, the amount of attribute uncertainty, and the amount of consumer self-confidence.[60]

A heart valve replacement would be considered a high perceived risk purchase, given the expense, the pain, and the possibility of life-threatening complications. In contrast, going to a dermatologist to treat a plantar wart has a relatively low perceived risk because it is a low-cost purchase with little discomfort and a fairly certain outcome. Consumers develop routines for reducing risk, such as decision avoidance, information gathering from friends, and preference for national brand names and warranties. Marketers must understand the factors that provoke a feeling of risk in consumers and provide information and support to reduce perceived risk.

5.  *Post-purchase behavior*: After the purchase, consumers may seek information that confirms its high value. Consumers may also experience dissonance stemming from noticing certain disquieting features or hearing favorable things about other brands—and will be alert to information that supports their decision. Marketers must monitor post-purchase satisfaction, post-purchase actions, and post-purchase product uses.

    The buyer's satisfaction with a purchase is a function of the closeness between expectations and the product's perceived performance.[61] If performance falls short of expectations, the consumer is disappointed. If it meets expectations, the consumer is satisfied, and if it exceeds expectations, the consumer is delighted. These feelings influence whether the customer buys the product again and talks favorably or unfavorably about it to others. The importance of post-purchase satisfaction suggests that product claims must truthfully represent the product's likely performance. Some sellers may even understate performance levels so that consumers experience higher-than-expected satisfaction with the product.

    Product or organization satisfaction, dissatisfaction, and loyalty influence subsequent behavior. Health care organizations can take positive steps to help buyers feel good about their choices. A pediatric practice can send warm introductory letters to new patients, solicit customer suggestions for improvements, offer child health information that will address common questions and concerns, and provide information using the channel the consumer prefers like text, email, or the practice website.

    One potential opportunity to increase frequency of product use arises when consumers' perceptions of their usage differ from the reality. For example, many people underestimate the time since their last preventive care visit to their physician or dentist. In this case, consumers must be persuaded of the merits of more regular usage, and any potential hurdles to increased usage must be overcome. In terms of the latter, product or service designs and packaging can make the product more convenient and easier to use. The pediatric practice can communicate regularly and build a relationship with customers explaining the need for routine vaccinations, physicals, and seasonal reasons for visiting the practice (illnesses in the winter and injuries in the summer). It can also offer more convenient hours to minimize the negative perception of waiting for the physician.

    Dissatisfied consumers may abandon or return the product, take public action by complaining to the organization, consult an attorney for a malpractice suit, or complain to government agencies and other groups. Private actions include not buying the product or warning friends. In these cases, the seller has done a poor job of satisfying the customer.

## THREE HEALTH CARE ENVIRONMENTAL TRENDS AFFECTING CONSUMERS

Three environmental forces affecting consumers are natural, economic, and political-legal. The corresponding trends are the increased prevalence of chronic diseases (natural), consumers paying more for health care (economic), and the growth of consumer health care accountability (political-legal). Market-driven health care organizations are analyzing these trends to leverage market opportunities and avoid market threats.

### *Natural Force:* Trend 1—Chronic Disease Prevalence is Increasing

Chronic diseases and conditions—such as heart disease, stroke, cancer, type 2 diabetes, obesity, lung diseases, and arthritis—are among the most common, costly, and preventable of all health problems.[62] Characteristics of chronic health problems are that they usually begin in middle age, last more than three months, can be controlled but not cured, and will benefit from early detection. About half of all adults in the U.S. (117 million people) have one or more chronic health conditions.[63] The top three chronic diseases are hypertension, high cholesterol, and upper respiratory disease (Figure 4.12).[64] A quarter of all adults have two or more chronic conditions, and the prevalence of multiple chronic conditions increases with age.[65]

The treatment of chronic disease accounts for 86% of U.S. health care costs.[66] An estimated 28% of people with two or more chronic conditions are responsible for 66% of U.S. health care spending. Nearly 75% of those age 65 and older have

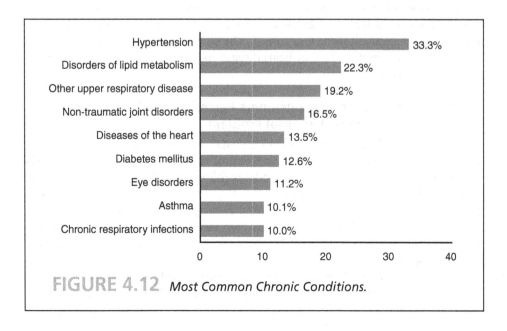

FIGURE 4.12 *Most Common Chronic Conditions.*

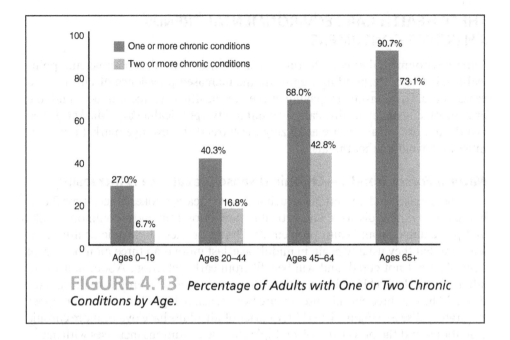

**FIGURE 4.13** *Percentage of Adults with One or Two Chronic Conditions by Age.*

multiple chronic conditions. Between 2000 and 2030, the number of people with one or more chronic conditions is expected to increase by 37%, an increase of 46 million people (Figure 4.13).[67]

Four health risk behaviors are responsible for most chronic diseases and conditions. They are a lack of exercise or physical activity, poor nutrition, tobacco use, and excessive alcohol consumption.[68] The CDC estimates that reducing these risk factors would prevent 80% of heart disease and stroke, 80% of type 2 diabetes, and 40% of cancer.[69]

### *Economic Force:* Trend 2—Consumers Perceive Health Care Costs as Their Foremost Financial Problem

Marketing research indicates that the high cost of health care was the most important financial problem consumers were facing in 2019. High health care costs were mentioned first by 17% of respondents followed by a lack of money or low wages by 11% and college expenses by 8%. High health costs were mentioned by 25% of respondents age 50 and 64 and by 23% age 65 and older.[70] The cost of health care for a typical family of four covered by an average employer-sponsored health plan increased 22% in five years from $23,215 in 2014 to $28,386 in 2019 (Figure 4.14).[71]

Consumer financial responsibility for health care has increased primarily because employers have shifted costs to employees. In 2009, employees' health insurance premiums averaged $3,515, and employers paid $9,860 for a total

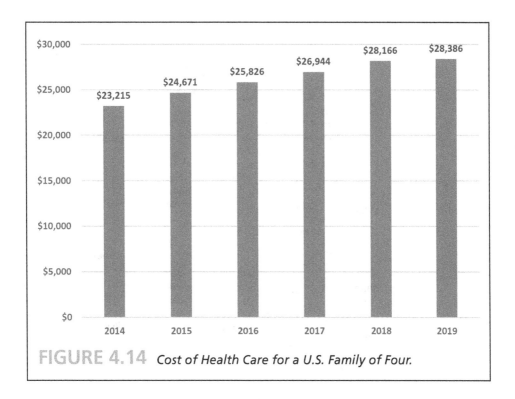

**FIGURE 4.14**  *Cost of Health Care for a U.S. Family of Four.*

of \$13,375. Total health care premiums increased 54% from 2009 to 2019. While the employer portion grew 48%, the worker portion was up 71% for the same 10-year period (Figure 4.15).[72] Employee co-pays and deductibles also increased.

The rising cost of health insurance premiums has resulted in increased demand for high-deductible health plans (HDHP) that have lower monthly premiums in exchange for larger deductibles. The percentage of all employees selecting HDHPs in 2014 was 20%, and the percentage increased to 30% in 2019 (Figure 4.16).[73]

### *Social-Cultural Force:* Trend 3—Consumers are Becoming More Engaged with Health Care

Consumers have traditionally been shielded from health prices and were unlikely to comparison shop for health services because insurance deductibles were low and provider networks were extensive. This has changed with increased consumer out-of-pocket spending and more narrow networks. Consumers have become price sensitive, interested in using the web to compare physicians and hospitals, and are increasingly deferring health services and prescriptions due to costs. A marketing research study found that 66% of consumers experience deep worry

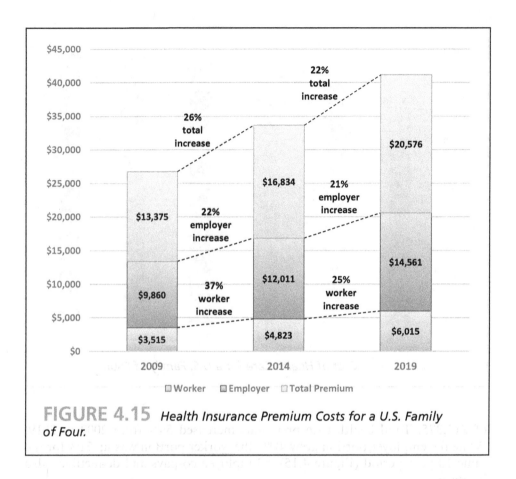

**FIGURE 4.15** *Health Insurance Premium Costs for a U.S. Family of Four.*

and stress when planning out-of-pocket health expenses. Deciphering health care jargon was a barrier for 69% of respondents, and 49% did not understand the cost implications of different health plan choices. Consumers also reported low levels of confidence in navigating the health system, and they wanted to receive help in making health decisions through one-on-one human interaction. Digital and self-service tools, however, were viewed as useful once consumers developed confidence and familiarity.[74] Wearable devices like Fitbit trackers and Apple Watches were found to improve daily health habits and personal accountability for 69% of consumers using them.[75]

Studies have also found that consumers who are more engaged with their health are less likely to have health problems and are more likely to report lower levels of physical pain, high blood pressure, and depression.[76] Health care providers—who receive value-based payments for better health outcomes, higher levels of quality, and population health measures—have clear financial incentives to motivate consumers to be more engaged and accountable for

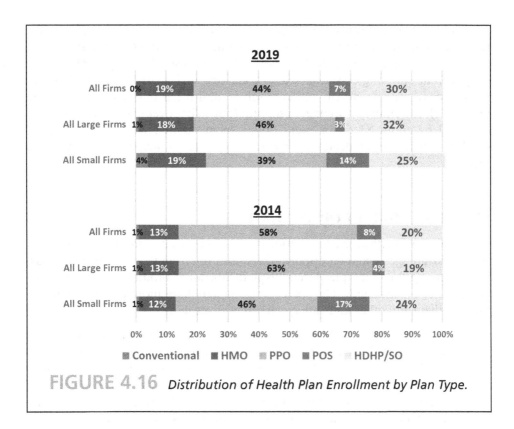

FIGURE 4.16   *Distribution of Health Plan Enrollment by Plan Type.*

their health. Employers also have financial incentives under the ACA to improve employee accountability and health. Employees who have low levels of health engagement cost employers 85% more in lost productivity. Additionally, employees identified as disengaged had 2.17 unhealthy days per month compared to engaged employees with 1.25 unhealthy days.[77] As a result, employers are investing in health care price comparison tools to help employees choose lower-cost health care alternatives as well as other tools to improve employee health.

Half of large employers with 200 or more employees, and 19% of all employers, offer employees health risk appraisals (HRAs). The purpose of a HRA is to identify and treat employee health risk factors at earlier stages. Questionnaires inquire about medical history, health status, and lifestyle. Biometric screening, another tool with increasing demand, is used to measure cholesterol levels, blood pressure, stress levels, nutritional patterns, and other health care risks. Fifty percent of large employers that offer HRAs, and 32% of employers offering biometric screening, reward employees with lower insurance premiums or lower cost sharing incentives for being more accountable.

The ACA also incentivizes employers financially for providing preventive health and wellness programs. These programs help employees lower blood pressure, body-mass index (BMI), and cholesterol levels.[78] The programs typically include smoking cessation, exercise classes, health education, meditation, yoga, access to gyms, nutritional counseling, and other options. An economic analysis of one employer wellness program found that overall employer medical costs fell by about $3.27 for every dollar spent on wellness, and the cost of employee absenteeism decreased by $2.73 per dollar invested in a wellness program.[79]

## STRATEGIC MARKET OPPORTUNITIES

Market-driven health care organizations are using innovative marketing strategies to take advantage of market opportunities resulting from these consumer trends. The following four examples briefly explain consumer product, price, channels, and promotion strategies. The succeeding chapters have more detailed explanations of these and other innovative marketing strategies.

1. *Product strategy*: The Mayo Clinic is focused on decreasing chronic disease prevalence and increasing consumer accountability and engagement through a product strategy focused on improving customer experience. Analyzing and managing customer experience is having a positive effect on brand meaning. Brand meaning is a primary influence on brand equity. Mayo is focusing on measuring and improving customer loyalty through an NPS program. Improved Mayo Clinic customer experience is leading to increased customer loyalty, stronger financial performance, and a higher level of brand equity.

2. *Pricing strategy*: A segment of consumers is responding to higher health care prices and increased accountability by researching and comparing prices before making health care purchases. The online company Healthcare Bluebook (healthcarebluebook.com) is supporting better pricing decisions by providing consumers, payers, employers, and health care providers with a pricing strategy health IT tool. Healthcare Bluebook lists physician and health system pricing information by location to help buyers compare different providers and save on out-of-pocket expenses. They also supply comparative pricing for medical tests, hearing aids, medications, and dental services.

3. *Channels strategy*: Another consumer segment who is willing to pay for personalized, immediate physician services is turning to ultra-elite concierge medicine practices. This channels strategy for Private Medical (privatemedical.org) in San Francisco, Silicon Valley, Los Angeles, and New York is to provide immediate care for families of adults, young children, teenagers, and even

grandparents in nursing homes—for a fee of $40,000 to $80,000 per year. Consumers may apply for care by referral only. The Private Medical value proposition is to outperform all other medical providers by "out-caring" them and by creating environments that lead patients and their families toward healing and peace of mind.[80]

The primary benefits are appointments, admissions, and other arrangements that are made rapidly, and the referrals are to the best physicians and hospitals in the U.S.[81] Consumers no longer need to navigate the health system alone. This is in contrast to the national average of 29 days for an appointment with a family care physician, up from 19.5 days in 2014. Specialists delays can be longer with a 32-day wait to see a dermatologist and a 21-day wait for the typical cardiologist.[82]

4.  *Promotion strategy*: Drug addiction is a chronic condition with more than 70,000 consumers dying from drug overdoses from illicit drugs and prescription opioids in 2017—a twofold increase in a decade. Overdose-related deaths have become the leading cause of death among consumers less than age 50.[83] As addicts have high mortality rates in health care settings, and addiction treatment can be costly, more states are turning to peer coaching promotion strategies where addicts in recovery meet with overdose victims.

    Coaches come to the hospital to discuss potential recovery options, but addicts need to be inwardly motivated to stay alive and have a plan. Only 20% of addicts accept a coach. For those addicts who want to continue using drugs, coaches offer advice on how to take drugs more safely and avoid overdoses and spreading diseases like HIV/AIDS or hepatitis. Coaches follow up with the patients for 90 days or more to support their progress.

## CHAPTER SUMMARY

Virtually all consumers use health care, but there is a wide range of health care demand. Consumer morbidity and mortality data, health care spending patterns, and changes in health status can help explain why health care is needed and who uses it. The top 10 causes of death are responsible for 74% of all deaths. There were significant decreases in deaths due to heart disease, cancer, unintentional injuries, chronic respiratory disease, and Alzheimer's disease from 2017 to 2018. Only 10 to 15% of an individual's overall health status can be attributed to health care services received, and health status is primarily determined by behavior, genetics, and social determinants like living conditions, access to food, and education.

Consumer health care behavior and purchasing are influenced by cultural, social, and personal factors. Cultural factors have the broadest and deepest influences. Family is the most important consumer buying organization in society, and family members constitute the most influential primary reference group. Personal characteristics include age and stage in the life cycle, occupation and economic circumstances, personality and self-concept, and lifestyle and values. Four key psychological processes—motivation, perception, learning, and memory—fundamentally influence consumer responses to various health care marketing stimuli.

Three of the most important consumer environmental trends are the increased prevalence of chronic diseases, consumers paying more for health care, and the growth of consumer health care engagement. The Mayo Clinic uses a customer experience-based branding strategy to reduce chronic disease prevalence and to increase consumer accountability and engagement. Healthcare Bluebook is a company offering consumers prices for local health care services to support value-based buying decisions. Ultra-elite concierge medicine practices are using innovative channels strategies to meet the needs of the wealthy who want high value and are willing to pay a high price. A number of states are using former addicts in promotion strategies that coach substance abusers who want to quit using drugs.

## DISCUSSION QUESTIONS

1. The Stimulus-Response Model explains how consumer health care behavior and purchasing are influenced by their cultural, social, and personal characteristics. You work in a county health department that is targeting lower-income consumers to prevent diabetes. You understand that it is imperative to have a distribution plan that takes into account cultural, social, and personal factors. How will you identify these factors in your target market? List the top three expected factors that will affect your plan and how you will adapt your plan to each factor.

2. Most needs for health care services and products seem tied to the physiological and safety needs shown in Maslow's hierarchy of needs pyramid. Describe the types of health care needs that could be related to the upper levels of Maslow's pyramid—the social, esteem, and self-actualization levels.

3. The obesity epidemic in the U.S. is responsible for many chronic conditions. Using the Five-Stage Model of consumer buying, outline how you would convince consumers to buy and use healthy foods to reduce obesity.

## CONSUMER MARKETING CASE: GETTING PEOPLE TO EXERCISE

Lack of physical activity is one of the four leading health risk behaviors responsible for most chronic diseases and conditions along with poor nutrition, tobacco use, and excessive alcohol consumption. Consumers who exercise regularly improve their physical and mental health, reduce obesity that can lead to or worsen chronic conditions, and reduce their health care costs. The problem is that only 16% of consumers exercise on any given day.[84] How can marketing be used to motivate consumers to exercise and improve their health?

According to the CDC 2018 Physical Activity Guidelines for Americans, consumers need to have physical activity each week that leads to improved aerobic fitness and muscle strengthening. Only 53% of consumers, however, meet federal physical activity guidelines for aerobic activity and only 23% meet the guidelines for both aerobic and muscle-strengthening activity.[85] A study conducted by the Annenberg School for Communication at the University of Pennsylvania tested how social media can be used as a cost-effective promotional strategy for large-scale physical activity interventions.[86]

A typical employee exercise program uses a range of promotional tools such as social media, brochures, posters, apps, electronic trackers, coaching, team activities, step challenges, and financial incentives. Penn researchers recruited 800 graduate students to enroll in an 11-week exercise program they called "PennShape."[87] This federally-funded, university-wide fitness initiative included weekly exercise classes, fitness coaching, and nutrition advice all managed through a website the researchers built.[88] The students could take running, spin, yoga, weight lifting, and other classes, and the top performers had the opportunity to win prizes based on the number of classes attended. What the participants did not know was that the researchers had segmented them into four groups to test how different kinds of social media content affected their exercise levels. This allowed the researchers to test four different motivations for behavior change. The four groups were individual control group, individual competition, team support, and team competition.

Participants in the control group could use the website and go to any class, but they were not aware of what other participants were doing. In the individual competition group, participants could see the exercise activity of five anonymous people on a leaderboard. Participants in the third group were put in teams of six, and they were eligible to win rewards based on their team's collective activity. This gave the teams an incentive to communicate with each other online and support fellow team members to exercise. The final group, team competition, had both competitive and supportive motivations. They could communicate with each other online, but they also saw a leaderboard showing how their team was performing against other teams.

The study results showed that it did not matter if participants were exercising in teams or as individuals, and competition by far was the most powerful motivator to get people to exercise. The control group exercised on average 20.3 times per week. The two competitive groups exceeded this level by 90% with members of the individual competition group exercising an average of 38.5 classes weekly and members of the team competition group averaging 35.7 classes. The most surprising result was that the social support team exercised far less than all other groups. The team support group averaged only 16.8 classes per week — less than half the exercise rates of the two competitive groups. Giving more online resources is often thought to increase performance, but giving the wrong kind of resources actually reduces performance.

A competitive environment puts people into an aspirational mindset, and participants are focusing on those who are exercising the most and are ignoring the others. The people who exercise the most make others want to exercise more, and this leads to a social intensification of participation on the entire group. Competitive groups frame relationships in terms of goal-setting by the most active members. These relationships help to motivate exercise because they give people higher expectations for their own levels of performance. A competitive setting results in each person's activity raising the bar for everyone else.

Social support messages actually result in the opposite effect. In a supportive environment, people become dependent on receiving messages and equal attention is to paid to everyone whether they are actively exercising or not. The presence of inactive people gives everyone permission to be inactive as well, and this creates a de-intensifying effect on the group. If people stop exercising, it gives permission for others to stop, and this can lead to an overall exercise decline.

The positive effects of social competition can also be used to motivate positive behaviors to improve medication compliance, diabetes control, smoking cessation, flu vaccinations, weight loss, and preventive screening. Lifestyle patterns can be difficult to change, but marketing strategies using social tools with appropriate content can be effective and have a high ROI.[89]

## CASE QUESTIONS

You are a health care marketing consultant and have been hired by IBM to improve employee health through increasing exercise. IBM employs a range of demographic cohorts including baby boomers, generation Xs, and millennials.

a) The Penn researchers found that using a competition-based social media strategy was most effective with students in their 20s. Do you think this strategy will be effective with all the different employee age groups at IBM? Explain how you will use marketing tools to support your answer.

b) PennShape was a short-term 11-week exercise program. IBM is intrigued by this research and wants to use a social media promotional strategy, but they are also interested in a longer-term exercise program. How would you determine if the PennShape program will be subject to "wear out?" If it is determined that PennShape cannot be extended long term, how would you make use of the Penn research to innovatively design a social media-based exercise promotion strategy for IBM?

c) How you would apply PATH consumer analysis to segment and target the IBM employee market? Use the PATH profiles and examples of attitudes toward exercise in Table 4.3 to further explain how you would motivate your target(s) to exercise.

# CHAPTER

# PHYSICIAN MARKETING

## LEARNING OBJECTIVES

In this chapter we will address the following questions:

1. Why should physicians consider strategic marketing to solve practice management problems?

2. What are the physician attitudes and behavior that affect physician marketing?

3. What are the most important environmental forces and trends facing physician practices?

4. How can physicians use innovative marketing strategies to solve practice management problems?

This chapter will explain how strategic marketing increases value for physicians, their patients or "customers," referral sources, and practice employees. It will also demonstrate how strategic marketing leads to improved practice financial performance, reduced risk, and higher market share. The chapter topics are physician views of marketing, physician market trends, physician attitudes and behavior, the most important environmental forces affecting physicians, and examples of physician management problems with strategic marketing solutions.

## PHYSICIANS ARE OFTEN SKEPTICAL OF MARKETING

The first hurdle in physician marketing is overcoming physician skepticism of the term marketing. Physicians typically have the transactional view of marketing and not the customer relationship view. Marketing is associated with promotional tactics like advertising, brochures, and sales. Physicians who try marketing tactics without data or analysis are often disappointed with the results. They also misconstrue the customer relationship approach to be "the customer is always right." If a patient asks a physician for a particular test or procedure, then the physician feels obliged to comply.

A more accurate understanding of the customer relationship view is when physicians and consumers build relationships and discuss the advantages and disadvantages of different clinical options. A study published in the *New England Journal of Medicine* found that when physicians listened attentively to patient questions, looked them in the eye, and then clearly and openly communicated potential care options, patients became more engaged with their health. Higher patient engagement leads to increased adherence to treatment guidelines and better clinical outcomes.[1]

One solution to this problem of marketing perception is comparing the physician clinical decision-making model to the strategic marketing decision-making model. When a patient presents with stomach pain, the physician asks a serious of questions about health history, duration of symptoms, and recent behavior. Lab, imaging, and other diagnostic tests may be ordered. If a peptic ulcer is diagnosed, initial treatment may include dietary changes and a prescription. A treatment plan is formulated, patient progress is tracked, and the treatment may be modified depending on the results.

Strategic marketers follow a very similar approach. An orthopedic physician explains to a marketer that patient referrals have been decreasing for an unknown reason. Secondary marketing research is analyzed including local market data, competitors, and practice volume and revenue data. Primary marketing is conducted with referral sources to understand how referrals are made.

The research finds that a competing physician practice has a new technology with superior clinical results and lower costs, there is a six week wait to next appointment, and the client's employees have low loyalty scores. A strategic mar-

TABLE 5.1  **Medical versus Marketing Decision-Making**

| Medical Decision-Making | Marketing Decision-Making |
| --- | --- |
| 1. Take medical history and conduct physical exam to understand patient complaint. | 1. Understand marketing problems through secondary marketing research. |
| 2. Order clinical tests and analyze results. | 2. Conduct primary marketing research to fill in information gaps. |
| 3. Analyze evidence to diagnose the medical problem. | 3. Analyze evidence to understand the marketing problem. |
| 4. Design a treatment plan to achieve a medical goal by treating the diagnosis. | 4. Design a marketing plan that will achieve the goals using a range of strategies and tactics. |
| 5. Implement the treatment plan. | 5. Implement the marketing plan. |
| 6. Track clinical results and potentially revise diagnosis or modify treatment. | 6. Track marketing performance and modify strategies and tactics to improve results. |

keting plan is developed in collaboration with the physician. The stated goal and objectives are to increase referrals and revenue by 15% and increase employee loyalty by 20%. The recommended strategies are to investigate the adoption of state-of-the-art clinical technology, improve scheduling efficiency, communicate these changes to referral sources, and better understand customer and employee loyalty drivers. The marketing strategies and tactics are then implemented, and the operations and financial results are measured and reported monthly.

The physician medical decision process and the marketing decision process are very similar. Both are evidence-based, analytical, and systematic (Table 5.1). Physicians who understand this similarity are more likely to adopt a customer relationship approach to managing their practice.

## PHYSICIAN MARKET TRENDS

The number of active U.S. physicians in 2019 was 1,005,295, an 18% increase over 2010 (Figure 5.1).[2] This included 479,896 primary care physicians practicing family medicine, internal medicine, and pediatric medicine. There were also 525,439

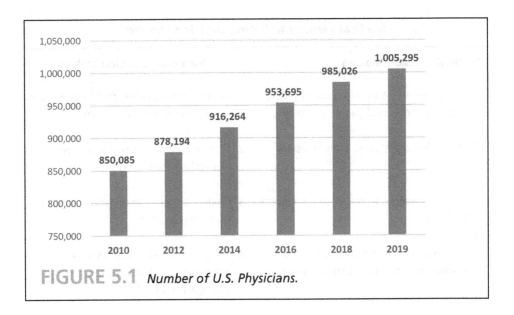

**FIGURE 5.1** *Number of U.S. Physicians.*

specialist physicians. The four states with the highest number of physicians were California (112,906), New York (89,500), Texas (64,602), and Florida (56,499).[3] The number of active physicians per 100,000 population in the U.S. increased to 277.8 in 2018, compared to 271.6 in 2016. Active physicians ranged from 449.5 in Massachusetts to 191.3 in Mississippi. The states with the highest number of physicians per 100,000 population were concentrated in the Northeast.[4]

Demand for physicians will continue to grow faster than the supply. Job growth for physicians between 2014 and 2024 is projected to increase 14.0%, while the national job growth projection is 6.5%.[5] By 2025, a shortfall of between 46,100 and 90,400 U.S. physicians is projected. The primary care physician shortage is expected to be between 12,500 and 31,100, and specialty care physician shortage is expected to be even greater, with 28,200 to 63,700 physicians.[6] These projections are based on the expected number of new medical school graduates, the aging of the U.S. population, the aging of the physician workforce, expansion of health insurance under the ACA, access to care to underserved groups, millennial work-life balance preferences, and the need to improve social determinants of health care such as smoking, diet, and exercise.

The median male physician age was 49.3 years and the median female physician age was 42.7 years in 2018.[7] There are 558,000 (61.6%) male physicians and 348,000 female physicians (38.4%). Thirty-three percent of all female physicians are millennials, while 19% of all male physicians are millennials (Figure 5.2).[8] As a group, millennials—born between 1981 and 1996—are interested in reducing their time spent in daily work compared to their boomer generation parents born between 1946 and 1964. Overall, physician gender is trending more female. Women

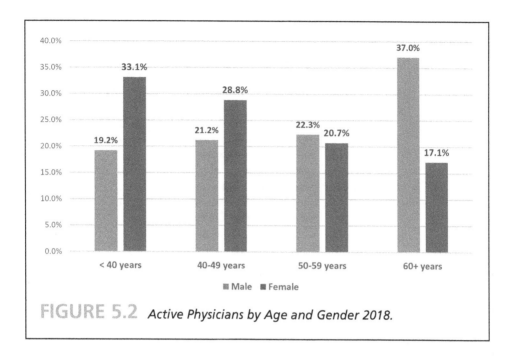

**FIGURE 5.2** *Active Physicians by Age and Gender 2018.*

comprise more than one-third of the active physician workforce, an estimated 46% of all physicians-in-training, and more than half of all medical students in the U.S. Male physicians are disproportionately represented in specialty fields with higher numbers of work hours, while female physicians are more common in primary care and tend to work fewer hours.[9]

The aging of physicians and the shift in gender could have a considerable impact on the physician workforce. The growing percentage of millennial female physicians is expected to shift overall physician preferences to more predictable schedules with a more even work-life balance. As younger physicians replace retiring physicians, a larger number of physicians will be needed to meet the increased demands of aging boomers. Additional clinical responsibilities will be transferred to nurse practitioners, nurse midwives, nurse anesthetists, clinical nurse specialists, and physician assistants.

Research from athenahealth, however, indicates stressful work environments may be taking a toll particularly on younger women. They are more likely than their male counterparts to report symptoms of burnout. In a 2017 survey of 1,029 practicing physicians, 54% of women under the age of 45 reported symptoms of burnout—emotional exhaustion, depersonalization, and sense of low personal accomplishment—compared to 31% of males the same age.

The average physician income in 2019 for a primary care physician was $237,000 and $341,000 for a specialist. Specialist income is higher because the procedures they perform are more highly compensated than the cognitive services

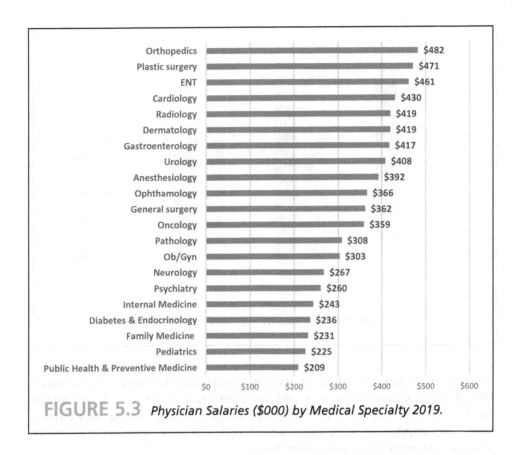

FIGURE 5.3   *Physician Salaries ($000) by Medical Specialty 2019.*

provided by primary care physicians—even if the primary care visits are compa-
rably measured using the metrics of time, risk, and skill. The average salary for
male primary care physicians was 25% higher than the average female salary, and
a male specialist salary was 33% higher than a female specialist. The highest paid
physicians in 2019 were orthopedics with $482,000, and the lowest paid were pub-
lic health and preventive medicine with $209,000 (Figure 5.3). When asked if they
felt fairly compensated, public health and preventive physicians had the highest
response with 73%. Infectious disease specialists and diabetes/endocrinology specialists had the lowest response with only 42% feeling fairly compensated.[10]

## PHYSICIAN ATTITUDES AND BEHAVIOR

Physician services are marketed to customers that include other physicians, consumers, employers, payers, and referral sources. Understanding the attitudes of
physicians and others that influence customer buying behavior is important for
developing effective marketing strategies.

### The Physician Training Culture

Attitudes and behavior are largely influenced by culture, social factors, and personal factors. Reference groups, such as medical school and residency instructors and fellow students, have a direct face-to-face as well as an indirect influence on these three elements. Students drawn to careers in medicine often have high intelligence, compassion, inquisitiveness, and sensitivity to others. They are also often driven, perfectionistic, goal-oriented, and prone to anxiety. The culture of physician training has a strong, and continuing, influence on how physicians think, feel, make buying decisions, and respond to marketing stimuli. Most medical training has traditionally encouraged rugged individualism, autonomy, authority, rigidity, and safety-seeking. They see themselves as members of a competitive, individually-focused, outcome-driven expert culture. Physicians use words like "I" or "me," but rarely "we" or "us." Teamwork and collaboration has not been emphasized. Physician training has begun to change, however, over the past 10 years to a more collegial model.

Medical school acceptance and graduation continues to be highly competitive. The four-year graduation rate for MD students was 90% in the late 1970s but dropped to 83% in the 1980s and to 81% in 2013.[11] While this intense environment conditions physicians to learn how to survive training, compete for a successful residency match, and build a practice, these traits can also lead to social isolation and burnout.[12]

Abraham Verghese, MD, developed an alternative medical training approach in an attempt to preserve the innate empathy and sensitivity that initially brings students to medical school.[13] Verghese's primary goal is to help students develop a deep personal relationship with the bed-ridden patient as opposed to focusing solely on data in a computer. As a professor at the Stanford University School of Medicine, Verghese integrated a formal humanities and ethics curriculum into all four years of medical school learning.

Renowned for his weekly bedside rounds, Verghese insists on examining patients without personal knowledge of their diagnosis to demonstrate the wealth of information available from the physical exam. His approach to diagnosing patients and in developing a caring, two-way patient-doctor relationship has value not only for patients and families but also for the physician. This innovative approach has led to the development of "The Stanford 25," a Stanford initiative designed to showcase and teach 25 fundamental physical exam skills and their diagnostic benefits to interns and residents.

### Physician Decision-Making

Studies have shown that in medical school and residency a didactic exercise usually requires 20 to 30 minutes for the senior doctor and students to arrive at a working diagnosis. In practice, however, a physician will interrupt a patient describing their symptoms within 20 seconds.[14] During this short period of time physicians employ pattern recognition—based on the medical history, physical examination, x-rays, or lab tests—to come up with two or three diagnoses. These shortcuts, or *heuristics*, are the essential working tools of clinical medicine that allow physicians to combine thoughts and actions. A heuristic is any approach to problem solving that uses a practical technique and is not necessarily optimal but is sufficient. Medical schools discourage heuristics and instead rely on systematic, didactic exercises both in the classrooms and at the bedside.

Regardless, heuristics have become the foundation for mature medical thinking. This is largely in response to the uncertainty, demands, and especially the limited time allotted to individual patients.[15] Decisions based on heuristics can save lives, but they can also lead to catastrophic errors. The move to value-based care—with financial incentives for quality measures, patient outcomes, and population health—has affected physician clinical decision-making. New decision-making tools include care standardization, algorithms, protocols, and clinical rules, all potentially influenced by the growth of artificial intelligence (AI). Since heuristics are part of the physician culture, it is not surprising that many physicians view value-based "cookbook medicine" negatively.

Physicians are likely to take a heuristic approach to marketing decision-making. To increase patient volume, a group of specialist physicians invested heavily in their practice website and in the sporadic use of four-color magazine advertising. When these marketing tactics did not yield results, they reluctantly decided to consider a strategic marketing approach. A systematic analysis of market and practice data found that 99% of patient volume came from professional referrals and 1% from their website. The print advertising spending had no effect on awareness, preference, or intent to use. A sales strategy was then implemented to build relationships with referral sources, and a customer loyalty strategy was used to increase referrer and consumer retention.

Physician culture also plays a role in health care cost decisions and end-of-life decisions. One-quarter of total annual Medicare spending is used by the 5% of U.S. patients who are in their final year of life. The physician culture is focused on extending life, and this includes targeting the hopeful "long tail" of patient survival statistics. Surgery, chemotherapy, and intensive care services are often ordered based on the chance of gaining time later. Since medical technology is capable of sustaining organs beyond mental awareness and coherence, physicians are unsure how or when to accept dying and give up on heroic measures. Evidence indicates, however, that spending in the last couple of months of life does not have much, if any, benefit.[16] Additionally, marketing research studies of patients with terminal illnesses indicate that their needs are not being met by accelerated care at the end of life. The studies showed that the highest priorities for patients with terminal illness were to avoid suffering, be with family, have the touch of others, be mentally aware, and not be a burden to others.[17]

Physicians are increasingly recommending hospice care. This is a cultural change because hospice care is not concerned with making a patient's life longer or shorter. Hospices employ nurses, physicians, and social workers to reduce pain and discomfort, maintain mental awareness, and give people time with their families. A clinical research study followed 4,493 Medicare patients with either terminal cancer or congestive heart failure, and it evaluated survival rates for a group of patients with traditional treatment and a second group who used hospice care. The study found that for breast cancer, prostate cancer, and colon cancer patients the two groups had the same survival time. Hospice care seemed to extend survival for some patients. Patients with pancreatic cancer gained an average of three weeks, lung cancer patients had an additional six weeks, and congestive heart patients lived another three months.[18]

## THREE HEALTH CARE ENVIRONMENTAL CHANGES AFFECTING PHYSICIANS

Three environmental forces—demographic, economic, and social/cultural—are forming trends that affect physicians. Demographically, physician practice patterns are limiting patient access to care. Economically, changing practice organizational structures and payment models are pressuring physician income. The cumulative impact of these and other environmental forces are resulting in negative social/cultural effects such as lower physician morale.

### *Demographic Force:* Trend 1—Reduced Access to Patient Care

The growth and aging of the population is the primary factor increasing demand for physician services. From 2014 to 2025, the U.S. population is projected to grow by 8.6%, from about 319 million to 346 million. Of the 75 million baby boomers born between 1946 and 1964, an estimated 3 million will reach age 65 every year from 2014 to 2034. This includes physicians, advanced practice providers, nurses, and other clinicians who are members of the boomer generation.

The population aged 65 and over is projected to increase by 41%, and the population under age 18 is projected to increase by only 5%. While older consumers have higher per capita consumption of health care than younger people, the more self-indulgent boomer generation will present even greater challenges to the health system. Compared to the boomer parents of the silent generation, the 50 million born between 1925 and 1945, boomers are proving to be less healthy than their parents. Research published in *JAMA Internal Medicine* compared the health of both generations and found that despite a longer boomer life expectancy, boomers had higher rates of hypertension, high cholesterol, diabetes, and obesity compared to their parents.[19] This demographic force will have a strong influence on how caregivers and policymakers manage the health care system in future decades.

Patient access to physician care is expected to decrease. Although the majority of physicians (54%) responding to a 2018 survey indicate they will continue practicing as they are, 46% of physicians indicate they will change their practice over the next three years. A national physician survey found that 80% are overextended or at capacity. Additionally, 46% of physicians plan to make changes including cut back on hours, retire, take a non-clinical job, become a contractor, work part-time, or switch to concierge medicine (Table 5.2).

The number of physicians exiting the workforce will be higher than the number of new physicians entering the workforce. In 2018, 17% of physicians indicated they will retire in the period 2021–2023 compared to 9% in 2012, the highest percentage recorded by this biennial survey. Retirements will reduce the number of physicians in the workforce by 136,000, while 85,000 physicians will complete residency and enter the workforce. This will result in 51,000 physician vacancies. Even if physicians do not retire at an annual rate of 6% by 2023, 32% of physicians are age 60 or older, and a wave of physician retirements can be anticipated.[20]

### *Economic Force:* Trend 2—Changing Physician Payment Models

Environmental disruptions include uncertain physician reimbursement, rising practice expenses, increased regulatory compliance, and the burden of mandated information technology. Physicians are increasingly moving from their own practice to employed settings with health systems and other organizations. A physician survey found that the percentage of physicians in independent practice decreased from 49% in 2012 to 31% in 2018. Physicians employed by a hospital or medical group increased from 2012 (44%) to the highest levels in 2014 (53%) and 2016 (58%) and then decreased to 49% in 2018 (Table 5.3).[21] Employment is attractive because it offers a stable income as well as the financial and technical

## TABLE 5.2   Physicians Reducing Patient Access

| Change in Practice Pattern | Percentage of Mentions |
| --- | --- |
| Cut back hours | 22.3% |
| Retire | 17.4% |
| Seek a non-clinical job within health care | 12.4% |
| Work locum tenens (contractor) | 8.4% |
| Work part-time | 8.5% |
| Switch to a concierge practice | 4.5% |

TABLE 5.3 **Physicians Identifying as Independent Practice Owners or Partners**

|  | 2018 | 2016 | 2014 | 2012 |
|---|---|---|---|---|
| Practice owner | 31.4% | 32.7% | 34.6% | 48.5% |
| Hospital or medical group employee | 49.1% | 57.9% | 52.8% | 43.7% |

support needed to manage new government, payer, and information technology requirements.

The population health management model, implemented through Accountable Care Organizations (ACOs) or other integrated systems, further supports this physician employment trend. ACOs provide coordinated care for entire population groups under a set budget. Physicians participating in these organizations are rewarded for achieving quality benchmarks and cost savings. This model is considered the bridge between fee-for-service and fee-for-value payment. In value-based models, physicians direct spending through care coordination and patient management. Extensive communication and collaboration is now needed by hospitals, primary care physicians, medical specialists, nurse practitioners, physician assistants, pharmacists, therapists, social workers, labs, and others that have traditionally operated in independent silos. A physician employment model can be more efficient and effective for improving clinical results.[22] Overall, physician-owned ACOs have performed better than hospital-owned ACOs.

Physician financial incentives, however, are lagging this trend. Merritt Hawkins, a national physician recruiting firm, tracked 3,131 physician and advanced practitioner recruiting assignments from April 1, 2018 to March 31, 2019. The compensation for 70% of searches offered a production bonus; and 56% offered a bonus based in whole or in part on quality measures such as patient satisfaction, adherence to treatment protocols, and outcome measures. This compares to 43% in 2018, and it is the highest percent of contracts offering a quality-based production bonus ever tracked by Merritt Hawkins. The remaining 30% of jobs offered a straight salary, an income guarantee, or other type of compensation. Average physician compensation based on value measures represented 11% of the physician's total compensation, an increase from 4% in 2017. Any incentive more than 10% of total compensation is judged to affect physician behavior or performance.[23]

In 2015, Congress took bipartisan action and passed the Medicare Access and CHIP Reauthorization Act (MACRA) to advance the move to value.[24] The objectives of the federal government are to improve outcomes, emphasize wellness, increase patient engagement, and provide more transparency through a single score that represents the value of physician care. Federal intervention was needed because providers have been slow to adopt value measures, transparency, and accountability. This legislation is viewed as the most significant Medicare change in 10 years. MACRA changes the way Medicare pays clinicians by establishing two tracks: the Merit-Based Incentive Payment System (MIPS) and the Advanced Alternative Payment Model (APM) track. Initially, most clinicians will be paid under the MIPS track. MACRA was fully implemented in 2019, but it is based on performance measures beginning in 2017. MIPS is expected to affect 9% of physician Medicare payments by 2022.

MIPS offers physician groups wide flexibility in selecting quality measures. Physicians will receive a composite score based on their performance in four categories: cost, quality, clinical practice management, and "advancing care information." They can choose six measures from a list nearly 300 choices. A single point above or below the national mean or median will result in a payment adjustment. Physicians will have incentives to work as a team, emphasize wellness, and increase customer engagement to optimize their scores. Additionally, physicians should be concerned about how the scores are collected, the reliability and validity of the data collected, and the weights used to create the composite score.

The quality data reported under MIPS is available to the public on the Physician Compare website.[25] Consumers can use MIPS information to select physicians instead of their traditional selection criteria that include the name of the medical school the physician attended, the number of years of practice, and malpractice claims history.[26] Older consumers with years of brand loyalty to particular physicians are not likely to switch physicians based on MIPS. Once MIPS is adopted by commercial payers, however, younger consumers—who are reliant on faulty but directional online reviews—are more likely to use MIPS for physician selection. MIPS quality information available online will also help employers, payers, and health systems select physician networks, and these decisions will strongly influence physician market share, referral patterns, and reputations.

### *Social-Cultural Force:* Trend 3—Low Physician Morale

Physicians are struggling to maintain morale levels. The primary source of professional satisfaction has been the patient relationship, according to 74% of physicians. This relationship as well as physician satisfaction are eroding due to reduced clinical autonomy, increased liability concerns, struggles for reimbursement, and the decreased time available to interact with individual patients. Research has found that 54% of physicians describe their morale as negative, 63% are pessimistic about the future of their profession, 49% would not recommend medicine as a career to their children, and 28% regret their choice to be a physician.[27] Surveyed physicians identified regulatory and paperwork burdens and loss of clinical autonomy as primary sources of dissatisfaction. Respondents spent 21% of their time on non-clinical administrative work. This time is equivalent to 168,000 physician FTEs *not* engaged in clinical activities. An estimated 72% of physicians reported that the added burden of third-party requirements detracts from the quality of care that they provide. Two RAND market studies confirmed that physicians are experiencing higher stress levels because they must design new patient care workflows and collaborate more with other clinicians.[28]

ACOs and patient-centered medical homes (PCMHs) are value-based physician organization structures that may seem threatening to physicians. ACOs are composed of primary care providers, specialists, hospitals, continuing care organizations, and other health care organizations. These different organizations are given financial incentives to collaborate, improve care, and reduce per capita costs. ACOs focus on preventive care and the management of chronic diseases. According to the National Association of ACOs, as of January 2020 there were 558 Medicare ACOs serving more than 12.3 million beneficiaries and hundreds more commercial and Medicaid ACOs serving millions of additional patients.[29]

A PCMH is composed of a cross-section of preventive and primary care providers who treat the comprehensive health needs of a specific population. They include primary care physicians, nurses, advanced practice providers, social workers, pharmacists, physical therapists, dieticians, and others. It typically takes more than two years of care coordination and management for a medical home to achieve its health outcomes objectives and to see a reduction in overall health care costs.[30] Another reason for physician stress is because as physicians become more efficient, they are working at the "top of their license" and seeing more intensive and complex patients.[31]

These value-based care models require physicians to rely heavily on electronic health records (EHRs) to collect, track, and analyze clinical and administrative patient data. Many physician practices have developed customized decision support and order sets within their EHRs. These tools prompt physicians and allied health professionals to follow new clinical protocols including pay-for-performance, episode-based, capitation, and shared savings models. Unfortunately, these new payment models that rely on a range of different types of quality data are overwhelming medical practices. A RAND market study found that improving outcomes and reducing costs is being hindered by requirements for data that are conflicting or not available.[32]

Physicians' physical or emotional exhaustion, frustration, and tension strongly influence their clinical judgments, actions, and motivation.[33] Unfortunately, few physicians will admit they have a diagnosis of major depression or that they are seeing a psychiatrist. In the physician culture, such an admission can be considered a sign of weakness. Physicians may feel that seeking psychiatric help will have a negative effect on their job status, prevent them from renewing their medical license, or raise their malpractice or health insurance costs.[34] Physicians are more likely to admit to burnout, a badge of courage in physician culture. Burnout is not listed as a mental illness in the *Diagnostic and Statistical Manual of Mental Disorders*.

Burnout can arise from such problems as being a driven perfectionist in an increasingly difficult medical system, personal problems like an unhappy marriage, or a head injury or other cause of mental illness. Burnout can also pose risks to patient safety, quality, and patient attitudes from not only the burned-out physician, but also from the organizational and environmental conditions causing the burnout. A physician who is less likely to be satisfied with work-life balance had at least one component of burnout from the Maslach Burnout Inventory:

- *Emotional exhaustion*: Feeling extremely tired or fatigued by their job

- *Cynicism*: Having a callous, uncaring, or hostile feeling toward patients and fellow workers

- *Inefficacy*: Feeling like they are not actually accomplishing anything worthwhile or making a difference at work

The Medscape National Physician Burnout & Suicide Report 2020 study found that burnout had decreased to 42% of physicians from 45% in 2015. Specialties that have been among the top in burnout over the past five years include critical care, emergency medicine, family medicine, internal medicine, neurology, and urology.[35] Burnout is also a major cause of physician suicide. Market-driven health care organizations are responding with innovative solutions. Atrius Health, a large physician practice in Eastern Massachusetts, is reducing burnout by developing "communities of practice." Clinical hubs are identified and restructured to break down barriers and better enable social relationships among care givers. This stronger sense of community has been found to reduce the social isolation that can lead to burnout.

## PHYSICIAN PRACTICE PROBLEMS AND STRATEGIC MARKETING SOLUTIONS

Strategic marketing can solve a wide range of physician practice problems. In this section, six marketing problems are solved with strategic marketing solutions.

### 1. *Marketing Problem*—Patient Health Needs Were Not Being Met in a Traditional Academic Medical Center Primary Care Practice

Rushika Fernandopulle, MD, an internal medicine physician at Massachusetts General Hospital in Boston, was frustrated. He was spending increasing amounts of time with hospital bureaucracy, ignoring phone calls and emails that did not relate to reimbursement, and most importantly he was spending less time with his patients. His frustration was compounded when he realized that his patients often could not solve their health problems because their social situations were usually the root cause.

### *Marketing Solution*—Create a Customer-Driven Physician Practice Culture to Meet Patient Needs.

A customer-driven organization is based on understanding customer needs, delivering products that are valued, and building long-term relationships. Management functions in traditional service organizations—such as operations, finance, marketing, human resources—are often inwardly focused and operate independent "silos." In a customer-driven organization, all management functions focus externally on the customer. Functions communicate with each other and collaborate to better serve customers. Three management imperatives for customer-driven organizations have been developed for the marketing, operations, and human resources management functions:[36]

1. Marketing imperative:
   a) Target the customers that the organization is capable of serving.
   b) Deliver an augmented product that meets customer needs for value, and develop profitable relationships with these customers.
   c) Customers recognize that their needs are being met. They are also aware that the product has a meaningful point of differentiation from competitive offerings.

2. Operations imperative:
   a) Create and deliver the specified service package to targeted customers.
   b) Select those operational techniques that allow it to consistently meet customer price, schedule, and quality expectations. Match processes to employee skills.
   c) Enable the organization to reduce its costs through continuing improvements in productivity.

3. Human resources imperative:
   a) Recruit, train, and motivate employees who can work well together for a compensation package that balances customer satisfaction, loyalty, and operational effectiveness.
   b) Employees will want to work for the organization because they value the organization's environment, they want to learn to interact in ways that add depth and dimension to their jobs, and they appreciate the opportunities to enhance their own skills.
   c) Service employees most value the ability to achieve results for customers. Internal quality in an organization is characterized by the attitudes employees have toward one another, how they serve each other inside the organization, and the pride taken in the products and services that they help to create and deliver.[37]

In 2012, Fernandopulle opened Iora Health, a primary care practice focused on the customer. Iora emphasizes keeping customers healthy as opposed to waiting for them to become sick. The goals of Iora are based on the value-based care model: improve clinical outcomes, reduce the per capita cost of health care, and actively manage the health of a defined patient population.[38] Keeping customers healthy and addressing the social problems that affect their health requires an engaged customer, but customer engagement requires more time and money than the traditional fee-for-service payment model allows. Fernandopulle chose a pricing strategy focused exclusively on a capitated payment structure to solve this problem.

Fernandopulle began by segmenting the payer market. An example of the marketing imperative is the targeting of payers that were interested in collaborative relationships with providers and in long-term patient outcomes. Early clients included a variety of self-insured employers such as Dartmouth College, the Freelancers Union, the New England Carpenters Fund in New Hampshire, and the Culinary Health Fund in Las Vegas. Eventually, two Humana Medicare Advantage plans in Seattle and Phoenix also became clients. While 5% of a payer's medical budget is typically allocated for primary care, Fernandopulle asks payers for 10%. He argues that increasing spending for primary care will result in a positive financial ROI because healthier consumers will spend substantially less on medical specialists and hospital admissions. Under capitated payment, payers give Iora a risk-adjusted flat monthly fee for each covered employee or member. In return, Iora accepts the risk for keeping its customers healthy. Iora customers have unlimited access to the primary care clinic visits without charges, co-payments, claims, or bills.

An example of the operations imperative is the employee "huddle" that takes place at every Iora clinic at 8:00 am. The huddle typically includes two physicians, two nurse practitioners, a full-time social worker, a front-desk receptionist, and eight health coaches. Participants preview the health of the patients with appointments that day and discuss the patients who *should* be having appointments. Appointments, tailored for individual patients, can be clinic visits, home visits, phone calls, video chats, or texts. Additionally, the operation of each Iora clinic is customized based on its local market. The customers in the Dartmouth College clinic have needs that are distinct from the needs of the self-pay, often undocumented Hispanic immigrants in the New York clinic. The only two Iora mainstays are the daily huddle and the use of the NPS that measures customer loyalty. It uses one question: how likely are you to recommend Iora to family or friends? Customer loyalty is the only customer measure correlated to financial performance (see Chapter 6 Hospital Marketing to understand how to implement an NPS strategy). Each clinic must review the NPS from the previous day in the daily huddle. Immediate action is taken to solve the operational problems identified.

An example of the human resources imperative at Iora is the importance placed on health coaches. While physicians are good at diagnosing and treating disease, health coaches are good at changing health behavior. Coaches live in the same community and speak the same language as their customers, and coaches interact with each customer at least twice a month. Dr. Fernandopulle modeled Iora health coaches after the *promotoras*, or community health workers, in the Caribbean and Latin America. Coaches are hired based on their customer service backgrounds and not necessarily on their medical experience. They are charged with finding innovative solutions to help customers adhere to healthy diets, coordinating free senior transportation to office visits or exercise classes, and creating incentives to ensure that customers don't miss dialysis appointments. For example, an Iora customer was not compliant with her diabetes oral medication. During a conversation with the customer, a coach learned that the tablets prescribed were difficult to swallow. The coach contacted the local pharmacy, and the pharmacist was able to substitute small tablets.

### 2. *Marketing Problem*—Cannot Recruit Millennial Generation Surgeons to a Traditional Small-Town Practice

Randy Ely, MD, started Ely Surgical Associates in 1988 in Burlington, North Carolina. In 2010, two of his original surgeons announced that they would retire in 2011. Burlington, a small city of 51,100, was also home to a 238-bed county hospital with a range of surgical cases. Dr. Ely decided to target millennial surgeons who were finishing their general surgery residencies to fill these two vacancies. The surgical volume was increasing, and the compensation was appropriate. Unfortunately, although he had interviewed several well-qualified candidates, none of the interviewees was interested in joining his practice. Dr. Ely decided to research the new physician market to solve this problem.

### *Marketing Solution*—Understand and Meet the Needs of Millennial Generation Surgeons.

The evaluation of an organization's strengths (S) and weaknesses (W) and the market's opportunities (O) and threats (T) is called a SWOT analysis. It's a tool for monitoring both the external and the internal environments. An organization must monitor key macroenvironment forces and significant microenvironment factors that affect its ability to earn revenue. Marketers need to track trends and identify related opportunities and threats. A marketing opportunity is an area of buyer need and interest that a company has a high probability of profitably satisfying. There are three main sources of market opportunities. The first is to offer something that is in short supply. The second is to supply an existing product or service in a new or superior way. The last source is a totally new product or service. A market threat is a challenge posed by an unfavorable trend or development that, in the absence of defensive marketing action, would lead to lower sales or increased expenses.

It's one thing to find attractive opportunities, and another to be able to take advantage of them. Each organization needs to evaluate its internal strengths and weaknesses. Clearly, the organization doesn't have to correct all its weaknesses, neither should it gloat about all its strengths. The big question is whether it should limit itself to those opportunities for which it possesses the required strengths, or consider those that might require it to find or develop new strengths.

Dr. Ely began to realize that the traditional approach to surgical practice needed to change in response to new environmental trends. Market demand for general surgeons was rising due to the demographic increase in the number of aging baby boomer consumers with chronic conditions. Unfortunately, the supply of medical students choosing general surgery was declining. The projected shortage of general surgeons was estimated to be between 23,100 and 31,600 surgeons by 2025.[39] One of the reasons underlying this trend was the 12% drop in general surgeon compensation from 2010 to 2012, the largest percentage decrease for all medical specialties.[40]

New social and cultural trends were also hindering Dr. Ely's practice because he was recruiting new surgeons who belonged to the millennial generation. In national surveys, millennials report that they have strong work ethics, but unlike boomers and generation Xers, millennials also have a strong preference for work-life balance. Surveys showed that what millennials most want is flexibility in where, when, and how they work. Millennials were likely to take a pay cut, forgo a promotion, or be willing to move in order to better manage work-life demands.[41] This generational change created a recruitment problem for physician practices. General surgeons practicing at community hospitals were traditionally obligated to accept emergency department call for unassigned surgical patients. Being summoned to the hospital at 2:00 am for a potentially uninsured patient contradicted millennial needs for work-life balance. Every surgical candidate Dr. Ely interviewed immediately lost interest in the job when they learned of the call responsibility.

The primary care physicians in internal medicine, family medicine, and pediatrics had faced a similar recruitment problem. Primary care physicians no longer had the time to treat patients in their clinics and also follow patients admitted to hospitals. This problem was solved by separating primary care into two subspecialties. A new physician position was created to solely treat inpatients, and they were called "hospitalists." Traditional office-based physicians limited their practice to patients who visited their clinics.

Dr. Ely decided to adapt the hospitalist model to general surgery. Two surgical hospitalists, or "surgicalists," could be scheduled for 12-hour shifts to provide 24/7 coverage for surgical patients presenting in the hospital ED. This scheduling innovation offered continuity of care for surgical patients, and it gave other hospital-based physicians a full-time surgeon readily available for consultations at any hour. Surgicalists benefited from predictable schedules that included one week of planned time off with no clinical duties every four or five weeks.

This innovative surgicalist strategy led to the recruitment of five new surgeons in Burlington in 2010. By increasing the number of surgeons in the overall community from three to eight, the hospital experienced a 20% increase in surgical volume. The surgicalist program was also instrumental in the recruitment of a thoracic surgeon and a bariatric surgeon. Burlington had never before been able to attract these surgical subspecialists, and without the responsibility for on-call emergency department coverage, the thoracic and bariatric surgeons could concentrate on building their subspecialty practices.

### 3. Marketing Problem—Value-Based Care Was Changing Vascular Medicine and Reimbursement

Farhan J. Khawaja, MD, an interventional cardiologist at Oklahoma Heart Institute (OHI), began to experience the change from volume to value reimbursement in the Tulsa market in 2013. Not only were reimbursement incentives shifting from increasing procedure volume to improved clinical outcomes, but vascular care medicine delivery was moving from inpatient to outpatient. Surgery was no longer the dominant approach for patients requiring vascular reconstruction for either obstructive occlusive or aneurysmal disease. Non-surgical, catheter-based therapeutic techniques were expected to increase by 7% to 10% annually for the next 5 to 10 years.[42]

### Marketing Solution—Identify a Market Opportunity, Design a Product, Test Market It, and Develop Marketing Strategies.

Analysis of changing environmental forces can lead to a market opportunity. A new product can then be developed to meet the needs of the target market. Different product benefits and attributes can be researched and validated using test marketing. Test marketing a new product can also measure the size of the market and assess the effectiveness of different marketing strategies. For example, organizations can see how consumers and channel partners react to pricing, channels, and promotion strategies and tactics. Important test market results include projections for product trial, first repeat purchase, adoption, and purchase frequency. Test market planning needs to consider who to target, the length of test market, what information should be collected, and what specific actions should be taken following the test.

Peripheral artery disease (PAD) affects 9 million patients annually, but it is often under-diagnosed and under-treated. PAD reduces blood flow in the legs, and it is usually caused by atherosclerosis. These are the same fatty plaques that clog coronary arteries and lead to heart disease. PAD symptoms include cramping, weakness, or numbness in hip, thigh, or calf muscles after walking or climbing stairs. Two million PAD patients are diagnosed with an advanced condition known as critical limb ischemia. Thirty percent of these patients have leg amputations and 25% die.[43] Diagnosing and treating PAD has been a problem because only about 25% of patients with PAD are aware that they have it. Most primary care physicians do not test for PAD, even if the patient has heart disease. Leg cramps and pain are often misdiagnosed as arthritis or muscle aches.[44]

Screening for PAD involves a simple test called the ankle-brachial-index (ABI) that measures blood pressure in the legs. This test costs between $60 and $117, and it is covered by Medicare.[45] The primary reason the ABI test has been not used more frequently is because the U.S. Preventive Services Task Force has not recommended the test due to insufficient clinical evidence.[46] Dr. Khawaja sensed, however, that diagnosing and treating PAD was a vascular medicine market opportunity due to the new emphasis on value, patient outcomes, and disease prevention. Dr. Khawaja started by analyzing OHI patient records. He found that only 7%, or 18 of the 250 vascular patients seen daily, had been assessed for PAD. He decided to conduct a PAD test market with current OHI patients. If the test market was successful, the PAD service line could then be expanded to the greater Tulsa area.

Dr. Khawaja assembled a multidisciplinary team including a vascular mid-level provider, an endovascular physician, a vascular surgeon, and a cardiovascular surgeon. He had OHI vascular inpatients complete a questionnaire, and he then segmented the patients based on the results. Patients who reported PAD symptoms were targeted for screening. These patients were screened the same day or next day using the ABI test. A positive ABI result led to an ultrasound evaluation by a vascular physician within 48 hours, and a positive result led to a vascular procedure. Follow-up appointments and surveillance testing were then scheduled. To support prevention, routine screening continued at intervals of six months and one year for ABI and ultrasound if the ABI was positive. Each patient's primary care physician was informed of the patient's progress throughout the course of diagnosis and treatment.

The PAD service line was expanded to non-OHI patients in 2014 based on the results of the test market. Dr. Khawaja implemented a marketing channels strategy to build relationships with referral sources and to coordinate patient care. He researched the vascular volume seen by Tulsa primary care physicians, orthopedists, pain management physicians, endocrinologists, and podiatrists. Dr. Khawaja scheduled personal meetings with these referral sources. He brought lunch to the practices, explained the benefits of the OHI PAD service line, and asked for referrals.

Dr. Khawaja supported his sales calls by distributing a simple, one-page PAD service summary with diagnosis codes, testing options, and a specially-designated referral telephone number. He arranged to lease ICAVL-certified mobile vascular laboratory ultrasound services to primary care physicians not affiliated with OHI and to key specialties with OHI over-read services. This provided PCPs with appropriate and reimbursable indications for ordering non-invasive vascular testing.

Dr. Khawaja targeted consumers with a promotion strategy to build awareness of PAD and preference for OHI. "Meet the Doc" community presentations were scheduled to generate patient self-referrals. The first PAD presentation drew 320 consumers, and 27 self-referred appointments resulted.

These marketing strategies resulted in OHI completing approximately 1,500 ABI and PAD ultrasound procedures in 2014. This was a 10-fold increase in the number of procedures completed in 2013. OHI-affiliated physicians referred 80% of these patients, and the remaining 20% were referred by physicians outside the organization.

In 2015, the OHI PAD service line was accredited by the Intersocietal Accreditation Commission. A regional media release announcing this accreditation was used to advance awareness of the PAD service line. As PAD assessments are increasing in the Tulsa market, clinical outcomes data will be collected, analyzed, and submitted to the U.S. Preventive Services Task Force to make the case for an ABI test recommendation.

### 4. Marketing Problem—Beverly Hills Cosmetic Dermatology Customer Experience Was a Product Weakness

Southern California is the hub of the U.S. entertainment industry and the home of Rodeo Drive luxury shopping. Personal appearance is important. To support the need for medical and surgical services, Beverly Hills has more than 50 cosmetic dermatology and plastic surgery practices within a 10-block area. Cosmetic dermatology customer experience was not meeting customer expectations because customers often felt that doctors were not spending enough time with them, and they felt rushed and hurried. As a result, customers complained openly and switched providers regularly.

### Marketing Solution—Develop a New Cosmetic Dermatology Practice that Puts Customer Needs First.

*Brand equity* is the marketing term used to define the value of a marketing advantage or disadvantage that a brand has compared to its competitors. Increasing brand equity is important because it leads to higher market share, revenue, profit, market capitalization, and consumer demand. Research used to develop the services branding model found that although an organization has more control over its *presented brand* (e.g., advertising, website) and *external brand communications* (e.g., publicity, word-of-mouth), these elements have only a secondary influence on brand equity.

*Brand meaning*, or reputation, has the primary influence on brand equity, and it is *customer experience* that primarily influences brand meaning. Customers and referral sources form an opinion about a medical practice with every interaction. Steps can be taken to improve customer experience by changing customer perceptions, administrative processes, employee attitudes, and the practice culture to meet or exceed customer expectations (Figure 5.4).[47]

Mark G. Rubin, MD, had spent five years providing cosmetic dermatology services while supporting an established Beverly Hills plastic surgery clinic. He was aware of the negative customer service perceptions, and Dr. Rubin decided to leverage this apparent market opportunity. He reasoned that an innovative cos-

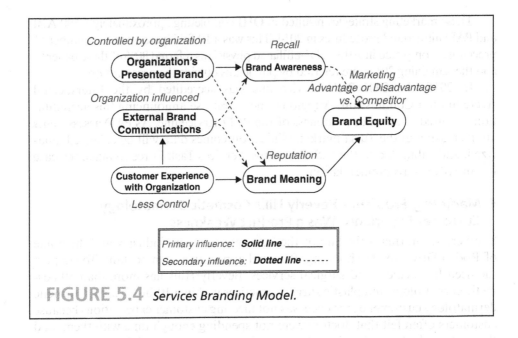

**FIGURE 5.4** *Services Branding Model.*

metic dermatology practice could successfully enter the ultra-competitive Beverly Hills market if it could radically change the customer experience.

Cosmetic dermatologists focus on a patient's appearance rather than treat skin diseases. They use precision laser, chemical peel, and micro-needling procedures to treat the skin, hair, or nails. Dr. Rubin founded the Lasky Skin Center based a brand strategy designed to exceed customer service expectations. An effective tactic supporting this strategy was longer customer appointments. The Lasky clinic began by scheduling new customers for 50% longer times, 45 minutes instead of the standard 30 minutes. Returning patients, usually seen for 15 minutes, were booked 100% longer with 30-minute appointments. These simple but meaningful innovations gave the Lasky staff more time to engage with patients, build relationships, and differentiate their practice.

This extended appointment system relies on a schedule that can be a challenge if customers are not punctual. If the practice day happens to veer off schedule, customers booked for succeeding appointments later in the day are phoned and asked if they could possibly arrive later to save them time waiting. Another incidental but valuable tactic is that the Lasky staff assists customers waiting longer than expected by personally walking to their parked cars to add coins to their parking meter. This is a small courtesy, but it helps customers avoid a $72 Beverly Hills parking ticket.

The Lasky staff is also trained to visualize and relate to each customer as if they were a member of their family. Using empathic and active listening, the staff takes ample time for each procedure. If a customer is later unhappy with the result of a procedure, they are encouraged to return so the staff can attend to what bothers them at little or no additional cost. Also, if a patient requests a new procedure that they have read about, but that is not likely to help them, the Lasky staff will explain this procedure in detail and will recommend medical options that are deemed more appropriate. This type of guidance further differentiates Lasky from other practices that may simply provide a requested procedure to appease a customer.

The Lasky clinic supports its superior customer service brand strategy with a premium pricing strategy. Lasky fees are higher than competitor fees, and these fees are clearly communicated to customers before service is rendered. To monitor pricing, Lasky regularly contracts with mystery shoppers to research competing cosmetic dermatology competitors. Pharmaceutical and medical device sales reps who call on Lasky and on competitors are also sources of customer experience and pricing information. When asked how they chose the practice, 95% of new Lasky customers indicate that the decision was based on positive word-of-mouth received from a current Lasky customer. The remaining 5% arrive at the practice through physician referrals. Only one or two patients a year chooses Lasky based on the practice website.

The Lasky Skin Center has grown from zero patients to a thriving practice with a 60-day new patient waiting list. The practice demonstrates that an effective brand strategy begins with a meaningful benefit, a valuable point of differentiation, and highly consistent tactical execution. Lasky plans to continue monitoring customer preferences and to innovate and do the "little things" that maintain a high level of marketing performance.

### 5. Marketing Problem—Organizations that Diversify by Offering New Products in New Markets Risk Failure

Organizations must offer new and innovative products to respond to changing market needs. Unfortunately, new products fail at an alarming rate, with new consumer products failing at a rate of 95%.[48] The most common reasons for product failure are (1) ignoring negative marketing research findings, (2) overestimating market size, (3) poor product design, (4) pricing is too high, and (5) unexpected competitor response. Diversifying into a new market with a new product entails a high level of risk.

Ansoff defined four strategies of product-market growth: market penetration, market development, product development, and diversification (Table 5.4).[49] A market penetration strategy attempts to increase market share with current products in existing market segments. This involves selling more products to established customers or by finding new customers within existing markets, often spending more on distribution and promotion, lowering price, or acquiring a competitor. With a market development strategy, an organization can expand into

TABLE 5.4  **Product-Market Strategy Matrix**

|  | **Current Products** | **New Products** |
|---|---|---|
| **Current Markets** | Market Penetration | Product Development |
| **New Markets** | Market Development | Diversification |

new markets with its current product line. It can target other market segments, other market channels, or new geographic regions or countries. This strategy is often successful when the organization has a unique product technology, lower prices result from higher economies of scale, and the new markets are similar to the current market segments.

A third product-market growth strategy is product development where an organization develops new products targeted to its existing markets. This can be accomplished by additional product research and development, or a joint venture or licensing agreement to distribute another organization's products. Finally, a diversification strategy is used to increase market share by introducing new products in new markets. This strategy has the highest risk because both product and market development are required. Diversification is often part of vertical integration strategy where an organization expands its business into other components of its supply chain. Another option is conglomerate growth where a corporation becomes a collection of businesses without any relationship to one another.

Crystal Run Healthcare is a 350-provider multispecialty practice in Middletown, New York, that was founded in 1996. The practice has evolved over the years and adapted to environmental changes including an ACO, a patient-centered medical home, and has entered into a number of risk-based contracts. In 2015, it decided to diversify and introduce a new health plan product in the health insurance market.

### Marketing Solution—A Strategic Marketing New Product Development Process Will Reduce the Risk of Failure.

Crystal Run Healthcare did not likely use this strategic marketing approach to develop their new health plan, but an eight-step new product development process could have been used to lower risk (Figure 5.5).[50]

1. *Idea generation* begins with identifying unmet market needs. Conducting 10 to 20 in-depth interviews with each target market segment can detect unmet needs or validate hypotheses. Crystal Run Healthcare could have interviewed self-insured employers in their geographic target to measure attitudes toward specific health plan benefits, features, distribution, and pricing. They could also

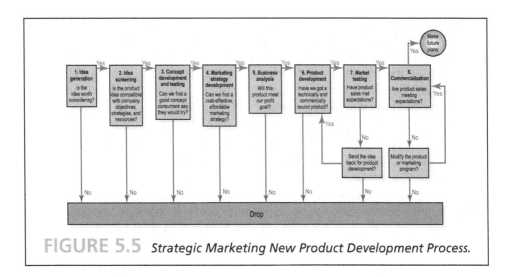

FIGURE 5.5 *Strategic Marketing New Product Development Process.*

have interviewed consumers to learn which product components are most important to them and how satisfied they are with each benefit and attribute.

2. *Idea screening* is used to rate and then rank an array of new product ideas. Examples of ratings are importance to target customers, competitive advantages, availability of investment capital, ROI, and in-house management expertise and experience. Crystal Run could have evaluated its health plan idea against starting a reference lab, adding a new medical specialty, opening a new office location, or another idea.

3. *Concept development* moves a product idea into a particular product concept. Each potential concept has a different set of targets and competitors. Important questions in this stage include who is the target customer, who will influence the purchase, how long is the sales cycle, and others. For example, Crystal Run physicians have reimbursement contracts with commercial insurers. How will reimbursement rates be affected if Crystal Run launches a product that competes with these health plans? *Concept testing* involves presenting the product concept to appropriate target customers and evaluating their reactions. Test results will indicate if there is sufficient market demand, confirm the best targets, and identify product substitutes and competitors. Crystal Run could ask self-insured employers to rate their new health plan product on solving a particular problem, filling an unmet need, product benefits importance and satisfaction, and likelihood of purchase.

4. *Marketing strategy development* follows a successful concept test and includes three sections. The first section begins with a description of target market size, structure, and behavior. This information is then used to develop a positioning strategy. The Crystal Run positioning statement could be "For

self-insured employers in the Hudson Valley, Crystal Run Health Plan can deliver higher value care because doctors understand medical outcomes and manage costs better than large commercial health plans." The second section includes first-year goals and objectives for sales, market share, and financial margin. The third section outlines the pricing, distribution, and promotion strategies along with the first-year marketing budget.

5. *Business analysis* comprehensively examines revenue, profit, and product cost forecasts for the portfolio of new products. The competitive landscape and the revenue and profit forecasts for the Crystal Run health plan would be compared to other new product candidates. This analysis would have quantified capital requirements, actuarial and sales expertise, investment in a health insurance information system, and other costs. Breakeven analysis and net present value analysis are then used to compare expected ROIs among the new products.

6. *Product development* transforms the product concept into a prototype if it passes the business analysis test. In the case of the Crystal Run health plan, a cross-disciplinary team of clinicians and managers could have translated customer requirements generated by market research into product attributes. The team then designs the work flows, customer paths, information requirements, pricing, channel and value-delivery networks, marketing communications, and all other strategies. Marketers are needed to continuously communicate customer preferences during this process.

7. *Market testing* of health care consumer goods, medical equipment, or medical services takes different forms. Glucometers for diabetics can be tested using in-home placement. New CT scanners are installed in selected practices for customer beta testing. Product manufacturers observe how test customers use the product, identify unanticipated problems, and develop customer training and maintenance services. The Crystal Run health plan could have been tested by working closely with one or two employers on a single chronic disease like diabetes. The health plan product could be expanded to other employers and possibly other conditions if the test market meets employer needs and achieves the projected financial objectives.

8. *Commercialization* involves rolling the product out to the target market. This will require the largest costs to date. The cost of introducing the Crystal Run health plan to the target market could easily exceed $100 million in the first year.

## 6. *Marketing Problem*—Value-Based Market Changes are Disrupting Practice Operations and Finances

Under traditional fee-for-service reimbursement, the primary physician practice's financial strategy focused on increasing physician office visits and procedures.

Value-based reimbursement, however, changed this volume growth strategy to one that rewarded improving clinical quality, patient outcomes, and population health. Some practices reacted by lowering their practice expenses in response to the reduction in value-based revenue. Reducing costs ultimately also reduced care quality and led to even lower value-based reimbursement.

Atrius Health is a large physician practice in the Greater Boston market with more than 740,000 adult and pediatric patients. It has 36 clinical locations, 50 medical specialties, and employs 900 physicians. Atrius had spent years standardizing processes, removing waste, and improving operational efficiency as a participant in the CMS Pioneer Accountable Care Organization program. With the continued growth of value-based care, Atrius began to question whether a comprehensive and innovative strategy may be needed.

### *Marketing Solution*—Develop an Innovative Product Strategy Based on Partnering with Other Providers and Customers.

Relationship marketing builds mutually-beneficial long-term relationships with key constituents. Relationship marketing can be used by physicians to build collaborative relationships with their customers and partnering with providers to reach the objectives of value-based care. The ultimate outcome of relationship marketing is the building of a unique organizational asset called a marketing network. A marketing network consists of the organization and its supporting stakeholders (e.g., customers, employees, suppliers, distributors, community members, and others) with whom it has built jointly profitable business relationships. By focusing on their most profitable customers, products, and channels, organizations capture a larger share of customer expenditures, increase customer loyalty and lifetime value, and improve financial performance.

An innovation refers to any good, service, or idea that is perceived by someone as both valuable and new, and innovations take time to spread through the social system. Innovation in marketing is critical. Traditionally, senior management hammers out the strategy and hands it down through the organization. Imaginative strategic ideas, however, exist in many places within and outside an organization. Management should encourage fresh ideas from three internal groups often underrepresented in strategy making: employees with youthful perspectives, employees far removed from organization headquarters, and employees new to the industry. Innovation is crucial for designing and implementing new, radical, care models.

Atrius Health created an innovative product strategy called "Care in Place" that targeted customers age 65 and older. Marketing research found that these customers highly preferred to remain in their home for health care, and this need is a core element of Care in Place. For example, when seniors call Atrius with a health problem, but do not have transportation to the practice, a visiting Atrius nurse arrives at the customer's home within two hours. The nurse has real-time phone access to a geriatric-trained nurse practitioner who can order in-home imaging, lab tests, prescriptions, and make treatment decisions. Atrius estimated that 44% of these customers would have been sent to a hospital ED by ambulance without Care in Place. In the first three months of the program, a total of $509,000 was saved in ambulance fees, ED visit fees, and other hospitalization costs.[51] This generated a positive return on the $97,000 investment Atrius made in developing "Care in Place." Atrius used eight steps to develop the Care in Place product strategy:[52]

***Step 1****: Establish an Innovation Center*

Atrius first created an Innovation Center, a new line management department with its own profit and loss to manage innovation initiatives. The underlying premise of the Innovation Center was understanding customer needs and wants. An analysis of customer needs prompts the development of personalized programs and innovative ways of working that in turn improves the experience of care and supports wellness.

***Step 2****: Create a dedicated multidisciplinary team*

A team of clinicians, engineers, designers, and operations specialists were selected based on divergence of thinking, a desire to disrupt the status quo, comfort with ambiguity, and functional competencies. This team was led by a physician who had a disruptive vision of care. An outside consultant with expertise in automotive product design trained and coached the team. Atrius committed to assigning full-time clinicians to the team because clinical credibility is critical to convincing other Atrius clinicians of the value of change.

***Step 3****: Probe customer needs*

To identify unmet and latent customer needs, ethnographic marketing research was conducted with seniors in their homes to holistically understand their situation. This research identified the strong desire of customers to stay in their homes for health care, and this insight became central to the Care in Place program. The care delivery status quo forced customers to leave home for office visits, trips to the ED, and to procedures from blood draws to X-rays to scoping procedures.

***Step 4****: Develop a complete understanding of the system*

The Care in Place team regularly met with over 60 different workgroups, managers, contractors, and departments within and outside Atrius to collect and analyze data. The primary purpose was to understand how care is delivered in every dimension to the senior target market. For example, a customer journey mapping project using 400 ED medical records found that nearly 50% of seniors did not need emergency care.

Nurses at different Atrius clinics routinely made referrals to the ED because customers could not travel to their physician's clinic or because appointment slots were full. Consumers age 80 and over had a 70% chance of being admitted to the hospital. Conversations with emergency physicians (EPs) revealed that many of these admissions were not medically necessary. Since the EPs had little understanding of the social environment at the customer's home, the EPs felt that hospital admission was less risky than discharging the seniors. The Care in Place team used this data to negotiate revised reimbursement rates with a health plan that covered 45% of Atrius seniors.

***Step 5****: Allow differing ideas to be considered*

It took four months to collect, analyze, and discuss all of the marketing and product research. The team continually brainstormed possible solutions based on customer problems, needs, and organizational constraints. They resisted the temptation of automatically selecting the easier solution. This thoughtful and systematic approach helped the team gain a deep understanding of why customers were using the hospital as well as potential alternatives.

***Step 6****: Allocate resources for rapid prototyping and market testing*

Innovation and operations teams work together to design prototypes and conduct test markets. The Care in Place team needed to prototype home visits with nurse practitioners. The first task was to convince a physician clinic to work with the team, and Atrius executives reinforced the importance of this test with the physician clinic. The Care in Place team worked with the clinic to create space in the clinic, order medical supplies, and access the nurse triage phone room. Additionally, the team contracted with two nurse practitioners in a per diem pool to do the prototype visits. The initial customer visits generated important learning, tested assumptions, and provided the feedback necessary to expand the model.

***Step 7****: Expand the model and process*

These projects tended to be research-based and required time to evolve. Project teams shared findings with executive management to help manage organizational expectations. As a result, the process added value to Atrius even before the new innovative care model had been completed. The Care in Place team led a series of town hall style meetings across the practice to identify potential future projects. Additionally, the team collected a range of customer perspectives from various sources and different types of customers. This feedback was organized into themes, such as "I feel rushed in my visit" and "Limited clinic hours don't work for me." These themes were then evaluated and ranked as customer priorities.

***Step 8****: Align innovation with enterprise strategy*

Care model innovation is very resource intensive, and it must be clear to employees throughout the organization that innovative thinking and programs are an integral part of enterprise strategy. Disruptive strategies need continuous executive buy-in for cultural acceptance and implementation. A critical lesson was that the innovation team director needed to be part of the practice senior leadership team.

## CHAPTER SUMMARY

Physicians are often skeptical of marketing before they understand that marketing can deliver value to customers by aligning market needs with medical services. Understanding physician attitudes, perceptions, and behavior is important for marketing physician services. Physician attitudes and behavior are largely influenced by medical school culture as well as social and personal factors. Medical training has traditionally emphasized the values of rugged individualism, autonomy, authority, rigidity, and safety-seeking. The value-based care market trend is responsible for supplanting these cultural attributes with teamwork, collaboration, and communication skills.

Three important environmental forces affecting physicians are demographic, economic, and social/cultural. Demographically, physician practice patterns are limiting patient access to care. Economically, changing practice organizational structures and payment models are pressuring physician income. Finally, the cumulative impact of these and other environmental forces are resulting in negative social/cultural effects like low physician morale and burnout.

Physicians have applied a variety of marketing tools to solve health care management problems, but most physicians did not realize that they were using strategic marketing. Examples are establishing a customer-driven organizational culture, analyzing environmental forces and participants, and test marketing. Additional physician marketing applications are improving the customer experience to increase brand equity, a systematic new product development process to reduce new product risk, and using a consensus approach based on market information to develop an innovative product strategy.

## DISCUSSION QUESTIONS

1.  A group of independent physicians and an academic medical center (AMC) are competing in the same market to offer endoscopy services. The physician group charges patients and third-party payers lower fees than the AMC. A regional health plan has contracted with the AMC but refuses to contract with the physicians. The physicians suspect that the AMC has used its bargaining power to influence the health plan. Is this unfair competition? What marketing strategies could the physicians use to secure a contract with the health plan?

2.  The Mayo Clinic brand is supported by employees who put patients first. There is a strong alignment between organizational values and employee attitudes that elevates the quality of care and lowers employee turnover. You have a new position as the vice president of human resources for a large multispecialty physician group in the Southeast. The group would like to change its culture to be like the Mayo Clinic. Outline the product marketing strategies and tactics your new practice will need to emulate the Mayo Clinic.

3.   A physician in private practice asks you, as a marketing consultant, how to attract more patients. The practice is serving about 10 patients a day and cannot run profitably unless the physician sees about 20 patients a day. What questions would you ask before starting to make suggestions?

## PHYSICIAN MARKETING CASE: CHANGING THE CHANNEL— A COUNTRY DOCTOR OPENS A TRUCK-STOP CLINIC

Every day, about 20,000 trucks pass through rural Raphine, Virginia, on I-81 in the Shenandoah Valley. As many as 1,000 drivers a night sleep at the local truck-stops, overshadowing the town of 1,976. The massive White's Travel Center truck-stop offers diesel, hot coffee and food, shopping, oil changes, and showers. Bobby Berkstresser owns the truck-stop, and as part of his plan to make it a destination, he asked local physician Rob Marsh, MD, to open a primary care clinic onsite in July 2012. The trucker lifestyle takes a toll on health due to long periods of being sedentary, poor eating habits, reduced quantity and quality of sleep, and the stresses of delivery times and traffic. Truck drivers get sick on the road, but many are never at home enough to have a primary care physician. Most just tough it out.

Now drivers can get a U.S. Department of Transportation-mandated physical, a flu shot, treatment for a sore back, and other medical services at White's Travel Center. Truck drivers are also required to take random drug tests. For one of his recent tests, driver Terry Jenkins had to park his truck in the lot of a big box store, take a taxi to hospital 20 miles away, wait a couple of hours there for test results, and then take another taxi back to his truck. Now Jenkins uses the truck-stop clinic for drug testing.

Marsh was raised in Middlebrook, Virginia (population 213), about 15 miles from Raphine and 50 miles west of Charlottesville. He was a highly-decorated U.S. Army Delta Force flight surgeon who barely survived the disastrous firefight in Somalia made famous by the book and movie *Black Hawk Down*. He returned to Middlebrook after his service and opened a family medicine practice to care for his friends, the many farmers in the community, and the people sitting in church alongside his family. Marsh's highest priority is developing relationships with his patients. Effective relationships rely on clear communication. He uses the form of communication individual patients prefer: personal face-to-face, telephone, text, or email.

Over the years, Marsh's community and his practice have changed. This area of the Shenandoah Valley was once dairy farm country, but dairy consolidation and mergers have reduced the options farmers have to sell their milk. As a result, the dairy farmer population is in decline. U.S. physician practice has changed as well. At the start of the 2010s, more than 60% of physicians were in solo practice. Now only 17% work alone, with 58% employed by hospitals and large medical groups. When Berkstesser suggested Marsh open the truck-stop clinic, Marsh saw it as an opportunity to expand his practice and adapt to a market need.

The truck-stop practice includes a physician assistant, medical students, and a nursing staff that includes his wife, Barbara. Marsh's nurses periodically set up in a room in the truck-stop restaurant, offering to check drivers' blood pressure while they wait for lunch. At other times, a nurse will go from cab to cab, dispensing flu shots. Marsh plans to add staff and expand clinic space so he can treat more patients. He already spends most nights making house calls and doing hospital rounds for his office practice patients. He often finds himself treating truck-stop patients at 8:00 pm, long after that clinic is supposed to close at 5:00 pm, so Marsh is thinking about keeping it open even later on some nights.

The locals can be seen at the truck-stop clinic by appointment only, but Marsh allows truck drivers to walk in. "I don't make no decision unless I can discuss it with him," said Chester Perry, a retired truck driver living in Raphine. Perry is recovering from a heart transplant. He and Marsh meet regularly in the small exam room at the truck-stop and discuss how best to manage Perry's dialysis while strengthening his heart. Marsh also visits Perry at the nursing home where he lives. It's a challenge nurturing ongoing relationships with most drivers because they come and go, but they do get doses of Marsh's warm, easy going manner, and personal approach. Using an electronic medical record system, Marsh can forward information from his exams to other health providers so drivers can get medication or follow-up care farther along their routes.

Many drivers pay Marsh in cash, providing a steady stream of income without the usual insurance reimbursement complications. Marsh hopes that long-term the truck-stop clinic will provide a financial cushion that will help him keep treating patients the way he prefers. "I'm a survivor—I'll make this work," said Marsh, age 60. "I'm willing to make those adaptations because I love what I do so much."[53]

*Watch the video*: www.usatoday.com/videos/news/nation/2014/12/24/20771265/

## CASE QUESTIONS

1. The retail clinics in Target stores employed clinical nurse practitioners, answered customer phone calls, and a front desk employee greeted customers and helped with their medical information. CVS acquired these Target retail clinics in 2015. CVS eliminated the front desk employee, removed the phone line to the clinic, installed a self-serve kiosk, and the nurse practitioner stays behind the closed exam room door.

    How does this CVS clinic experience differ from White's Travel Center truck-stop clinic customer experience? Which clinic do you expect to deliver better health care? How do think the CVS clinic will affect the Target NPS and customer loyalty?

2. How do the following three environmental trends affect the office-based practice and the truck-stop practice being run by Rob Marsh?

   a) Reduced access to patient care
   b) Changing delivery and payment models
   c) Increased physician burnout.

3. Marsh has found a marketing opportunity by "changing the channel." As a health care marketing consultant, you have been hired to advise Marsh on further expanding family medical practices to other truck-stops. Use the marketing strategies of targeting, positioning, product, price, channels, and promotion to explain your answer.

   a) Target—Define and size the market. How many truck-stops are within 25 miles of Raphine? If Marsh decides to expand his truck-stop clinics, what should he do about his office-based clinic?
   b) Positioning—Develop a positioning for Marsh's truck-stop clinics.
   c) Product—How does customer experience affect the brand equity of the Marsh truck-stop clinic? Since Marsh IS the brand, how can he replicate the customer experience? Should Marsh use the NPS to increase brand equity? Why?
   d) Pricing—Identify and describe a pricing strategy for truck-stop clinics.
   e) Channels—This could be the most innovative strategy for Marsh. How can he defend against competitors?
   f) Promotion—The takeover of Target retail clinics by CVS Minute Clinic had important communication flaws. How can Marsh expand and effectively manage communication with the target market?

# CHAPTER

6

# HOSPITAL MARKETING

## LEARNING OBJECTIVES

This chapter will answer the following questions:

1. How did marketing management become an important hospital management function?

2. What are the most important hospital trends taking place in the hospital market?

3. How have hospitals reacted to these market trends?

4. What are three environmental forces and associated trends affecting hospitals?

5. How are hospitals using strategic health care marketing to solve problems?

The first U.S. hospitals in the eighteenth century were essentially almshouses supported by religious organizations or government. Physicians donated their time and hospital costs for nurses and staff tended to be low. Today, hospitals represent one-third of U.S. health care expenditures, and most hospitals are continuing to struggle financially. The focus of this chapter is on understanding how strategic health care marketing can assist hospitals in increasing value and brand equity through better alignment with market needs. As background, the size and characteristics of the hospital market are analyzed. Next, three important market forces affecting hospitals are explained. The remainder of the chapter explores a range of hospital management problems and how strategic marketing has led to solutions. The chapter begins with a review of the role of marketing in hospitals.

## EVOLUTION OF HOSPITAL MARKETING

Hospital marketing was traditionally viewed exclusively as a communications function. This coincides with marketing's nearly universal, strong, top-of-mind associations with promotional tactics like advertising, public relations, and selling. Strategic marketing, however, is considerably more comprehensive. It is based on the analysis of environmental changes, identification of market opportunities and threats, the development of marketing goals, and the creation and implementation of effective marketing mix strategies to reach the goals. The evolution of hospital marketing was primarily the result of economic environmental forces.

### *Public Relations Tactics*

Hospital marketing began with public relations tactics. Marketing in most hospitals had its beginnings in the development and distribution of publications. Examples of internal hospital publications targeted to employees and physicians are newsletters, service line or department brochures, and internal social media content. External publications targeted to consumers, payers, the media, and other external audiences include press releases, publicity features, annual reports, and external social media content. In academic medical centers, publications also communicate new clinical research findings to physicians, researchers, and consumer audiences.

Many hospital publications departments expanded and became public relations departments. A public is any group that has an actual or potential interest in or impact on an organization's ability to achieve its objectives. Public relations includes a variety of programs to promote or protect an organization's image or individual products. The hospital public relations manager, often someone with previous experience with a media company, was familiar with media operations and interests, and had established media contacts they could leverage. Additional examples of hospital public relations activities include lobbying government representatives, speech writing, event planning, sponsorships, public service activities, corporate identity development, and even fund raising.

Crisis communications capabilities are a critical, but not often used public relations activity. Managing local media communications reactions to medical mistakes or administrative problems can be handled by an in-house public relations team. Hospital crises that attract national or international attention usually need external public relations counsel and resources. In 2014, Texas Health Presbyterian Medical Center in Dallas experienced a crisis when an Ebola patient was discharged from the hospital ED and died just after his readmission. Compounding this problem, two nurses treating the patient also contracted Ebola, and the National Nurses United union publicly criticized the hospital.

The Texas Health Presbyterian public relations department was overwhelmed by media inquiries, and the hospital hired New York-based public relations firm Burson-Marsteller to help respond to the media. Burson-Marsteller began by developing talking points and training the hospital's media spokespeople. Burson-Marsteller helped Texas Health Presbyterian produce a pro-Texas Health Presbyterian video of smiling nurses praising their managers. They also organized a "rally" of staff carrying pro-hospital placards outside the ED to positively influence television news crews. To counter fears that patients might stay away, the hospital used social media with the hashtag "#PresbyProud" to issue rebuttals to allegations about its safety practices. A YouTube video was created to reassure the public and proactively thank them for forgiving the errors. Burson-Marsteller also arranged a CBS News *60 Minutes* feature segment designed to create positive public opinion associated with the problem.

### DRGs Set the Stage for Strategic Hospital Marketing

The Medicare program began using Diagnosis-Related Groups (DRGs) in 1983.[1] A DRG is a statistical system of classifying any inpatient stay into groups with predetermined payments. The DRG classification system divides possible diagnoses into more than 20 major body systems and subdivides them into almost 500 groups for the purpose of Medicare reimbursement. The value of hospital strategic marketing increased because this prospective payment system replaced hospital billing based on full charges. The move to fixed payments included financial incentives for hospitals to understand and manage service line costs. DRGs also created competition among hospitals for customers and for market share.

Strategic marketing was adopted by more progressive hospitals to analyze environmental forces and market trends, understand local market needs, and manage customer perceptions to increase market share and revenue. The definition of a hospital "customer" included not only patients and consumers, but also market influencers such as physicians, hospital employees, payers, government, and others. Marketing planning focused on evidence-based strategies for building brand equity through effective targeting, positioning, product, pricing, channels, and promotion strategies. Other less market-driven hospitals simply changed the name of the public relations department to the marketing department.

## Fundamentals of Hospital Marketing Effectiveness

Many hospital marketing departments have struggled to identify their role in the organization and to realize a positive return on marketing spending. A group of academic medical centers from the top 20 U.S. News & World Reports, "Honor Roll of Best Hospitals," decided to address these issues by participating in a marketing research study of hospital marketing effectiveness.[2] The 11 academic medical centers (AMCs) in the study sample are in Table 6.1. Each hospital sponsoring the study contributed its top 10 marketing challenges as the basis of the research discussion guide.[3] Interviews with AMC marketing departments were conducted in-person and by telephone by Health Centric Marketing Services, a health care marketing research company.

A leading indicator of marketing effectiveness was organizational design. The study found that the strongest influence on marketing effectiveness was having the chief marketing officer report directly to the chief executive officer. An executive position allowed the chief marketing officer to influence high-level management decision-making, to share responsibility and accountability, and to represent the AMC's strong commitment to strategic marketing. The AMC study participants without this type of organizational structure gave their AMCs a "neutral" rating for being market-driven. They also rated marketing ROI and accountability as only "somewhat important."

Another aspect of organizational design was combining all marketing functions under one division. This structure was the basis for the most effective inte-

## TABLE 6.1   AMC Marketing Effectiveness Study Sample.

| | |
|---|---|
| Barnes-Jewish Hospital | Tufts—New England Medical Center |
| Brigham and Women's Hospital | University of California—San Francisco |
| Duke Health System | University of California—Los Angeles |
| Emory Healthcare | Vanderbilt University Medical Center |
| Johns Hopkins Medicine | Yale—New Haven Hospital |
| Northwestern Memorial Hospital | |

gration and management of these functions. Three AMCs (#7, # 9, and #10 in Table 6.2) had strategic and tactical responsibility for product, channels, and promotion of these functions. They also had a dotted line connection to the finance division for pricing. These AMCs added competitive information and product data to support payer contract negotiations that were led by the AMC chief financial officer. Five AMCs' marketing divisions also had responsibility for strategic planning. AMCs with divided strategic planning and marketing departments often had difficulty sharing market data and collaborating. AMCs #4, #7, #8, # 9, and #10 (Table 6.2) were able to avoid this conflict.

Integration of marketing functions with operations, human resources, and finance led to effective product and brand strategies. Every interaction between a hospital employee and a patient-customer or physician-customer affected the value of the customer experience. Having the marketing division actively collaborate with the hospital operations, human resources, and finance divisions was essential to ensuring that all hospital employees understood the customer perspective. Collaboration was highest among AMCs that used matrix management structures. Although marketing often led these cross-functional teams, merely having marketing participate with these teams was beneficial. A marketing manager was often assigned and located in the AMC human resources departments. The purpose was to help human resources recruit and hire AMC employees who were a good fit for the AMC customer experience culture.

There were weak linkages in many AMCs between brand awareness and customer preference, loyalty, satisfaction, and retention. A best practice was to integrate consumer prospect databases and customer databases to compare these variables for non-customers and customers. Several AMCs followed this practice for inpatients but not for outpatients. One AMC uses mystery shoppers to compare these measures between their AMC and its competitors.

A channels strategy best practice was to have a physician liaison sales department within the marketing division that builds relationships with referring PCP and specialist physicians. This capability included a call center that received and indexed calls from both referring physicians and from consumers. The call center had access to physician schedules, and it could directly page an AMC physician if a referring physician had a question. The physician liaison sales staff also made multiple touches with referring physicians throughout the patient referral process, and the sales staff visited the referring physician offices several weeks after each patient discharge to receive feedback. Another channel strategy was having a marketing division channels specialist build direct relationships with payers. This representative provided consumer market preference data and other data to brokers and MCO medical directors.

An integrated marketing communications best practice was consistently projecting and evaluating marketing spending ROI. The difficulty is often in identifying creative and media strategies that are measurable and cost-effective. An AMC

TABLE 6.2 AMC Marketing Functions.

| Function | AMC 1 | AMC 2 | AMC 3 | AMC 4 | AMC 5 | AMC 6 | AMC 7* | AMC 8 | AMC 9* | AMC 10* | AMC 11 |
|---|---|---|---|---|---|---|---|---|---|---|---|
| Strategic planning | | | | ● | | | ● | ● | ● | ● | |
| Market research | ● | ● | ● | ● | ● | | ● | ● | ● | | ● |
| Market analysis | | ● | ● | ● | ● | ● | ● | ● | | ● | ● |
| Production marketing | ● | | ● | | ● | ● | ● | | | | ● |
| Health policy planning | | | | ● | | | | | | | |
| International marketing | | | | ● | | | | | | | |
| Managed care contracting | ● | | | | ● | | ● | ● | ● | ● | |
| Consumer call center | ● | | ● | | ● | | | | | ● | |
| Physician call center | ● | | | | ● | | ● | | ● | ● | |
| Physician channel development | ● | ● | | | ● | | ● | ● | ● | ● | ● |

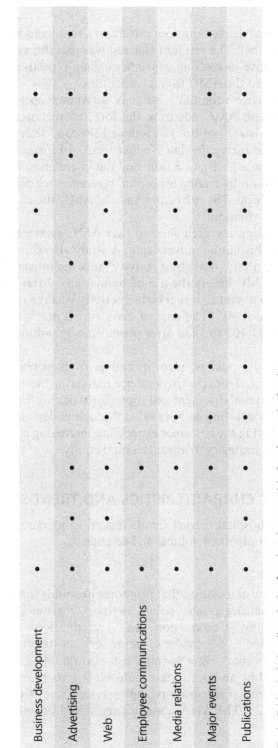

Business development

Advertising

Web

Employee communications

Media relations

Major events

Publications

*Single division includes all marketing functions (except pricing) and strategic planning.

tested bus wraps and bus shelters outdoor advertising that included a designated telephone response number. The result of this test was that the wraps and shelter signage were cost-effective in meeting consumer calling objectives. This promotional tactic differentiated the AMC from competitors.

A second cost-effective promotion strategy was newspaper and television banner advertising. These AMC ads took the form of rectangular newspaper print ads placed in consistent positions as well as 15-second television spots that aired at consistent times during the day. Neither media ad format used graphics. The ads asked consumers a health question, and they were given the opportunity to respond to the question by calling a hospital consumer telephone number or visiting the hospital website. The call center and the AMC site captured the consumer demographic information.

Advertising marketing research showed that AMC awareness and preference increased due to this banner advertising. A study also showed that 2% of the AMC patients said that "marketing activity" was the most influential reason for choosing the AMC before the use of banner ads. After using the banner ads for two years, 8% said that marketing activity was the most influential reason for selecting the AMC. The cost of acquiring a marketing-influenced patient dropped from $1,103 to $433 after promotion spending was shifted to banner ads.

The ACA changed hospital payment incentives from increasing volume to increasing value, so the need for effective strategic marketing has never been more important. Value-based reimbursement and strategic marketing both have increasing value at their core. Marketing delivers value through understanding customer needs and wants, improving the customer experience, increasing customer loyalty, and creating innovative strategies to advance brand equity.

## HOSPITAL MARKET CHARACTERISTICS AND TRENDS

This section examines hospital market trends related to market size, segmentation, and inpatient and outpatient volume and revenue.

### Hospital Market Size

The AHA, a professional association that promotes hospitals through providing information and influencing public policy, defines "registered" hospitals as accredited by the Joint Commission on Accreditation of Healthcare Organizations or certified as a provider of acute services under Title 18 of the Social Security Act. Alternatively, a hospital can also qualify as registered if it is licensed as a hospital by an appropriate state agency, its primary function is to provide diagnostic and therapeutic patient services, and it meets 10 AHA operational requirements. The AHA classifies registered hospitals as general, special, rehabilitation, chronic disease, or psychiatric.[4] The total number of registered hospitals was 6,146 in 2018.[5]

### Hospital Market Segmentation

Registered hospitals can be segmented by *type* of hospital. The AHA segments hospitals as community, nonfederal psychiatric, federal government, and other hospitals. Community hospitals are all nongovernmental, short-term general, and special hospitals. They include academic medical centers and teaching hospitals if they are nonfederal short-term hospitals. Special hospitals include those that specialize in obstetrics and gynecology, otolaryngology, rehabilitation, orthopedics, or another medical specialty. Other hospitals include nonfederal long-term care hospitals and hospital units within an institution such as a prison hospital or school infirmary. Long-term care hospitals have an average length of stay of 30 or more days.[6]

Community hospitals represented 85% of registered hospitals, nonfederal psychiatric hospitals were 10%, federal government hospitals were 3%, and other hospitals were 2% in 2018 (Table 6.3).[7]

Since 1975, the number of hospitals has steadily declined by more than 14% from more than 7,100 hospitals to just over 6,100. The most dramatic decline occurred between 1990 and 2000.[8] In 1984, there were 2,780 rural hospitals that represented 48% of total community hospitals.[9] Rural hospitals have struggled with increasing

TABLE 6.3 **2018 Hospital Type Segmentation.**

| Hospitals | 2018 | % |
|---|---|---|
| Registered hospitals | 6,146 | 100 |
| Community hospitals: | 5,198 | 85 |
| Nongovernmental not-for-profit | 2,937 | 48 |
| For profit | 1,296 | 21 |
| State and local government | 965 | 16 |
| Nonfederal psychiatric hospitals | 616 | 10 |
| Federal government hospitals | 209 | 3 |
| Other hospitals | 123 | 2 |

costs and decreasing market size. The number of rural hospitals decreased by 34% to 1,821 in 2018 and represented 35% of total hospitals. Urban hospitals increased by 11% to 3,377 and represented 65% of total hospitals.[10]

Hospitals can also be segmented by the *number of licensed hospital beds*. The AHA reported an estimated total of 1.4 million hospital beds in 1975 and 924,100 in 2018, a decrease of 34%. The most dramatic decline occurred between 1995 and 2000 with a steady total loss of slightly less than 100,000 beds.[11] Overall, the number of beds per 1,000 population was 4.6 in 1975, and it dropped by 53% to 2.4 by 2016.[12]

Comparing the percentage of community hospitals segmented by the number of beds between 1975 and 2015, 6 to 24 bed hospitals increased by 67%. This was likely related to the 38% decrease of hospitals with 50 to 99 beds (Figure 6.1). The 25 to 49 and 500 and over bed segments remained unchanged, and remaining segments decreased (Figure 6.1 and Table 6.4).[13]

Smaller and rural hospitals are being most affected by inpatient occupancy declines. The number of rural community hospitals declined nearly 8% between 2017 and 2013, to 1,875, while the number of urban hospitals increased nearly 2% during that time to 3,387.[14] Hospitals with 6 to 24 beds lost 38% and hospitals with 25 to 49 beds lost 25% occupancy. Large hospitals with over 500 beds lost only 10%. As hospital occupancy declined from 75% in 1975 to 63% in 2014, excess hospital capacity rose (Figure 6.2 and Table 6.5).[15]

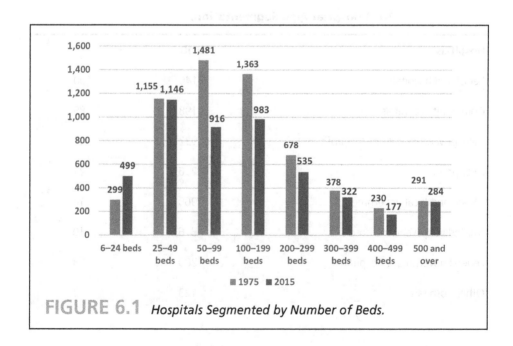

FIGURE 6.1 *Hospitals Segmented by Number of Beds.*

TABLE 6.4 **Community Hospital Bed Comparison.**

| Hospitals by Number of Beds | 2015 | 1975 | Index vs. 1975 |
|---|---|---|---|
| 6–24 beds | 499 | 299 | 167 |
| 25–49 beds | 1,146 | 1,155 | 99 |
| 50–99 beds | 916 | 1,481 | 62 |
| 100–199 beds | 983 | 1,363 | 72 |
| 200–299 beds | 535 | 678 | 79 |
| 300–399 beds | 322 | 378 | 85 |
| 400–499 beds | 177 | 230 | 77 |
| 500 beds or more | 284 | 291 | 98 |
| Total | 4,862 | 5,875 | 83 |

### *Hospital Volume and Revenue Trends*

Innovations in technology such as minimally-invasive surgery and advanced anesthesia techniques have led to increases in outpatient procedures and decreases in hospital admissions. Traditional inpatient procedures such as joint repair and cataract removal have moved to ambulatory surgery centers and outpatient departments. Patients recovered more quickly from these surgical procedures, and there was growing demand from payers for value-based payment and increased demand for convenience from consumers. The data illustrate the continued slow bleed of patients out of hospitals. Hospital admissions per 1,000 population decreased 12% from 119 in 1999 to 105 in 2018, and the number of inpatient days decreased 20% from 704 to 567.[16] Meanwhile the number of community hospital outpatient visits per 1,000 population increased 5% from 1,817 to 1,907.[17]

The change from inpatient to outpatient utilization has had a negative effect on hospital revenue. The AHA's 2019 Hospital Statistics report showed hospitals' 2017 outpatient revenue represented 49% or $472 billion, and inpatient revenue was 51% or nearly $498 billion.[18] Although outpatient visit volume was relatively flat year-over-year, net outpatient revenue increased 6% between 2016 and 2017. Expenses increased 5% to $966 billion from $920 billion.

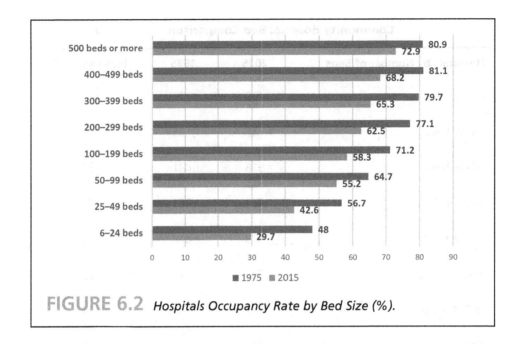

FIGURE 6.2 *Hospitals Occupancy Rate by Bed Size (%).*

TABLE 6.5 **Community Hospital Occupancy by Bed Size (%).**

| Hospitals by Number of Beds | 2015 | 1975 | Index vs. 1975 |
|---|---|---|---|
| 6–24 beds | 29.7 | 48.0 | 62 |
| 25–49 beds | 42.6 | 56.7 | 75 |
| 50–99 beds | 55.2 | 64.7 | 85 |
| 100–199 beds | 58.3 | 71.2 | 82 |
| 200–299 beds | 62.5 | 77.1 | 81 |
| 300–399 beds | 65.3 | 79.7 | 82 |
| 400–499 beds | 68.2 | 81.1 | 84 |
| 500 beds or more | 72.9 | 80.9 | 90 |

Inpatient revenue was 66% of total hospital patient revenue in 1999, and outpatient revenue was 34%. By 2017, the percentage of outpatient revenue had increased to 49% and inpatient revenue decreased to 51% (Figure 6.3).[19] The primary reasons for the growth of outpatient revenue were higher outpatient visit and surgery volume, price increases, and the shift of procedures from lower cost physician office settings to higher cost hospital outpatient settings.

Interestingly, overall hospital profits were a record-setting $88 billion in 2017, which was a 13% increase over 2016 and 27% higher than 2013. Operating revenue increased just 4.6% in 2017 due mainly to flat utilization, but non-operating revenue—primarily investment income—jumped 92% in 2017 following the 103% increase in 2016.[20]

## THREE HEALTH CARE ENVIRONMENTAL FORCES AFFECTING HOSPITALS

Hospital market trends and market behavior have been strongly influenced by three health care environmental forces: (1) Economic forces have resulted in accelerating the erosion of hospital financial margins, (2) social and cultural forces are increasing consumer engagement in personal health care decision-making, and (3) technological forces are leading to disruptive innovation by new competitors in the health care market.

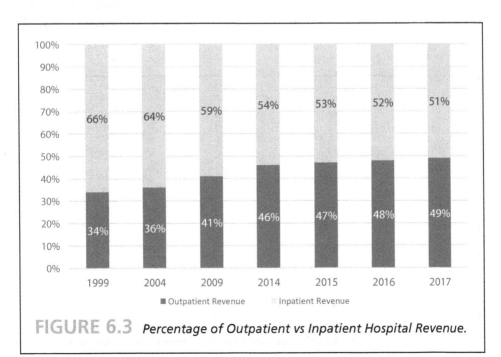

FIGURE 6.3  *Percentage of Outpatient vs Inpatient Hospital Revenue.*

### *Economic Force:* Trend 1—Hospital Financial Results are Likely to Continue Trending Lower

The hospital-centric health care approach of treating disease is being transformed into a proactive emphasis on preventing disease and injury. Moving from acute care to population health and chronic care management has clearly led to financial problems for hospitals. The ACA mandated fee-for-service payment reductions and projected that hospitals would lose $260 billion in Medicare payments between 2013 to 2022 (Figure 6.4).[21]

Total margins and operating margins for community hospitals have been analyzed using the most recent data available from the AHA in 2020 (Figure 6.5). From 1999 to 2016, total margins ranged from 4.6% to 8.3%, and operating margins were 2.0% to 7.4%.[22] Hospital operating margins declined 21% from 2018 to 2019, according to tracking firm Kaufman Hall. Smaller hospitals and those in the Great Plains region performed the worst financially.[23]

The analysis of hospitals with negative total and negative operating margins from 1999 to 2016 was also completed by the AHA. The percentage of community hospitals with negative total margins ranged from 23% to 33% for the period. The percentage with negative operating margins ranged from 26% to 42% (Figure 6.6).[24]

The financial research also cited poor patient volumes and revenues and higher-than-expected labor and nonlabor expenses for the decrease. Although marketing research predicts that market demand for hospital orthopedics, neurosurgery, and spine surgery services will increase, organic market growth will represent only 20%

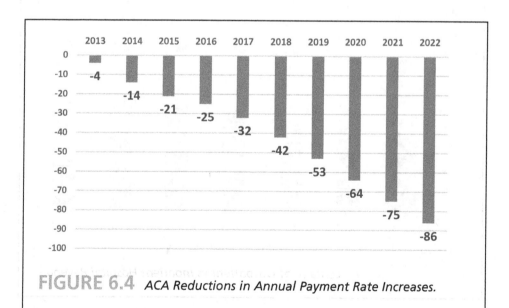

**FIGURE 6.4** *ACA Reductions in Annual Payment Rate Increases.*

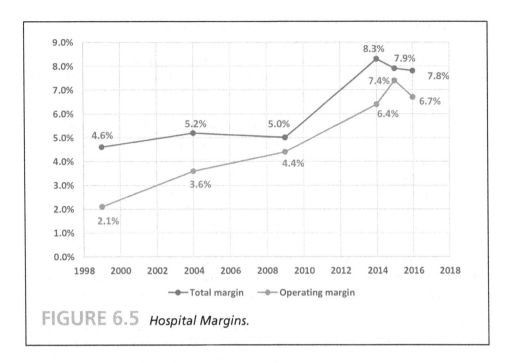

FIGURE 6.5  *Hospital Margins.*

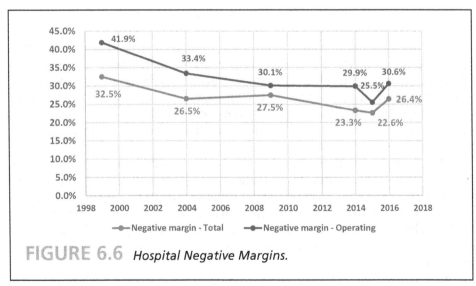

FIGURE 6.6  *Hospital Negative Margins.*

of the volume needed to sustain positive hospital financial margins. The remaining 80% of volume will have to be taken from market competitors.[25]

Hospital executives recognized the problem and their most pressing goal mentioned in a 2018 survey was to improve financial margin performance. To improve margin trends, hospitals need to increase total revenues without increasing costs, reduce total costs without reducing revenues, or achieve a combination of revenue increases and cost reductions. Executives most mentioned three strategies for improving margins: sustain cost control (62% mentions), identify more opportunities for expense reductions (57% mentions), and increase revenue growth from nontraditional sources (56% mentions).[26] Becoming more market-driven was not among the top strategies.

The Congressional Budget Office (CBO) analyzed hospital labor productivity and found it was a weakness. If hospitals were able to increase productivity by 0.8% per year from 2018 to 2025, it would be in line with average U.S. economic productivity growth. Unfortunately, even with average U.S. productivity the percentage of hospitals with negative profit margins would increase to 41% by 2025 and the average hospital profit margin would fall to 3.3%. Alternatively, if hospitals improved their productivity by only 0.4%, then the percentage of hospitals with a negative profit margin would increase to 51% in 2025. The average hospital profit margin would also drop to 1.6%. If hospitals were unable to increase their productivity or to reduce cost growth in some other way, then 60% of hospitals in 2025 would have negative profit margins and the average hospital profit margin would fall to −0.2%.[27]

Reduced hospital revenue and margins have also led to lower credit ratings. There were 41 downgrades and 12 upgrades in 2017, a ratio of 3.4-to-1. This compares to 2.8-to-1 and 2-to-1 in 2008 and 2009, respectively. The 2017 ratio was also higher than in 2016 with 32 downgrades and 21 upgrades, or a 1.5-to-1 ratio, according to Moody's. More than 60% of 2017 downgrades were among small- to medium-sized hospitals and health systems with less than $1 billion in operating revenue. Twelve of the downgrades in 2017 were in Ohio and Pennsylvania where Moody's said health systems were bogged down by lagging economies, aging demographics, a difficult payer environment, and competitive service areas. In Pennsylvania, half of the state's rural hospitals operated at a net loss in 2016, and in Ohio 61 hospitals have low or negative operating margins.[28]

The factors primarily responsible for the downgrades were reduced revenue and cash flow resulting from lower inpatient service demand and higher expenses. In FY 2016, the overall hospital annual expense growth rate was 7.2% and the revenue growth rate was 6%. Consumers with high-deductibles and payers employing financial incentives reduced hospital revenues by moving from higher-priced hospitals to lower-cost freestanding imaging centers, urgent care centers, and retail clinics.

At the end of 2017, Moody's predicted declining cash flow for hospitals and declared a negative financial outlook for the hospital industry.[29] Moody's attributed the increase in expense growth to rising pension contributions, labor costs, and pharmaceutical costs. In 2018, Moody's Investors Service further revised its nonprofit and public health hospital financial outlook from stable to negative based on the expectation that operating cash flow would contract by 2% to 4%

over the next 12 to 18 months. Further compounding this revenue problem was the projection that hospitals would lose $260 billion in Medicare payments from 2013 to 2022 through mandated Medicare payment reductions.[30]

### Social-Cultural Force: Trend 2—Consumer Engagement with Hospitals is Increasing

Consumers are more motivated to be engaged with health care services primarily because their out-of-pocket spending and health care accountability have increased. Engaged consumers are actively seeking health information, are more deeply involved in the process of their care, decide how best to fit care into their lives, and take action on decisions. Research also shows that higher levels of engagement are linked to better clinical quality and outcomes. Engaged consumers benefit hospitals because value-based care payments increase with improved quality, outcomes, and population health.

Hospitals have not been customer-driven organizations, and the dominant organizational cultural perspective has been the operations imperative. The role of operations is reactive and cost-oriented. Service is delivered with a focus on standardization, and quality is defined from an internal perspective. There are tight rules for customers, and frontline managers control workers. The marketing imperative, however, is a better fit for increasing consumer engagement: target the "right" customers and build relationships, offer solutions that meet their needs, and define quality packages with a competitive advantage.[31] Hospitals that can transition from the operations imperative to the marketing imperative by delivering value and building relationships will increase consumer engagement and improve clinical and management results.

*Hospital selection* has changed with increased consumer engagement. Traditionally, most consumers relied on a physician referral when deciding which hospital to use. A 2007 survey found that 34% of consumers surveyed said that they relied completely on their physicians for hospital selection decisions, and 12% said their physician had the majority influence. By 2013, the decision-making process reversed with 26% of consumers completely responsible for the hospital decision and 38% had majority influence (Figure 6.7).[32]

Increased consumer engagement with a hospital is nurtured through positive experiences, and a customer's experience with an organization has been shown to be the most important factor for increasing brand equity (see Figure 5.4 in Chapter 5 Physician Marketing). More than cost or clinical quality, experience determines whether a customer will be loyal to a hospital.

Rather than focus on customer experience and measure loyalty using the NPS, hospitals have stressed customer satisfaction. The reason is that hospitals are mandated by CMS to use the Hospital Consumer Assessment of Healthcare Providers and Systems (HCAHPS, pronounced *h-caps*) to measure patient perceptions of safety and satisfaction. The ACA added HCAHPS performance to the calculation of value-based incentive payments in the Hospital Value-Based

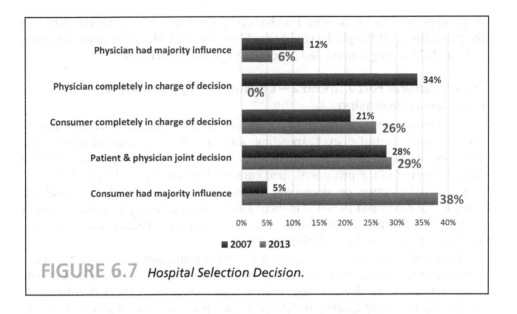

FIGURE 6.7  *Hospital Selection Decision.*

Purchasing Program beginning with October 2012 discharges. HCAHPS scores that fall below a specified threshold result in Medicare financial penalties.

A study by the *International Journal of Health Care Quality Assurance* found that although there is a statistically significant link between satisfaction and loyalty, satisfaction's effect on loyalty was relatively small. In fact, a large increase in satisfaction (measured by a one-half point increase in satisfaction on a five-point Likert scale) resulted in only a 1.2% change in loyalty. The link between satisfaction and loyalty is even weaker for hospitals with high satisfaction scores.[33] A study by the Health Research and Educational Trust found that a simple one-paragraph word-of-mouth email from a family member relating a personal experience at a hospital had nearly the same impact on consumers' decisions to use a hospital as the HCAHPS report.[34]

The average HCAHPS survey has a 33% consumer response rate. A convenience survey like HCAHPS needs at least a 70% response rate to minimize nonresponse bias and be considered statistically valid and reliable. The reasons for this low level of HCAHPS survey response are the number and types of questions, the time required to complete the survey, and receiving the survey up to six weeks following discharge.[35] A study of hospitals with at least $10 million in annual revenue identified the financial results of increasing HCAHPS scores compared to increasing customer loyalty scores as measured by the NPS. The average hospital that focused exclusively on improving HCAHPS performance was able to increase annual revenue by $424,000. The average hospital that invested the resources necessary to improve customer loyalty by a modest 10% increased revenue by an average of $22 million.[36]

Hospitals benefit from a clear understanding of how their *pricing* impacts the perceived value of their brand. Consumers view hospital pricing as critically important, and an estimated 56% of consumers attempt to find out their out-of-pocket costs before receiving care.[37] Studies have also shown that meeting this consumer need will improve both the consumer experience and hospital financial margins. Prices vary widely across hospitals. While an MRI for a knee can cost $700 at one hospital, it can cost $2,100 at another hospital in the same market. Consumers have not been able to identify comprehensive prices for their particular medical situation. Perhaps more importantly, patients' out-of-pocket costs often depend on the specifics of their insurance plan and the prices that are negotiated by their insurer, meaning the listed prices do not reflect what they actually pay.

In a survey of hospital finance managers, 62% mentioned negotiating their hospital prices by benchmarking competitive market rates. Unfortunately, this traditional approach does not consider consumer price sensitivity. Half of the survey respondents mentioned using financial analysis to measure how different prices affect hospital volume, revenue, and profit. Far fewer, however, used a cost-to-serve analysis or measured price risk by payer, service line, or clinical service. Only 11% made use of marketing research to understand consumer demand elasticity. Six percent of hospitals mentioned that they did not have a pricing strategy (Figure 6.8).[38]

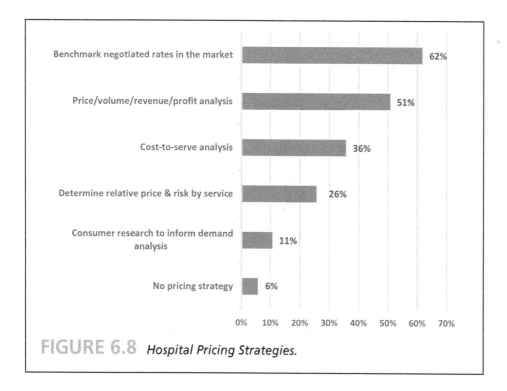

FIGURE 6.8 *Hospital Pricing Strategies.*

Many hospitals have been slow to respond to the need for pricing information. Nearly a quarter of hospital survey respondents were not using any price transparency strategies. Less than half responded to consumer price requests within a defined period of time, and only 10% list prices online (Figure 6.9). Many hospitals understood that lack of pricing information was frustrating for consumers, but they did not think that pricing was a priority for consumers in their particular market.[39]

Giving consumers a specific price will not only increase the likelihood of hospital selection, it will also improve hospital billing, collections, and margin results. The payment experience presents an either strongly positive or negative opportunity for hospitals. A consumer survey found that 55% of respondents were sometimes or always confused with hospital bills, and 61% were surprised by out-of-pocket costs. This finding underscores the importance of using pre-service pricing information to accurately set expectations.

Emory Healthcare, a nine-hospital system based on Atlanta, Georgia, sends consumers a pre-service financial statement to explain and confirm pricing. The statement identifies each part of the billing statement, shows the detail and total amount of expected overall and consumer payment, uses consumer-friendly language, and includes a space for staff to add any relevant notes based on consumer conversations.[40]

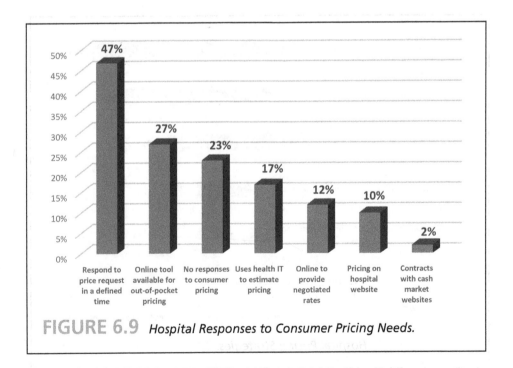

FIGURE 6.9  *Hospital Responses to Consumer Pricing Needs.*

St. Luke's Health System in Boise, Idaho, decided to develop a billing program from the consumers' perspective. St. Luke's contracted for an online payment platform that emails consumers bills and enables them to directly pay online. The system also consolidates bills for all family members and electronically matches them to the payers' explanation of benefits. This system resulted in a better payment yield, lower delinquency rates, lower outstanding balances, and a significant improvement in consumer experience scores.[41]

Consumers can also access hospital prices online through the websites Healthcare Bluebook (healthcarebluebook.com), Guroo (guroo.com), FAIR Health (fairhealthconsumer.org), and others. Walgreens, Walmart, Target, and other retailers are investing in lower-cost and conveniently located primary care walk-in clinics to exploit the market opportunity for lower priced and more convenient outpatient and non-hospital-based services.[42]

Hospital price disclosure has always been part of the ACA, but under guidance from the government, hospitals were only required to provide charges to consumers upon request. This changed in January 2019 when CMS made it mandatory for hospitals to make public their "standard charges" for all "items and services." Many hospitals complied by publishing their chargemasters. The typical chargemaster is a list of over 20,000 procedures, lab tests, supplies, and medications and is different in every hospital. Publishing the chargemaster is analogous to a car dealer disclosing list prices for the cost of each auto part on the sticker. Examples were a cardiology procedure listed as "HC PTC CLOS PAT DUCT ART" for $42,569 at Vanderbilt University Medical Center, "Embolza Protect 5.5" for $9,818, and a "Visceral selective angio rad" for $5,538, both at Baptist Health in Miami.[43]

In reaction, CMS proposed in November 2019 that hospitals report more detailed pricing information based on payer-specific negotiated rates. CMS also asked for at least 300 self-selected common "shoppable" items and services, with 70 items specified by CMS. Additionally, hospitals include costs for associated ancillary items and services that the hospital provides in tandem with the shoppable service, and they must communicate this information in a manner that is "consumer-friendly." This proposed regulation is scheduled to be effective in January 2021. Shortly after the rule's release, however, the AHA, Association of American Medical Colleges (AAMC), and Children's Hospital Association (CHA) jointly announced they would be filing a lawsuit challenging the new requirements.[44] Concurrently, CMS announced that health plans have to provide cost-sharing information to enrolled individuals through an online tool on their website and in paper form. Health plans would also have to disclose negotiated rates for in-network providers and historical out-of-network allowed amounts.

These hospital and health plan proposed rules rely entirely on legal authority under the ACA. Interestingly, this action is one of several examples of the Trump administration leveraging provisions of the ACA to achieve some of its major health care priorities, while simultaneously arguing in court that the entire ACA law is invalid.[45] The Supreme Court will hear Texas v. United States—now popularly known as California v. Texas—during its fall term in 2020.

Consumers regularly rate their ability to *access* care as their top health care priority. Hospitals that employ primary care physicians should be aware that a physician clinic is typically the first point of entry to a hospital for a consumer with a non-emergent medical problem. Since 44% of initial primary care appointments occur after business hours and on weekends, research supports that consumers chiefly want more convenient hours, an easily reached location, walk-in appointments, and lower cost (Figure 6.10).[46]

Many hospitals, however, continue to focus on traditional approaches to access such as outpatient and ambulatory surgery centers, urgent care centers, and imaging sites. More innovative approaches to access—including retail clinics staffed by nurse practitioners and physician assistants, video visits, e-visits, and concierge primary care—are less common (Figure 6.11).[47]

Consumers often face three barriers to primary care access: the clinic is closed, there are no available appointments, or the location is inconvenient. Aurora Health Care, with a 1,600-physician-employed group in Milwaukee, Wisconsin, expanded hours to ensure they have availability when consumers want care. Aurora focused on adding "family hours" in mornings, evenings, and weekends. Each physician was required to offer at least eight family hours each month but not more hours overall. Aurora found that the adjusted schedules resulted in a net increase in appointment availability and a 10% increase in annual patient visits.

Mercy Medical Center in Des Moines, Iowa, also developed an innovative strategy to solve the problem of no appointment availability by converting urgent

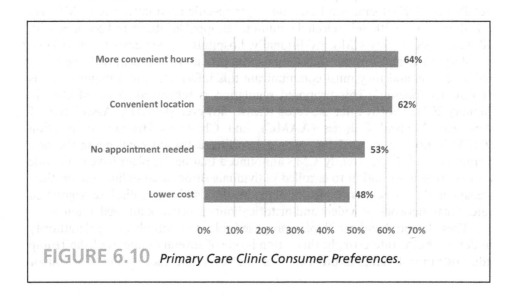

**FIGURE 6.10** *Primary Care Clinic Consumer Preferences.*

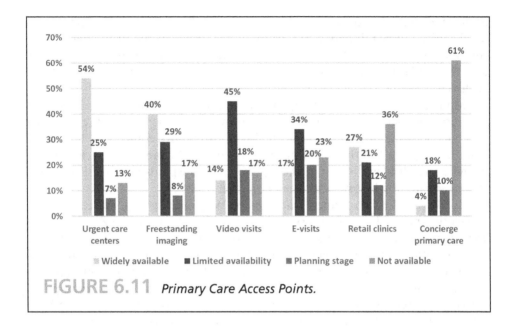

**FIGURE 6.11** *Primary Care Access Points.*

care visits to physician referrals. Mercy urgent care centers are located adjacent to hospital-owned physician offices and all physician offices are networked and share schedules. A consumer visiting a Mercy urgent care center who needs a primary care or specialty physician referral, is immediately scheduled for an appointment with a Mercy physician with same-day or preferred day availability. This strategy has also been effective in converting episodic urgent care visits to sustained relationships with primary care physicians.

Several hospitals have also supplemented their physician practices with convenient care retail clinics to solve the problem of an inconvenient location. Kaiser Permanente recognized the need to build retail clinics, but they did not want to dilute their brand name by affiliating with a retailer. Kaiser partnered with Target to offer co-branded services that extend beyond the Target retail clinic's capabilities. The Kaiser Permanente Target clinics, located in Target stores in Southern California, are staffed by Kaiser nurse practitioners but also offer telemedicine access to Kaiser's urgent care physicians, pediatric care, well-woman care, family planning, and chronic illness management. These innovative clinics have also expanded Kaiser's market reach to consumers who are members of competitive health plans.

### *Technological Force:* Trend 3—Innovation and Health IT are Disrupting Hospital Care

Several large technology-enabled business and care models are disrupting the hospital market. A new health care management company named Haven was formed by Amazon, JPMorgan, and Berkshire Hathaway to improve their employee health and decrease costs. CVS Health acquired Aetna to combine pharmacy, retail clinic, and health plan expertise to more seamlessly and profitably manage consumer health care. IBM Watson Health acquired Truven Health Analytics and uses Watson Health's cognitive capabilities to derive insights from Truven's 8,500 health care clients.

Many smaller innovative companies have also created services and products that target unmet consumer needs for improved customer experience, convenience, and accurate pricing. Imagine Health is a disruptive company with a stated vision to "rip the health system open at its core and change America forever." Imagine Health identifies the highest performing hospitals and physicians, and then negotiates the best rates for their employer clients.

Zocdoc can help consumers who need primary care, specialty care, and mental health services. It is a free service that identifies physicians by ZIP code, lists user reviews, and allows consumers to book an appointment online. Virtuwell, another option for online diagnosis and treatment, has consumers complete an intake form with symptoms and questions that is then reviewed by a nurse practitioner. The nurse practitioner responds with a treatment plan and a prescription, if needed. The cost is $49 and health insurance is accepted. A full refund is offered if Virtuwell cannot treat the problem or if the consumer is dissatisfied.

Hospitals have three primary marketing strategies for competing with these and other disruptive innovators: (1) collaborate with new health care market entrants, (2) change the hospital's business model and culture to be more market-driven, or (3) invest internally in the development of an innovative service or product. Five hospital organizational imperatives are needed to either collaborate with new entrants, turn consumer health experience into a competitive advantage, or create a new and innovative offering:

1. Hospital executive management must buy in and commit to this change.

2. Innovation, supported by financial incentives, needs to be part of the strategic plan.

3. An adequate budget and cross-disciplinary teams need to be established.

4. Maintain the consumer perspective while identifying problem solutions.

5. Use a proven new product development process with specific go/no decision points.

An example of a collaboration with new health care market entrants is an innovative channels strategy to improve medical product distribution. Amazon is partnering with Xealth (xealth.io), a digital prescribing platform, as well as with health systems Providence Health & Services (Seattle) and the University of Pittsburgh Medical Center. Amazon Prime will be used by physicians and other health care providers to recommend and deliver bundles of medical products to patients' homes before discharge. Amazon product distribution resources will save time for providers and for consumers who commonly call if they misplace or forget their discharge instructions. This new channels strategy could be broadened to include other health systems, and it could be used to distribute prescription drugs using the Amazon acquisition, PillPack (pillpack.com), a "smart" full service online pharmacy.

An example of a partnership dedicated to improving consumer experience is the Piedmont Now app developed by Atlanta-based Piedmont Healthcare and Gozio Health (goziohealth.com). Consumers use this mobile wayfinding platform that provides step-by-step directions to any destination within Piedmont's hospitals, urgent care centers, and physician offices. It uses a smartphone-based, indoor positioning, and wayfinding platform specifically designed for hospitals and health care systems. Piedmont Now reduces the stress involved in arriving at appointments on time in a new location. The app also gives consumers mobile access to electronic health records and a "save my spot" urgent care center reservation function.

Partnering with an external company may help hospitals communicate price and make access more convenient, but hospitals can also increase value by leveraging their own product strengths by becoming market-driven. A strong hospital point of differentiation is the integration of different types of health care and management. Hospitals offer comprehensive clinical services, maintain complete health records, and can personalize interactions and coordinate care across the health care continuum. In order to take full advantage of these product strengths, hospitals must understand and meet consumer expectations. For example, consumers expect to know a procedure price in advance, make an appointment outside of business hours, talk to a provider without having to travel, have their appointment start on time, and understand their bills and pay them easily.

Using market sensitive, multidisciplinary management and clinical teams to design and implement these consumer strategies is critical to success. According to a research study of hospital consumer marketing tools, 85% of hospitals responded that they have done survey research. This a start, but it is also important to understand if the survey research accurately reflects the market perspective and if the research conclusions can actually be implemented. This study also found that other consumer marketing tools often used in other industries are underused by hospitals (Figure 6.12).[48]

A hospital internal investment in the development of an innovative service or product is higher risk but it can also have a higher reward. Nearly half of people diagnosed as having HIV never establish regular care, and this can lead to serious and potentially lethal illness. The University of Virginia School of Medicine created the PositiveLinks (positivelinks4ric.com) smart phone app to address serious gaps in health care for people living with HIV. The app has improved consistency in physician visits at both 6 and 12 months of care. Additionally, the percentage of people with "undetectable HIV viral loads"—a key outcome for individuals living with HIV—increased significantly for users of this intervention.

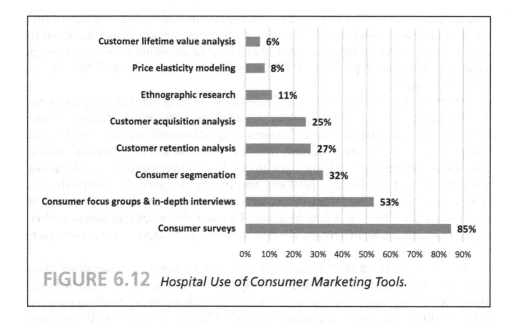

**FIGURE 6.12** *Hospital Use of Consumer Marketing Tools.*

PositiveLinks was developed with significant input from people with HIV. The app offers a powerful mix of engagement, social interaction, and access to care providers. It provides appointment reminders, important health information, and offers daily questions about stress, mood, and medication adherence. In addition, it features a virtual support group where users can interact anonymously to ask questions, share their stories, and find strength through community with others with HIV.

In a clinical paper outlining their findings, the researchers credit the app's collaborative design and integrating the principles of warm technology. Cold technology is impersonal, isolating, and not concerned with feelings or emotion. In contrast, warm technology is personal, facilitates human contact, and shares emotions. This innovation was not just a typical app but also a pathway to human contact.[49]

## HOSPITAL MARKET BEHAVIOR

Hospitals struggling with lower inpatient demand and declining financial performance have reacted by joining health systems, acquiring physician practices, merging with other hospitals, and reducing numbers of employees.

### Hospital System Growth is Accelerating

The National Bureau of Economic Research (NBER) Center of Excellence defines a health system as two or more health care provider organizations that have (1) common ownership, (2) a contractual arrangement such as an ACO, or

(3) an informal arrangement such as common referrals. ACOs typically have the most complex structures since they include groups of physicians, hospitals, and other health care providers who coordinate the value-based care of Medicare patients.

Independent hospitals and smaller health systems face competition from out-patient services offered by large provider practices and ambulatory surgical centers. They react by forming or joining larger systems to improve economies of scale, decrease expenses, and attain higher reimbursement rates from payers. An example of a horizontally integrated hospital system is two or more hospitals operating under the same brand name. Alternatively, a health system can be a vertically integrated organization consisting of hospitals, physician practices, and post-acute care facilities.

There were 637 health systems in 2018, and they represented 70% of community hospitals and 45% of physicians. Health system characteristics are wide-ranging. Systems ranged from 1 to 167 hospitals. The medians were 2 hospitals, 301 physicians, and 406 hospital beds. The typical health system also included a median of 119 primary care physicians. The 10 largest health systems are profiled in Table 6.6.[50]

### Acquisition of Physician Practices is Also Growing

A second hospital growth strategy has been to purchase physician practices in the hospital's market area. Practice acquisition benefits hospitals by increasing access to patient admissions and referrals. A strong majority of newly trained physicians (91%) would prefer to be employed and few seek an independent, private practice setting.[51] Physician who are hospital employees or contractors have a stable income and can delegate responsibilities for practice management. Unfortunately for hospitals, fewer desirable physicians are becoming available, practice acquisition deals are attracting more regulatory scrutiny from the FTC and IRS, and competition from other hospitals and physician networks for physician practices is raising the stakes.[52]

Purchasing physician practices actually began in the 1990s. Novant Health was one of the many hospitals nationwide that implemented this vertical integration channels strategy. The Winston-Salem, North Carolina based health care system believed that they could gain market share, increase operational efficiency, and ultimately reduce overall health care costs by participating in as many components of the health care system as possible at that time. The integration of medical practices included an estimated 800 physicians. Like many hospitals, Novant experienced financial and management challenges, but unlike some other hospitals, it persevered and made changes based on its commitment to its physician integration strategy.

Understanding that its physician practices needed to be managed more like a multispecialty group than as a hospital clinic, Novant adapted and placed decision-making for these practices back in the hands of the physician

**TABLE 6.6** The 10 Largest U.S. Health Systems in 2018.

| Health System | Hospital Beds | Physicians | Ownership | States |
|---|---|---|---|---|
| HCA Healthcare | 36,873 | 14,604 | Public | 20 |
| Ascension Health | 17,577 | 11,419 | Religious | 15 |
| Trinity Health (MI) | 15,319 | 11,236 | Religious | 18 |
| Community Health Systems | 15,023 | 4,817 | Public | 20 |
| Tenet Healthcare | 15,006 | 7,580 | Public | 10 |
| Catholic Health Initiatives* | 11,026 | 5,965 | Religious | 14 |
| Providence St. Joseph | 9,696 | 12,638 | Religious | 7 |
| Lifepoint Health | 9,060 | 2,993 | Public | 29 |
| Kaiser Permanente | 8,982 | 24,955 | Nonprofit | 3 |
| Adventist Health System | 7,700 | 2,558 | Religious | 9 |
| Dignity Health* | 7,288 | 8,553 | Religious | 3 |
| UC Health (CA) | 3,292 | 10,147 | Govt. | 1 |
| Partners Healthcare | 2,690 | 7,802 | Nonprofit | 2 |
| MedStar Health | 2,413 | 9,131 | Nonprofit | 2 |
| Mt. Sinai Health | 2,226 | 10,400 | Nonprofit | 1 |

*Catholic Health Initiatives and Dignity merged to form CommonSpirit Health in 2019.

groups. Network management leaders with strong practice management experience were hired. Physician compensation was tied to patient activity instead of a straight salary. Novant also formed a joint venture with the physicians to address the increasing costs of medical malpractice insurance. This "risk retention group" provided more competitively priced malpractice insurance to the medical staff. Over time, this approach to vertical channels integration improved financial results and allowed Novant to invest in additional clinical and management resources, such as new medical equipment and physician recruitment.

### *Hospital Mergers and Acquisitions are at Record Level*

A third hospital reaction to volume and financial declines has been to consolidate market position through mergers and acquisitions of other hospitals. Acquiring hospitals have benefitted by controlling more of their markets. The hospital being acquired gets access to additional management resources, purchasing discounts, and better access to investment capital. Although the number of mergers had increased to 115 in 2017, the supply of investment capital to fund these transactions has been tightened and deal scrutiny by the Federal Trade Commission, IRS, and Department of Justice has been intensified (Figure 6.13).[53]

Mergers and acquisitions have had both a positive and negative impact on credit quality. Diversified health systems may be able to spread financial risk

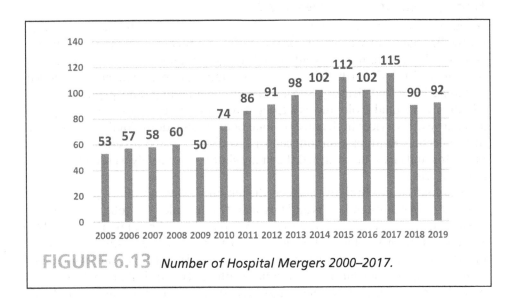

FIGURE 6.13  *Number of Hospital Mergers 2000–2017.*

across multiple cities or states to subsidize hospitals with lower levels of financial performance. Baptist Health South Florida, however, acquired Bethesda Healthcare System in 2017 and was then downgraded. Similarly, the University of Pittsburgh Medical Center health system was downgraded after its merger with Pinnacle Health System.

Since hospital mergers have the potential to cause price increases, lower credit ratings, and reduce the incentive for hospitals to improve quality of care, some hospitals are choosing to enter an affiliation instead. System affiliation is becoming an increasingly popular option for hospitals that wish to increase financial and clinical capacities by collaborating with another organization while maintaining their own brand identity. Affiliation, rather than merger, also avoids Federal Trade Commission scrutiny regarding market price increases.

Englewood (NJ) Hospital and Medical Center entered into a clinical and academic affiliation with Hackensack (NJ) University Health Network. Englewood is collaborating with Hackensack on a number of projects including the creation of a regional cardiac surgery program. Kootenai Health in Coeur d'Alene, Idaho, joined the Mayo Clinic Care Network in Rochester, Minnesota. Kootenai was able to improve quality of care by gaining access to various Mayo Clinic resources such as the AskMayoExpert database and electronic consulting that connects Kootenai physicians with Mayo Clinic physicians to consult on diagnoses, care management, and therapy.

### Employee Layoffs are Widespread

A fourth hospital response to lower revenue has been to lay off employees. High-profile Brigham and Women's Hospital, which is affiliated with Harvard Medical School, offered voluntary buyouts to 1,600 workers and announced it would lay off staff in 2017. Other hospitals are also planning to eliminate clinical services including labor and delivery, substance abuse counseling, and psychiatric care. Children's Hospital Colorado is expected to drop preteen psychiatric programs and telehealth services in the face of state budget reductions. Methodist Hospital in Henderson, Kentucky, announced 61 layoffs and closed a pediatric inpatient unit. Hospitals have also warned they may shut down entirely as revenue shrinks and costs rise.

Catholic Health Initiatives, one of the nation's largest nonprofit providers, cut nearly 900 jobs through layoffs and buyouts. This included 620 jobs at hospitals in Texas and another 250 in Kentucky. Another large hospital in Texas, MD Anderson Cancer Center, laid off about 800 employees after losing $267 million in its last fiscal year. Layoffs have resulted from a variety of financial reasons, with some relating to poor business decisions. Catholic Health Initiatives lost money on its in-house insurance business, and MD Anderson cited the high cost of rolling out a new electronic health records system.[54]

The layoff trend has been accelerated during the Covid-19 pandemic. Dallas-based Baylor Scott & White Health announced in late May 2020 that it was laying off about 1,200 employees, nearly 3% of its workforce. Baylor Scott & White spent $85 million to prepare for and respond to the pandemic, and it also saw patient volume declines between 50% and 90%, depending on the site of care.[55] Layoffs have a negative effect on hospital culture, and the hospital employee culture has been found to have an impact on patient mortality rates.[56]

## HOSPITAL PROBLEMS AND STRATEGIC MARKETING SOLUTIONS

The primary reasons that hospitals are stuck in neutral are that (1) they have developed a complex and highly variable portfolio of assets, (2) there is strategic uncertainty about how to leverage those assets, and (3) there is cultural reluctance to take calculated risks that upset the status quo. Hospitals are focused on solving problems related to decreasing financial margins, improving consumer engagement, responding to disruptive innovations, and others. Strategic marketing can help solve these problems. The following six examples explore how different hospitals have or could use strategic marketing to overcome these challenges.

### 1. *Marketing Problem*—The Cleveland Clinic Found it Needed to Improve Employee Engagement to Earn Value-Based Incentives from CMS.

CMS announced a 1% holdback of Medicare inpatient DRG reimbursement, beginning in 2012, to fund a financial incentive pool. Hospitals could earn their holdback, plus a value-based incentive bonus, through improving their performance on 12 clinical process outcome measures and on eight patient experience measures.

The Cleveland Clinic analyzed its clinical results (e.g., infection rates), patient perceptions (e.g., satisfaction scores), and employee engagement (e.g., lower employee turnover, higher productivity) in preparation for earning incentives.[57] The health system discovered that superior clinical outcomes and more positive patient perceptions had strong correlations with high employee engagement scores. Unfortunately, aggregate Cleveland Clinic employee engagement scores ranked below the 40th percentile according to a national health care benchmarking database.

### *Marketing Solution*—Use Hospital Employee Marketing Strategies to Increase Employee Engagement.

Cleveland Clinic conjectured that if they could improve employee engagement, then better clinical outcomes, patient experience scores, and reimbursement would follow. The first step was to identify employee engagement best practices. This included helping employees to understand what engagement is, what are the benefits, how to be engaged, and how to improve engagement.

Second, Cleveland Clinic initiated cultural change and a more inclusive management style. All 42,000 employees were invited to attend focus group sessions to discuss employee and consumer engagement. These focus groups were small, diverse, half-day sessions. It was the first time that a mix of all types of Cleveland Clinic employees—from food service workers to volunteers, to physicians—met together. They talked about organizational culture, values, priorities, and vision. Physicians learned that they had more impact on employee and consumer engagement than they realized. An important discovery was that administrative and other non-clinical employees really wanted to feel part of the care team that delivered and improved patient health at Cleveland Clinic.

In order for the health system's top management to effectively transform the culture, they needed to build on the Cleveland Clinic's reputation for world-class outcomes by communicating the "how" and the "why" behind having a culture of strong employee engagement. The "Cleveland Clinic Experience" employee marketing strategy was created to make each of the 42,000 hospital employees a "patient caregiver" regardless of their job title. Employees were educated on what it meant to be a caregiver. Managers and teams created employee engagement plans with accountability measures designed to hone employee competence and confidence. Employees were then coached to meet their engagement objectives by their managers. Managers were also given access to substantial financial incentives to support increased engagement in their units and departments.

Cleveland Clinic also created its own "pulse" surveys to determine if managers were working on, and making progress on, their action plans. This accountability measure effectively channeled feedback to managers throughout the year and kept the executive team informed about how the organization was progressing and what areas needed improvement. Overall employee engagement scores increased in the first year of the program, and HCAHPS data showed an improvement in the hospital's patient safety and experience ratings.

Some Cleveland Clinic teams, however, were not improving. The human resources department began a special effort to educate and coach managers in the bottom 25% of employee engagement. Cleveland Clinic stepped up employee recognition by implementing Caregiver Celebrations, special events where high performing caregivers were recognized by their peers and managers. Cleveland Clinic created new training opportunities and introduced the concept of employee engagement and coaching to their remote facilities.

Managers became accountable for their employee engagement scores in a way that was less tactical and score-oriented than it had been. The value of employee engagement became both more institutionalized and conversational with the emphasis on communicating and understanding the importance of being engaged and less about data and reports.[58] Employees contributed to "MyTwoCents," an online forum to provide feedback and make suggestions for improvements. More than 6,000 ideas were submitted, over 800 new ideas were implemented, and 4,500 employees throughout the enterprise participated in 150 projects. These submissions resulted in cost savings of over $2.5 million and in projected future savings of $3.5 million.

Clinically, another offshoot of the program was a radical redesign of the organization around disease symptoms instead of departments or service lines. For example, consumers presenting with a headache may need to be seen by a psychologist, a neurologist, or a neurosurgeon. Cleveland Clinic created a neurologic system in a neurologic institute where consumers are evaluated for headaches in a central location. Different neurological providers are now within close proximity and more effectively confer with each other immediately.

This fundamental organizational change was made throughout the enterprise and saved consumers time moving between departments, increased management efficiency, reduced costs, and improved employee engagement.[59] Internally marketing the "caregiver culture" at the Cleveland Clinic was a disruptive innovative. This employee marketing strategy resulted in enhanced employee engagement, a positive consumer experience, and improved financial results.[60]

### 2. *Marketing Problem*—Hospital Financial Margins are Being Reduced by the Elimination of Reimbursement for Hospital Care Complications and "Never Events."

Annual mortality studies routinely find that medical errors are a top cause of death in the U.S.[61] CMS instituted a policy that eliminates reimbursement for hospital-acquired conditions such as certain infections, advanced bed sores, or fractures. These are examples of preventable medical errors—like performing surgery on the wrong side of the body—that should never happen. The list of "never events" covered under the CMS payment policy can be organized into three categories: surgical events, medical products and devices, and case management.

### *Marketing Solution*—EBD Product Augmentation Strategies Improve Clinical Outcomes and Reduce Errors.

An augmented product, by definition, exceeds customer expectations and takes place at the fourth product level. Hospitals can use product augmentation strategies to differentiate their inpatient and outpatient products, reduce costs, improve outcomes, and increase value. Choosing the particular product attributes need not be based on luck, convenience, or engineering suggestions. Hospitals can use *conjoint research analysis* to begin the process of creating an augmented product.

Conjoint research measures consumer preferences for alternative product benefits and attributes. Targeted consumers are surveyed and asked to rank product attributes based on paired comparisons. Analyzing the resulting data shows which product benefits and attributes represent the highest consumer value. For example, Wellington Hospital in New Zealand used conjoint research with adolescents to understand their inpatient hospital preferences. The two most preferred product elements were locating the adolescent unit adjacent to the pediatric area and not near adult patients. The second most important element was having the capability for using their mobile phones.[62]

Evidence-based design (EBD) can also be used to support a product augmentation strategy. EBD is an interdisciplinary approach to hospital product development that integrates space planning, human factors, social psychology, sustainability factors, and esthetics to develop a facility that is responsive to user needs. Hospital EBD best practices were explained in the "Fable Hospital" model developed by health care design leaders in 2004 and was updated in 2011 with "Fable Hospital 2.0."[63] While large, quiet, private hospital rooms with plenty of natural light and artwork may seem like expensive luxuries, EBD research indicates that these and other architecture and design features can actually improve patient care, reduce health care expenses, and generate a financial return on investment within three years.

Because CMS and other payers are no longer reimbursing hospitals for the costs of hospital-acquired infections, patient falls, and certain medical errors, hospitals are adopting EBD design strategies to help avoid these problems. Dublin Methodist Hospital in Columbus, Ohio, was designed to be calming and healing. Dublin used EBD to build intimate family spaces and private rooms with natural light and gardens. There is no overhead paging, and special ceiling tiles are used in common areas to absorb sound. Among the documented clinical outcomes were lower rates of hospital-acquired infections and patient falls. Hospital management calculated that the cost of the EBD elements represented only 2.5% of the total project cost of $150 million.

Another example is the $1 billion Palomar Medical Center in California opened in August 2013. This hospital has 288 single-bed rooms and was designed to expressly comply with the Fable Hospital 2.0 EBD concepts. Forty percent of patient rooms are technologically capable of being instantly converted to an intensive care unit allowing for the escalation or reduction of care as needed. This removes the need to transport patients throughout the hospital and reduces the risk of handoff errors or infections.

Faucets in each patient room start running water when infrared devices signal that a person has entered a room. This reminds physicians, nurses, and visitors to wash their hands and reduces infection. Additionally, there are no central nursing stations. Nursing activities take place at small workstations outside each room. This arrangement reduces medical errors by allowing nurses to note patient charts while simultaneously observing and talking with patients. Nurses also save time and increase productivity because large supply closets are located adjacent to patient rooms.[64]

The University Medical Center of Princeton New Jersey had outgrown its building, and management made the decision to replace it. The new hospital design began by building a single mock patient room using *ethnographic marketing research*. Ethnography comes from anthropology and collects empirical, sensory information gathered from observation and experience. The purpose of ethnographic research is to capture insights about a group of people, a culture, or an individual. Observation and questioning are two ethnographic research methods used to identify deeper behavioral insights from participants.

Nurses and physicians spent months moving Post-it notes around a model room set up in the old hospital. It was a single room, had a big foldout sofa for guests, a view outdoors, a novel drug dispensary, and a repositioned bathroom. Equipment was installed, and hypothetical medical situations were simulated by the staff. Eventually, actual hip and knee replacement surgical patients were moved in from the old surgical unit to compare the old and new rooms. After months of testing, patients in the model room rated food and nursing care higher than patients in the old rooms, but in fact the meals and clinical care were actually the same.

The most important product development conclusion was that patients in the model room asked for 30% less pain medication. Reduced pain has been found to have a cascading effect on healing. The orthopedic patients in the model room had faster recovery times and were able to move quickly to begin advanced rehabilitation. These shorter stays and reduced costs also led to fewer accidental falls and infections.

The researched model room configuration was replicated throughout the new $523 million, 636,000-square-foot hospital. Ratings of patient satisfaction then rose to the 99th percentile, an increase from the 61st percentile in the old building. All of the rooms are singles because ethnographic research found that patients sharing rooms did not communicate important information with their physicians—and shared even less information if the other patient in the room had guests. Ample space is given to patient visitors because the presence of family and friends has been shown to also hasten recovery. A large window with natural lighting and a view outdoors have been considered patient morale boosters since the 1930s.

The newly built rooms were also designed to be "same-handed" instead of mirrored. In most hospitals, adjacent rooms are mirrored and share a head wall behind each bed that has all the equipment and attachments built into it. Mirrored rooms are common because they cost less to construct and take up less space. They require that everything including the position of the bed, the IV tubes, and the call buttons be reversed, from right to left or from left to right, in every other room. All same-handed designed rooms position equipment uniformly, and nurses and physicians make fewer mistakes when they reach for buttons or equipment.

Nurses routinely sort drugs from a single dispensary for all patients on a floor, and this process is prone to error. Another simple error-reducing idea incorporated into the new University Medical Center of Princeton was a double-door lock box used to store patient prescriptions in each room. Pharmacists can unlock the box to deliver drugs from the hall directly to specific patient rooms. The box can be unlocked by nurses from inside the patient room to retrieve drugs as needed.[65]

### 3. *Marketing Problem*—A Hospital Was Losing Market Share Due to Changes in Consumer Health Care Behavior and Market Growth.

WellStar Health System in Marietta, Georgia, is a five-hospital integrated delivery system that serves over 1 million residents in the northwest Atlanta metropolitan area. Outpatient market share analysis for its 762-bed main campus WellStar Atlanta Medical Center (Midtown) was decreasing in outlying areas. Further analysis found that traffic conditions were contributing to this decline.

INRIX provides transportation analytics around the world, and metro Atlanta was the eigth most congested city in the world with the average driver wasting 70 hours annually in traffic congestion.[66] Traffic volume in the WellStar market area had reached the point that residents would not drive to the main hospital campus if they could use alternative health services closer to their home or work locations.

### *Marketing Solution*—A Product Concept Test and Marketing Research Led to Increased Outpatient Access and Market Share.

WellStar's marketing research identified two market opportunities for outpatient services. A new continuing care retirement community was being developed in eastern Cobb County, WellStar's primary market. The second opportunity was the financial incentives of the Affordable Care Act for outpatient care. To take advantage of these market opportunities WellStar decided to further research market demand for an outpatient "health park" in East Cobb.

This product concept was a major departure from the traditional approach of locating outpatient services either on or adjacent to a hospital campus surrounded by individual physician offices that were widely dispersed. The health park product concept included a range of medical, diagnostic, and therapeutic services in a centralized, natural setting. Coordination between primary and specialty physician services would be enhanced because the offices would be in a single location and used the same electronic health record (EHR). The health park concept would also support population health management by delivering low-acuity wellness and disease prevention services. Finally, a health park would include evidence-based ambulatory health care design elements such as sensitivity to local neighborhood needs, convenient arrival and service access through "wayfinding," welcoming visual aesthetics, natural lighting, and noise reduction.

WellStar began measuring consumer demand for a health park with a quantitative consumer marketing research survey. Consumer demand and current availability for eight health park-based medical and surgical services were tested with a sample of 693 East Cobb residents using online and telephone interviews. The survey indicated strong interest in all of the health park services with the exception of a moderate interest in a sleep center (Figure 6.14).[67]

Based on this research, WellStar formed the East Cobb Community Advisory Committee to build relationships with local community groups and residents and to further understand community health needs. Building relationships is not only an effective strategy for increasing brand equity, but local relationships have value in and of themselves. Hospital employees typically reside in their hospital's primary market, and every encounter between employees and community members is an opportunity for a positive experience. Relationships offer a competitive advantage over virtual competitors as well as those that do not have a local com-

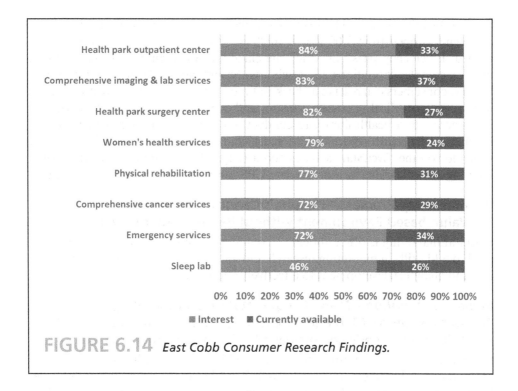

FIGURE 6.14 *East Cobb Consumer Research Findings.*

munity presence. Several months later, WellStar purchased a 23-acre parcel of East Cobb land that had a natural buffer of wetlands and streams, open green space, and the capacity for walking trails to enhance health and healing. Land and architectural building design options were shared with the East Cobb Community Advisory Committee, and the Committee ranked their design preferences.

WellStar then conducted qualitative marketing research to further confirm the alignment between market needs and health park services. Three focus groups were conducted with three target markets: seniors, women aged 25 to 64, and East Cobb residents who recently moved to the community. The research found that consumers continued to strongly support a single, convenient location for a broad range of medical and outpatient services. Additionally, they had very high expectations for physician clinical and communication skills and having providers spend ample time with patients.

The research also uncovered that consumers viewed the term "lower long-term health care costs" specifically as lower insurance deductibles, co-payments, and co-insurance. Consumers were very concerned, however, that this lower-cost care would also limit their access to care. Seniors especially felt that joining high-quality care with lower-cost care were two contradictory ideas. Convincing consumers of the value of preventive care and that more health care is not always better care would be a challenge for WellStar.

The WellStar East Cobb Health Park opened in September 2014. The urgent care clinic is open from 7:00 am to 10:00 pm every day, and no appointment is needed. Emergency physicians staff the clinic and treat routine ailments, illness, injuries, complex lacerations, for newborns through adults. Using the urgent care website, consumers can reserve a check-in time or find a doctor. There are primary and specialty medical practices, a bistro, and a pharmacy. The Health Park also offers access to a health library to conduct research by condition, patient demographics, or by health service. Additionally, contact information and directions are provided to other WellStar facilities and a range of community education events covering worksite wellness, heart screens, CPR, and several community health clubs.

### 4.  *Marketing Problem*—Hospitals Cannot Compete in a Value-based Environment without Being Market-Driven.

Hospital marketing is often limited to communications. Hospital marketers may need to add skills in marketing research and analysis, product management, pricing, and channels development to effectively compete.

### *Marketing Solution*—Market Segmentation and Targeting are Two Basic Strategic Marketing Tools that Can Help Hospitals Meet Customer Needs and Increase Their Financial Margins.

Market segmentation identifies the demographic, psychographic, financial, clinical, and other characteristics of a hospital's total available market. For example, hospitals can segment *wholesale buyers* in order to target large groups or organizations and segment *retail buyers* to target individuals. Hospitals need to understand how their wholesale and retail market segments make buying decisions and what services these different purchasers need and want.

1. Segmentation and Targeting Wholesale Buyers

Hospitals begin the wholesale market segmentation process by identifying different commercial health plans, self-insured employers, and population health organizations in their market area. The next step is to speak with individuals responsible for making organizational health care decisions, understand their specific needs, and learn how the organizations make hospital buying decisions.

Kaleida Health is an integrated health system in Buffalo, New York, that is collaborating with Blue Cross Blue Shield of Western New York in a bundled payment program for heart surgery. Bundled payments offer reimbursement under a single comprehensive fee for all hospital and physician services provided to a patient, and the hospital and physicians are held financially accountable for all of a patient's care. This includes care before a procedure, the procedure itself, and the outcomes following hospital discharge. The physicians and the hospital share in the savings, and in the additional costs of avoidable medical problems, for each heart case. Bundled payments incentivize all providers involved to clearly communicate, avoid unnecessary tests and treatments, coordinate care, base decisions on medical evidence and best practices, measure outcomes, and ensure that complications do not result in discharged patients being readmitted to the hospital.

A second wholesale segment is self-insured employers that may need care coordination and worksite health services. Self-insured employers take direct financial responsibility for the costs of their employees' medical claims. The percentage of private sector employees covered in a self-funded plan was 61% in 2018, and employers are increasingly interested in reducing costs of high priced health services.[68] Pepsico, Lowes, and Walmart have entered into national bundled payments agreements that offer higher patient employee volume in return for lower provider prices.

Walmart's Center of Excellence (COE) Program has more than 1.1 million covered lives, and it began contracting with six hospital systems nationwide for heart, spine, and transplant services in 2013. The Walmart COE program covers these services at 100% including travel, lodging, and an expense allowance for the patient and a companion. The hospitals were selected based on their documented levels of quality, potential for cost-savings, and convenience for Walmart employees.

Research data shows about 30% of spinal procedures are unnecessary. The Walmart national spine COEs are Mayo Clinic facilities (Arizona, Minnesota, and Florida), Mercy Hospital Springfield (Missouri), Virginia Mason Medical Center (Washington), and Geisinger Medical Center (Pennsylvania). The selected hospitals have a culture of following evidence-based guidelines, and they financially incentivize physicians and surgeons to use a comprehensive and medically conservative approach with surgery as the last option.

A third hospital wholesale buyer segment consists of different population health organizations. Population health is a proactive, continuous process that manages both clinical care and costs.[69] Market segmentation and targeting are at its core. The primary goals of population health are improving and maintaining health to reduce the need for medical services, decrease hospital admissions, and eliminate readmissions especially for chronically ill consumers. Population health is based on calculating consumer risk scores and segmenting consumers by health care needs. A risk score represents the likelihood that an individual will experience a particular health outcome based on clinical data and lifestyle indicators like smoking, exercise, obesity, and others. Large datasets of consumer risk scores are analyzed and segmented using algorithms to chart how those factors influence ultimate outcomes. Examples of the targeted outcomes are hospital admissions, readmissions, emergency department visits, or the likelihood of developing heart disease, diabetes, cancer, or another disease.

Payers and providers use risk scores to estimate costs, target interventions, gauge a patient's health literacy and lifestyle choices, and try to prevent patients from developing more serious conditions resulting in additional spending and worse outcomes. An example of a population health study is the Framingham Risk Score for cardiovascular disease. This decades-long study of thousands of consumers by the National Heart, Lung, and Blood Institute uses risk scores to predict the likelihood of a cardiovascular disease diagnosis within 10 or 30 years.[70]

A hospital can target payers for value-based population health contracts by forming (1) a population health service organization (PHSO), (2) a clinically-integrated network (CIN) or (3) an ACO. PHSOs collaborate with local health stakeholders to assess their community's health needs and then lead the process to fill those gaps.

The primary PSHO community health assessment tool is a quantitative consumer marketing research study. This study is used to segment and target consumers based on social determinants of health and health needs such as post-acute and home health services, care coordination, telemedicine, and preventive care. The AtlantiCare—Geisinger health system in New Jersey developed a PHSO to manage patient navigation services. This service advises consumers with decisions related to complex cancer care, or whether to go to the ED or an urgent care center. The PHSO is also partnering with Medicare Advantage plans to manage and market nontraditional hospital services such as adult daycare, home-based palliative care, and transportation for medical appointments.[71]

A clinically-integrated network, or CIN, is essentially a collaboration among physicians and hospitals to develop clinical initiatives to improve local health care service quality and efficiency. CINs are recognized by the Federal Trade Commission as a safe harbor for joint management and pricing of health care services. CINs negotiate payments with payers, have patient data sharing systems, and track population health to improve quality and reduce cost.

The LCMC Healthcare Partners is a CIN developed by the LCMC Health system in New Orleans. LCMC Health includes Louisiana Children's Hospital, Touro Infirmary, three community hospitals, and physician clinics. About 30% of the health system's patient population receives medical services through value-based contracts. Nearly 900 physicians are participating in the CIN including 270 primary care physicians. In its first year in 2018, the LCMC CIM generated $3.6 million in gains from value-based contracts through improved quality performance and shared savings.[72]

ACOs were mandated by the ACA to manage population health. They include local physicians, hospitals, and other health care providers focusing on the health of a prescribed population. The Heartland Regional Medical Center ACO (St. Joseph, Missouri) was one of the first ACOs to join the Medicare Shared Savings Program (MSSP) in 2012. Heartland operates 63 clinics and the community's only hospital. It won a Malcolm Baldrige National Award for Quality in 2009 for having a culture that demonstrates continuous community health performance improvement. Heartland was one of only four ACOs that chose the MSSP two-sided risk model with a larger share of savings (60% vs. 50%) and larger risk of losses.

The ACO oversees care for 135,000 Medicare patients as well as members of three commercial health plans. Its first-year objective was to make rapid changes by enhancing EHR quality reporting at the point of care and enabling physicians to identify patients' unmet medical needs. A health IT team built a data dashboard that opens to a comparison of how a patient's care compares with evidence-based standards, and it flags gaps in care such as missed cancer screenings and lab tests for patients with chronic conditions.

The data analytics team then built a system to automatically generate lists of at-risk patients, including those with multiple chronic conditions and those deemed to be at rising risk because of elective surgery or an acute condition. The software mines hospital and emergency department records, medical charts, and billing data to find patients with total treatment costs in the top 15% of ACO patient spending.

Care managers then follow up with at-risk patients on the daily list by phone, through office visits, and in some cases, by visiting patients in their homes. The ACO's marketing strategy also includes educating physicians about new quality improvement priorities and providing them with quarterly performance reports to help them identify deficiencies. As a result, Heartland reduced overall spending by roughly 15% in the first year of the program. The ACO received a $2.9 million performance bonus representing 60% of the total savings from CMS.

The most important reasons for Heartland's success was effectively communicating and educating providers about the goals of the ACO, developing an effective care management program, and using data to monitor areas for improvement. Heartland engaged physicians, managers, and hourly wage employees by restructuring their financial incentives to support the new quality measures. It also increased patient engagement by communicating with Medicare beneficiaries about the benefits of the ACO model through newsletters and by creating community through activities like walking groups.

## 2. Segmenting and Targeting Retail Buyers

The retail market segmentation and targeting processes for consumers and referring physicians are similar to the wholesale buyer process. The population of the consumer market and physician market are important for estimating segment size. Both markets will vary by primary care, specialty care, inpatient care, outpatient care, and the numbers and locations of hospital competitors.

A common approach to estimating the primary hospital consumer market is to analyze patient origin by ZIP code. The primary market is defined geographically by the ZIP codes associated with 75% of total hospital volume. The size of the hospital market is the aggregate populations of these ZIP codes. The size of the physician market is calculated by counting the number of primary and specialty physicians in these ZIP codes. The list of physicians should be supplemented with other physicians who refer patients to the hospitals but who have practices located in other ZIP codes.

Consumers can be segmented by location, demographics, payer type, psychographics, customers and non-customers, and other characteristics. A conjoint survey was used to develop a value-based segmentation of a hospital consumer market (N=756). Respondents were screened for a hospital experience within the previous five years for cancer, cardiac, gastrointestinal, obstetrics, or orthopedics. Using paired-comparisons, consumers were asked to rank the importance of ten hospital attributes:

| | |
|---|---|
| 1. Clinical outcomes | 6. Patient satisfaction |
| 2. Physician recommendation | 7. Recommendation from friend or family |
| 3. Specialization in medical condition, | 8. Convenient location |
| 4. Out-of-pocket cost | 9. Amenities |
| 5. Pre-service price information | 10. Facility appearance |

Each consumer was then assigned to the segment with their highest average attribute importance score. Through the application of value-based segmentation to conjoint survey results, hospitals can understand which clusters of their consumer market gravitate toward different value propositions and how best to communicate with them (Figure 6.15).[73]

Physician segmentation is often analyzed by researching each physician's total number of patient hospital referrals, referrals by hospital, referrals to other physicians, patient referrals by health plan, and hospital revenue generated by referrals. Many hospitals employ physician liaisons to target referring physicians for incremental patient referrals. Physician liaisons usually have nursing backgrounds, strong physician communication skills, and call on physicians to build relationships. Based on a survey conducted by the American Association of Physician Liaisons, liaisons could be more effective. The survey found that liaisons met with physicians only 27% of the time that they called on practices, and most meetings were 15 minutes or less.[74]

Sentara Healthcare System, an eight-hospital system in the Tidewater area of Virginia, used secondary marketing research and sales to increase physician referrals. Sentara had an open medical staff, and most physicians referred their patients to multiple hospitals. They first identified the top 200 physicians by hospital admissions by ZIP code using quarterly admissions data supplied by the Virginia Hospital & Healthcare Association. Sentara then analyzed these physicians by hospital referrals and identified 70 physicians who referred at least 50% to 60% of their patients to Sentara hospitals. These 70 physicians were further analyzed

Value-Based Consumer Segmentation

| | "The clinicals"<br>Quality | "The values"<br>Price |
|---|---|---|
| Objective | • Physician excellence<br><br>• Clinical outcomes<br><br>• Medical condition specializations | • Pricing available before visit<br><br>• Out-of-pocket cost amount<br><br>• Value of outcomes/price |
| Subjective | "The high-touchers"<br>Reputation<br><br>• Patient satisfaction & loyalty<br><br>• Friend or family recommendation<br><br>• U.S. New & World Reports "Best Hospitals" ranking | "The atmospherics"<br>Facility<br><br>• Convenient location<br><br>• Level of amenities<br><br>• Appearance |
| | *Care-focused* | *Care-peripheral* |

FIGURE 6.15  *Value-based Consumer Segmentation.*

using data from the hospital internal billing system to update admissions data to analyze patient revenues.

The 70 physicians were then qualitatively analyzed and ranked by a cross-disciplinary team of Sentara managers including the director of referral sales and development, vice president of strategy, planning representatives, and service line directors. The physicians were evaluated based on the strength of their relationship with Sentara, their quality of care data, and the projected long-term financial value of each physician relationship.

This consensus-based approach reduced the target to the 35 physicians with the highest potential for increased referrals at Sentara. This number of physicians was manageable for the Sentara physician sales people to target for more referrals. The result was that targeting increased revenue for these physicians by 38% from $26.8 million to $36.9 million.[75]

Innovative hospitals are moving beyond physician referral and volume marketing and are focusing on physician performance improvement. For example, 500-bed Monmouth Medical Center in Long Beach, New Jersey, analyzed quality and cost data for congestive heart failure patients and their affiliated physicians. The data sources were from hospital billing, cost accounting, medical outcomes, and physician practice pattern reports.

These data were then examined in the context of specific cardiovascular DRGs to target patient cases with above average congestive heart failure lengths of stay, significant variability in care, and below average outcomes. Monmouth used this data to target and assist 44 physicians—who had five or more congestive heart failure cases—to help them improve their clinical outcomes and patient reimbursement.[76]

### 5.   *Marketing Problem*—Hospitals are Now Competing for Market Share Based on Value. How Do Hospitals in the Same Market Differentiate Themselves to Gain Share?

Hospitals can segment the market and target different wholesale and retail buyers, but there will inevitably be direct competition. One approach is to merge with other area hospitals, and another is to increase promotion spending to become the "share of voice" market leader. Both of these strategies have potentially high levels of financial risk.

### *Marketing Solution*—Create and Implement a Hospital Positioning Strategy.

Completion of segmentation and targeting strategies prepare hospitals for the development of product positioning strategies. The purpose of positioning is to communicate a single product benefit that meets a target need and is differentiated from competitors.

The standard positioning format includes a target market, a product, the frame of reference or product category, a primary benefit that data show is valuable to the target, and a differentiating attribute that supports the benefit. The positioning strategy is consistently implemented through marketing communications and the customer experience.

> To (the target market), the (product) is the brand (frame of reference) that (primary benefit) because (key differentiating attributes).

A medical device, pharmaceutical, or health information system company that markets a physical product needs a different positioning for each product. Johnson & Johnson uses the positioning "For heartburn sufferers, PEPCID AC® is the brand of OTC drug that works in 15–30 minutes to reduce stomach acid production because it contains an H2 blocker." Hospitals and other entities that market services, however, position the organization and individual products.

Hospital wholesale buyers and retail buyers want different benefits and will need different hospital positionings. The development of a positioning strategy begins with consumer research to understand different perceptions of the hospital. Engaged consumers are having a stronger influence on hospital selection. The health care information sources most valuable to consumers in making a hospital buying decision are recommendations from friends and family, online information, and reviews from other consumers. Rankings for the most important hospital selection attributes are participation in the consumers' insurance network, quality of care, staff expertise, the cost/value ratio, staff friendliness, and advanced technology.[77]

Healthgrades consumer marketing research found that ease of accessibility and appointment availability were the two highest priorities for consumers with lower acuity problems such as flu or a sore knee. Specialty physician quality ratings were most important for consumers with higher acuity problems such as abdominal or head pain.[78] A *Journal of Patient Safety* found that if consumers were given safety and cost data, 97% of consumers chose the safer hospital regardless of cost.[79]

The semantic differential is a marketing tool that can help a hospital begin the development of a positioning strategy using a five-stage process[80]:

1. *Explore a comprehensive list of hospital dimensions*: Researchers need to ask a sample of consumers to identify all the dimensions or characteristics that come to mind when they think about a particular hospital. If a respondent suggests "quality of medical care," this dimension is coded using a five-point or seven-point bipolar adjective scale, with "inferior medical care" at one end and "superior medical care" at the other. Other examples of dimensions consumers may mention include the range of hospital services offered, condition of the buildings, level of customer service, size of the hospital, and research versus community orientation.

2. *Edit the list of relevant dimensions*: The number of dimensions mentioned could be large, and the list should be evaluated and grouped based on similarity and frequency of mentions.

3. *Administer the instrument to a sample of respondents*: The respondents are asked to rate one dimension at a time. The bipolar adjectives should be randomly arranged so that the unfavorable adjectives are not all listed on one side.

4. *Averaging the rating results for each dimension*: Each hospital's image is represented by a vertical "line of means" that summarizes average perceptions of that hospital (Figure 6.16). Hospital A is perceived as large, modern, friendly, with superior medical care. Respondents view Hospital B as being the most specialized medically, with the most modern facilities, and having a high level of customer service. Hospital C, in contrast, is seen as small, dated, impersonal, and with comparatively inferior medical care

5. *Evaluating the variance*: Each hospital's line of means does not reveal the level of variability for each dimension. How many respondents perceived that Hospital B had the most modern facilities? Did the respondents have an actual

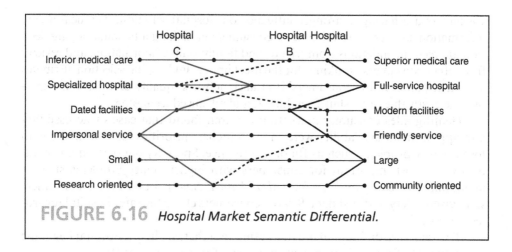

**FIGURE 6.16** *Hospital Market Semantic Differential.*

customer experience at this hospital and how long ago? It is also important to understand the demographics of the respondents. For example, if a hospital is specializing in maternity and other women's health needs, then the perceptions of men age 50 and older may not be relevant to their positioning.

### Examples of Three Hospital Positionings

These examples are the high-quality care positioning, the convenience positioning, and population health positioning.

### 1. High-Quality Hospital Positioning

The high-quality positioning is focused on best-in-class care and being a "destination" hospital or health system. In most local markets there is one hospital that has the evidence-based clinical outcomes and cost-effectiveness data to support this positioning, and this is usually an academic medical center. The high-quality positioning requires an extensive clinical care partner network that supports an equally strong care continuum. This network includes primary care physicians, specialist physicians, and post-acute care service providers including rehabilitation, home health, assisted living, and skilled nursing organizations.

The high-quality hospital positioning is attractive to wholesale purchasers such as health plans, employers, and ACOs. These purchasers expect real-time access to admission, discharge, and transfer data in order to monitor and influence care delivery decisions. Data sharing, mutually defined standards of care, and coordinated discharge planning are needed to effectively manage their patients. Consumer preferences for high-quality care partners is also important. Examples of hospitals with a high-quality care positioning are found in the annual *U.S. News & World Report* Best Hospitals rankings. The 2019 rankings compared more than 4,500 medical centers across 25 specialties, procedures, and conditions, with165 hospitals nationally ranked in at least one specialty. The Honor Roll ranked the top 21 hospitals in the U.S. overall. Best hospitals were also ranked by state and by metropolitan statistical area (MSA).[81]

## *U.S. News and World Reports*

### *Best Hospitals Honor Roll 2019–2020*

1. Mayo Clinic
2. Massachusetts General Hospital
3. The Johns Hopkins Hospital
4. Cleveland Clinic
5. New York-Presbyterian Hospital-Columbia-Cornell
6. UCLA Medical Center
7. UCSF Medical Center
8. Cedars-Sinai Medical Center
9. NYU Langone Hospitals
10. Northwestern Memorial Hospital
11. University of Michigan Hospitals—Michigan Medicine
12. Stanford Health Care—Stanford Hospital
13. Brigham & Women's Hospital
14. Mount Sinai Hospital (NY)
15. UPMC Presbyterian Shadyside
16. Keck Hospital of USC
17. University of Wisconsin Hospitals
18. Tie: Hospitals of the University of Pennsylvania-Penn Presbyterian
18. Tie: Mayo Clinic Hospital (Phoenix)
20. Tie: Houston Methodist Hospital
20. Tie: Yale New Haven Hospital

2. Convenience Hospital Positioning

A convenience-based positioning aligns with consumers' needs for hospital services such as maternity, diagnostic testing, rehabilitation, physical therapy, and urgent and emergency care. Consumers also want competitive prices, easy access, and personalized services. Convenience is often a strength of community hospitals with a number of ambulatory satellite offices. Competitors will be other community hospitals in the market as well as national retail clinics at Target, CVS, and Walmart and concierge medicine practices such as MDVIP.

A hospital needs a unique, valuable competitive advantage to differentiate itself from market competitors. Online scheduling can be a differentiator that allows hospitals to acquire more patients. A Healthgrades study found that about 80% of consumers prefer online scheduling across both primary care and specialties. The consumers who most prefer online scheduling book more appointments and tend to be younger, more affluent, and higher-educated. When given a choice between physicians with similar experience, proximity, availability, and patient satisfaction ratings, the vast majority of consumers (81% for PCPs, and 77% for specialists) choose the physician who provides online scheduling.[82]

Benefis Health, a rural 220-bed health system in Great Falls, Montana, uses online scheduling from Experian Health. The patient scheduling tool is a data-driven scheduling platform that improves patient access. About 50% of Benefis appointments are now booked online after business hours, and this percentage is increasing. Hospitals can analyze their appointment data to further improve access. Additionally, Benefis combines scheduling with the Experian Health mobile patient financial tool. Patients use this tool to receive an accurate price estimate based on their insurance plan. Patients can also choose to make an advance payment or other payment arrangements.[83]

3. Population Health Hospital Positioning

A third hospital positioning focuses on integrated population health management. This hospital positioning is effective in targeting health plans, ACOs, and employers interested in value-based health care contracts. The hospital needs to first segment and target a comprehensive network of ancillary providers. These organizations will be evaluated to potentially partner with the hospital for preventive, ambulatory, and post-discharge services. Each partner needs to be accountable for measuring quality outcomes and for sharing financial risk and savings. Additionally, this network of providers needs to use a common health information system to share a wide range of patient information.

Once this infrastructure is in place, the hospital needs to be able to estimate health outcomes and costs for its market. This analysis should cover incidence of specific diseases, health risk factors, and current utilization costs. A forecast is then prepared to project how costs can be reduced for specific diseases and conditions and how health outcomes can be improved.

Before entering risk-based contracts with wholesale buyers, a hospital must segment and analyze three consumer health segments: heavy users, escalating users, and potential users. Hospital care managers will be assigned to heavy users to actively monitor their chronic conditions. Escalating users will be managed through medical homes that nurture close personal relationships with consumers, especially those with chronic conditions. Potential users will be targeted for preventive services including health education programs, networking and social media groups, and online virtual primary care.

Hospitals can adopt the population health management positioning incrementally. For example, organizing a care network that contracts with one employer to provide one or two related medical specialties has been shown to be effective in gaining population health management experience, improving outcomes, and generating savings.

Kaiser Permanente has a long track record for integrating the Kaiser Foundation Health Plan, the Kaiser Foundation Hospitals, and the Permanente Medical Groups with population health management tools. Kaiser Permanente started Thrive Local, a new social network initiative in 2019, by partnering with health IT company Unite Us. The purpose of Thrive Local is to more effectively connect the 12.3 million Kaiser patients with the community services such as housing, food, and transportation. The program will enable providers and caregivers to seamlessly match an individual's social needs with the appropriate services from within a robust network of nonprofit, public, and private resources. The network of resources will be integrated into Kaiser Permanente's EHR system.[84]

### 6. *Marketing Problem*—Hospitals are Interested in the Financial Benefits of a High Net Promoter Score, but They are Struggling to Increase Loyalty, Revenue, and Margins.

It is a simple task to ask customers the NPS question "How likely are you to recommend our hospital to family and friends" on a scale of 1 low to 10 high. Many hospitals have added this Recommend question to a patient satisfaction or other marketing research study, but no further action was taken.

### *Marketing Solution*—Develop and Implement a Net Promoter Operational Program.

Most hospital satisfaction research lacks credibility, has not led to changes in business processes, and has not led to increased satisfaction. Net Promoter is an operational change management program and not a research project. A research project creates insights for a group of managers, but an operational program will engage the entire hospital in improving customer relationships.

An operational approach begins with understanding which customer data and internal processes can be used to create change across the hospital.[85] Hospital Net Promoter programs are effective if they (1) have a customer-driven organizational culture, (2) use a Net Promoter loyalty roadmap, (3) map the customer experience, (4) conduct ongoing marketing research, and (5) create a comprehensive customer experience strategy.[86]

1. Is Your Culture Really Customer-Driven?

The NPS is an ideal tool to help create a customer-driven culture. It accounts for both rational and emotional customer behavior, and it can provide results in real-time. The results enable employees to act quickly on what they can learn from customers. A study of organizations that are using NPS found that 68% of executives said that their organization was highly customer-driven. Unfortunately, only 15% of those organizations actually demonstrated customer-driven behavior.[87] An NPS program can help align customer expectations, perceptions, and experience, but an organizational transformation is often needed to create customer-driven behavior[88]:

a) Customer experience is embedded as a core cultural value.

b) Executive management visibly leads the Net Promoter program.

c) A customer loyalty strategy has been developed, communicated, and accepted by all employees.

d) Line management drives activities based on customer feedback.

e) Employee goals and incentives are tied to customer experience.

Potential roadblocks in reaching these goals are employees and executives who may be skeptical that loyal customers actually determine business results. They may believe that customer loyalty is the organization's "next big idea" and interest will eventually fade. Employees may also feel threatened that their authority may be eroded. These impediments may be avoided by beginning with a pilot Net Promoter program in a department with less complicated customer problems and high financial payouts. The pilot can build credibility and organizational momentum by making relatively simple customer experience improvements and reporting surprising loyalty insights.

Cancer Treatment Centers of America (CTCA) is a specialty hospital chain that has made advances aligning customer expectations, perceptions, and experience. CTCA was founded in 1988 on the principles of "patient-empowered medicine." With facilities in Chicago, Philadelphia, Tulsa, Phoenix, and Atlanta, CTCA patients experience a personalized, integrated, and coordinated approach to cancer care. Lab turnaround times are the fastest in the industry, physicians are required to quickly return patient phone calls, and a travel planner arranges patient transportation to appointments. In addition to chemotherapy, radiation, and immunotherapy, patients receive non-traditional services like laughter therapy, massages, and organic food.

The CTCA NPS ranges from the high 80s to the low 90s and compares favorably to the average hospital NPS of 55.[89] The CTCA culture supports this high level of loyalty, and four principles are followed to maintain focus on patients. *Real-time consumer feedback* is gathered and clearly communicated so front-line employees can use it to make better decisions and enhance the customer experience. All customers complete surveys including NPS ratings at discharge, and focus groups are conducted weekly and observed by staff at various levels across departments.

The best feedback is worthless if there is no *follow-up*. Every customer receives a call after discharge, employees are contacted following weekly focus groups to resolve patient problems, and clinicians meet three times per week to resolve problems in their areas. Board member meetings begin with patients presenting a specific customer experience, and the meeting does not continue until the problem is resolved.

*Employees are trained* and given the tools needed to meet customer expectations. Employees are screened during hiring to ensure that they have the customer attitudes needed to succeed at CTCA, and all employees attend a two-day orientation that uses an innovative cross-departmental curriculum to improve employee understanding of different roles needed to create loyal promoters.

Finally, it is important to *measure loyalty often*. Patients are surveyed throughout their experience because the more often reports are released the more chances there are to try new approaches to learn if they improve results. CTCA understands that employee loyalty supports customer loyalty. Employees complete a NPS survey annually, and senior executives and board members review the results in employee town hall style meetings to fully understand the reasons for the scores. Employees and departments are analyzed to see which have the highest percentage of promoters. CTCA uses their patient tracking system to identify which employees had contact with each patient. This data shows, for example, which oncologists are generating the most promoters. The approaches used by these physicians are analyzed, and then the outstanding physicians train other CTCA physicians.[90]

## 2. Develop a Net Promoter Loyalty Plan

A customized Net Promoter loyalty plan guides the development of the program and focuses on operational and structural improvements. The plan is designed to enhance customer experience and loyalty one customer at a time. These improvements can be rapid, involve fewer cross-team relationships, and use fewer organizational resources.

A customer calls a hospital to complain about a billing statement that was due before an extended medical procedure had been completed. An example of an operational improvement is when the billing manager apologizes, empathizes with the situation, and extends the payment due date to support service recovery. The customer has been changed from a detractor to a promoter.

Structural improvements take more time and have a greater impact on customers. These changes deeply affect organizational processes and employees in areas such as product or service delivery, pricing, distribution channels, and R&D. They involve more data, cross-functional team coordination, information technology, and an additional investment in time. The hospital in the example here can achieve a structural improvement if the projected financial benefit of increasing the number of promoters is more than the costs of reduced cash flow and the expense of modifying the billing software.

The following Net Promoter roadmap summary has seven sections, and the timeline to fully execute the plan is typically one to three years depending on the hospital's culture.[91]

### *Net Promoter Loyalty*

#### *Plan Summary*

(1)   Executive engagement and proof points—Develop an economic argument for the association between increased loyalty and increased revenue and profits.

(2)   Customer strategy and organizational context—Segment customers, identify customer touch points, and assess touch points for high financial value and potential improvement.

(3)   Internal communications and clear accountability—Implement a closed-loop process for operational improvements requiring focused communications in areas with the most impact. Empowered front line employees need to know what actions they can take and how to follow up with detractors and promoters.

(4)   Operational quick-win improvements—Rapidly complete small-scale service and loyalty improvements that will build momentum for cultural change.

(5)   Track record of trustworthy data—Collect trustworthy data that support an understanding of structural improvements and opportunities. NPS data need to be statistically valid and reliable before employee incentives are determined.

(6)   Strategic investments—The executive team can use trustworthy data to support investments. Data analysis provides confidence for making structural improvements.

(7)   Assesstment and ongoing improvements—Regularly evaluate the Net Promoter program to measure results and effectiveness. Performance is compared to goals and objectives, ROI forecasts, and incentives are reviewed and strategic options reassessed. Estimate the potential impact of reducing the cost to serve, forecast increases in long-term revenues and margin, and determine the level of loyalty and NPS needed to support the financial projections.

3. Map the Customer Experience

Understanding how hospital customers make purchasing decisions and the critical customer-hospital touch points are the crux of the loyalty plan. Build a model around what matters to specific customer segments based on a complete hospital experience. Hospitals are accustomed to defining the customer experience from the inside out, and they begin the improvement process by examining how individual internal departments operate. A more effective approach reverses this and views customer experience from the outside-in. This begins by researching how promoters make purchasing decisions.

Marketing communications influence hospital awareness, preference, and buying. Evaluating perceptions of brand communications will identify what messages are being received and how promoters are interpreting them. Analyze the consumer perceptions and attitudes related to specific communications including websites, referral sources, social media, and customer reference groups. Compare pre-purchase consumer brand attitudes to actual customer attitudes. The objective is to do a gap analysis between consumer expectations and customer experience for service touch points such as scheduling, registration, specific hospital services, facilities, billing and collections, and others.

In addition to attitudinal data, customer experience needs to be segmented by demographics and behavioral perspectives. One health system found that respect was especially important to less educated, lower-income patients and those who had frequent hospital stays. A higher percentage of men and the elderly ranked compassion as extremely important, while more educated and younger patients responded that being kept informed was a critical requirement for loyalty.[92]

Hospital customer experience can be a mix of rational ideas and emotional feelings, and NPS probes both elements. Hospital customers may be under stress due to health concerns, but they will forgive less than perfect service if hospital employees are authentic and care about them. Identify the customer experience characteristics most important to each segment. A Bain & Company NPS research study found that promoters in a market recommended a hospital largely based on compassion and respectful care and care responsiveness. Detractors were most likely *not* to recommend a hospital due to lack of care responsiveness and a comfortable and convenient environment (Figure 6.17).[93]

4. Conduct Ongoing Customer Marketing Research

Customer experience is subject to change, and it needs to be continuously tracked through marketing research to stay current. Use ethnographic research techniques to observe actual customer experiences in progress. Conduct in-depth structured interviews with customers and employees who shared the experiences. Identify expectations and missed opportunities on behalf of both customers and employees.

Ascension Health, a large health system in St. Louis, established a customer loyalty baseline by conducting extensive research with over 1,800 patients. The information revealed that patients have specific expectations and needs around the clinical, environmental, and emotional aspects of their hospital experience. This research study led to an ongoing customer analysis process to identify and improve specific customer experiences.

An Ascension inpatient was given a NPS survey shortly after being admitted and diagnosed with adult-onset diabetes. Her NPS was an unenthusiastic 5 on the 0 to 10 scale. A nurse manager who reviewed her survey went to the patient's

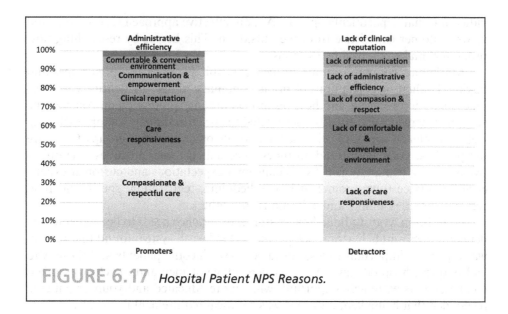

**FIGURE 6.17** *Hospital Patient NPS Reasons.*

room and learned that she was very troubled by the diagnosis, unsure about what she could eat at the hospital and when she returned home. The nurse manager then arranged for a dietitian to have a bedside consult to explain how best to change her diet. All Ascension patients are given a second NPS survey before discharge, and the diabetic patient NPS improved from detractor to promoter with an NPS of 10.

5. Create a Comprehensive Customer Experience Strategy

A customer experience strategy can be successfully implemented if a hospital uses research to build a model of what matters to their customers, makes operational changes to eliminate customer experience pain points, and designs innovative processes that deliver value from the customer's perspective. Research indicates that measuring the performance of different end-to-end customer "journeys," as opposed to individual touch points, is statistically linked to economic outcomes.[94] For example, an organization may be 80% successful at each customer experience stage, but only 30% of customers will have an overall positive experience.

## CHAPTER SUMMARY

Hospital marketing has evolved from a focus on publications and communications to a strategic management function covering all of the elements of a marketing plan. The size of the hospital market has been decreasing, and hospital margins are declining due to reimbursement changes. Hospitals are faced with becoming more accountable for outcomes, increasing quality improvements, and for managing population health. Many hospitals have responded to market forces by joining health systems, acquiring physician practices, and participating in mergers and acquisitions.

Hospital patients have evolved and become consumers because they are paying more for their health care, are interested in a better customer experience, expect more convenient access to care, and need understandable pricing. Disruptive companies using innovation have entered the hospital market, and this trend is further decreasing hospital financial margins.

Hospitals can use strategic marketing to increase reimbursement and improve clinical quality by increasing employee engagement; adopting evidence-based design; researching and meeting market needs; and applying segmentation, targeting, and positioning strategies. Market-driven hospitals are developing comprehensive NPS programs and re-evaluating operational processes and systems that improve customer experience, loyalty, and financial performance.

## DISCUSSION QUESTIONS

1. Hospital marketers are the primary channel between the environment and the hospital. What could local hospital marketers have done to monitor and recommend actions to reduce the threat of the Covid-19 pandemic to their hospital?

2. Some organizations that have developed successful Net Promoter programs recommend that they be led by executives from operations or finance divisions but not from marketing. Recommend how a hospital Net Promoter program should be led and the reasons for your recommendation.

3. All three community hospitals in a major market use the benefit of "high-quality care" as the basis of their positioning strategy. As a newly-hired health care marketing consultant for one of these hospitals, how would you develop a differentiated strategic positioning?

4. Research studies have shown that surgery patients in rooms with more natural lighting took less pain medication. Their drug costs were 21% less than for equally ill patients assigned to darker rooms. How could a hospital use this study to enhance its product design strategy and to market its surgery services to patients, physicians, and payers?

5. You are a hospital marketing vice president, and your team has identified a market opportunity for a new "men's health" product line. How would you organize the marketing function for this new program? What obstacles might you face? Who would you need to get involved to make the program a success? How would you evaluate its success or failure (in both economic and non-economic terms) after it has been rolled out?

## Hospital Marketing Case: A Struggling Rural Hospital is Revived through Market-driven Leadership, Innovative Thinking, and Technology in Remote Idaho

Mimi Rosenkrance, 58, was on her cattle ranch getting ready to vaccinate a calf. Unfortunately, the 1,000-pound mother cow decided that was not going to happen. She charged, knocked Rosenkrance over, and repeatedly stomped on her. Rosenkrance was dizzy, nauseated, had bruises spreading on both her legs and around her eye, and almost passed out. Her son called for a volunteer ambulance to drive her to Lost Rivers Medical Center, a small rural hospital in Arco, Idaho.[95]

The 14-bed hospital serves Butte County and covers an area half the size of Connecticut. Butte's population was only 2,597 in 2020, down from 2,893 in 2000. Although Lost Rivers has only one physician and three beds in its emergency department, Rosenkrance's customer experience was extraordinary. She immediately had a CT scan for a potential brain injury, X-rays for broken bones, an IV to replenish her fluids, and her ear sewn back together. Lost Rivers does not have a pharmacist, but Rosenkrance was prescribed and received the painkillers she needed.[96]

An estimated 16% of the U.S. population lived in rural areas in 2000, and 14% lived there in 2016. Rural hospitals in the U.S. have been closing at a rate of about one per month since 2010. The percentage of consumers on Medicare and Medicaid in rural areas is higher than in urban areas, and older and lower-income consumers typically require more intensive and expensive care.

Physicians are especially in short supply in rural areas, and physician recruitment in Idaho (population of 1.74 million in 2018) was particularly difficult. The state ranks 49th in physicians' per capita, and it is one of five states without a medical school. Lost Rivers faced all of these problems. The nearly 60-year-old hospital had dilapidated facilities, low morale, and reluctant patients. Lights were dangling from wires, a physician kept a diapered pet goat in the building, and horses were brought in routinely for X-rays. The hospital owed millions in back taxes and penalties, had filed for bankruptcy in 2010, and was on the verge of closing in 2013.

The resurgence of Lost Rivers Medical Center was largely due to new leadership that same year. Brad Huerta, a former administrator at Portneuf Medical Center in Pocatello—and an adjunct faculty member in health care administration at Idaho State University—was hired by the hospital board as CEO. Huerta was told on his first day by the outgoing CEO that $170,000 was needed for payroll by Friday, and the hospital bank account had just $7,000. His first task was to quickly secure a line of credit for payroll. Huerta then reduced the bloated headcount and began a campaign for a $5.6 million bond issue to support Lost Rivers. The bond passed by a two-thirds majority, and Lost Rivers was able to emerge from bankruptcy.

Huerta's primary strategy to rebuild Lost Rivers was grounded in changing the culture, innovation, and technology. He instituted a new philosophy: If it doesn't happen at a "real" hospital, it doesn't happen at Lost Rivers. Huerta saved money and built community by asking Arco residents to help renovate clinic exam rooms. Huerta brought in more rotating specialists to support cardiology, orthopedics, mental health, gastroenterology, and women's health. He started using telemedicine to connect the hospital to experts elsewhere, and is now planning to open a surgery center and a long-term care rehabilitation wing.

The pharmacy relies on technicians and students from Idaho State University to fill prescriptions, and their supervisor is a pharmacist at the University who checks their work remotely. Patients who want to talk to the pharmacists use a small private room with a phone and video link. To bring in more revenue, Huerta applied for grants to create the first Level IV trauma center in Idaho. Lost Rivers now gets paid more for the high-acuity emergent care it was already providing. The hospital also now has a helicopter pad for emergencies that cannot be handled at Lost Rivers.[97]

Huerta ensured that Lost Rivers adopted an EHR prior to the January 1, 2016 federal government deadline to qualify for a $650,000 government bonus. Lost Rivers used the EHR to increase the speed of collections, scrub claims to find revenue that would otherwise have been lost, and moved medical records to a cloud-based system that did not require more information technology employees.

Lost Rivers posted an $800,000 profit in 2015 and had the highest level of hospital patient satisfaction in Idaho. Despite Huerta's efforts, however, the long-term success of Lost Rivers is not guaranteed. He has to concentrate on retaining the customers the hospital has and continue to give them a reason for returning. So far, however, the market driven-approach seems to be working.[98]

## CASE QUESTIONS

1. Retaining customers is a challenge for rural hospitals. According to the U.S. Census Bureau, the average lifetime value of an individual health care consumer is $1.4 million, or $4.3 million for a family of four.[99] Another study found that consumer outmigration cost one-half of U.S. hospitals 10% of annual revenue and one-fifth of hospitals 20% of revenue.[100] Since outmigration is a particular problem for rural hospitals, what consumer loyalty marketing advice could you give to Brad Huerta? What can Lost Rivers do as a local stakeholder to influence population growth?

2. Hospital ad spending was an estimated $4.9 billion in 2017, and it was estimated to grow 1.8% annually.[101] Unfortunately, measuring ad spending ROI has been difficult.[102] A new Lost Rivers Medical Center board member sug-

gested that the hospital consider an advertising campaign. As the Lost Rivers vice president of marketing, how would you respond?

3. The marketing imperative has three parts: target the right customers and build relationships, offer solutions that meet their needs, and define quality packages that are differentiated and have a competitive advantage. How did the Lost Rivers CEO Brad Huerta implement the marketing imperative? What else could Huerta do to further implement the marketing imperative?

# CHAPTER

# MARKETING HEALTH TECHNOLOGY

## LEARNING OBJECTIVES

In this chapter we will address the following questions:

1. What are the characteristics of the medtech and health IT markets?

2. What are the most important environmental forces and trends that marketers need to manage?

3. How can health technology companies benefit from strategic marketing?

4. How can marketing tools be used to solve problems for medtech and health IT companies?

The World Health Organization defines health technology as the application of organized knowledge and skills in the form of devices, medicines, vaccines, procedures, and systems to solve health problems and improve quality of lives.[1] The traditional role of marketing in health technology companies has been to support the sales team and implement marketing communications. Innovation was limited to product enhancements developed in the R&D department.

Recent health care market changes have resulted in health technology companies adopting strategic marketing to align their offerings with customer needs. The purpose of this chapter is to explain health technology market characteristics, explore the market forces affecting health technology companies, identify market threats and opportunities, and show how strategic marketing can be used to solve health technology company problems.

## HEALTH TECHNOLOGY MARKET CHARACTERISTICS

Understanding the health technology market definition, size, and product segments is important for developing effective marketing strategies. This chapter focuses on medical devices (medtech) and health information technology (health IT) companies. Medtech products prevent, diagnose, and treat illness, disease, and injury. Health IT collects, stores, and transfers health care clinical, financial, and operations data and information. Consolidation of hospitals and value-based care have increased demand for electronic health records (EHRs) to support better clinical decisions and reduce medical errors. As of 2017, 97% of hospitals and 86% of office-based physician practices were using electronic health records.[2]

The Food & Drug Administration (FDA) regulates health technology. In the 1960s and 1970s, Congress increased oversight over medical devices by passing the Medical Device Amendments to the Federal Food, Drug, and Cosmetic Act. In 1982, the organizational units at the FDA that regulated medical devices and radiation-emitting products merged to form the Center for Devices and Radiological Health (CDRH).[3] The CDRH established the Digital Health program, which seeks to better protect and promote public health. The FDA is also working with the FCC and Office of the National Coordinator for Health IT (ONC) to propose strategies to regulate health IT. The FDA is particularly interested in the safety of medtech products that integrate health IT components.

### Medtech Products and Markets

*Definition*: The FDA defines medical devices, or medtech, as any instrument, apparatus, implement, machine, contrivance, implant, *in vitro* reagent, or other similar or related article. Medtech products are used to prevent, diagnose, and treat illness or disease. All medtech devices, equipment, and supplies are approved and regulated by the FDA. Medtech products are primarily developed using mechanical and electrical technologies that detect, measure, restore, correct, and rehabilitate areas of the body to improve health. Examples are simple tongue depressors and bandages and more complex programmable pacemakers, sophisticated imaging systems, dialysis machines, orthopedic implants, and others.

Unlike pharmaceuticals, medtech products do not achieve their intended use through chemical reaction and are not metabolized in the body.[4] Medtech companies are increasingly adding electronic systems to their devices to collect, transmit, and analyze data. These data are being used in mathematical and statistical applications to improve medical decision-making. Medtech products that include both a device and a drug—like a drug eluting cardiac stent—are classified as compound technology. The FDA has developed a special review process for these products.

*Medtech market size*: The medtech market is growing rapidly. The global medtech market is projected to grow from $387 billion in 2016 to $522 billion in 2022.[5] Global medtech revenue increased 4.3% from 2016 to 2017, but net income declined by 7.2% from $16.1 billion in 2016 to $14.9 billion.[6] The U.S. is the world's largest medtech producer with approximately 18,800 manufacturing facilities registered with the FDA. U.S. medtech revenue was $156 billion in 2017 representing 40% of global market revenue of $390 billion, and it is expected to grow to $208 billion by 2023.[7]

The U.S. is also the world's largest consumer of medtech products with annual imports surpassing $55 billion. The value of imported medtech products has also steadily increased resulting in a trade deficit. The top global medtech companies by revenue have headquarters in the U.S. and Western Europe, but China and other Asian countries are increasing their global market share (Table 7.1 and Figure 7.1).[8]

TABLE 7.1 **Top 10 Global Medtech Companies Billion $, 2016.**

| Rank | Medtech Company | Revenue | Specialization |
|------|-----------------|---------|----------------|
| 1. | Medtronic Ireland | $29.36 | Cardiac and vascular; minimally-invasive renal & surgical products; spine, brain, & pain therapies; and diabetes therapies. |
| 2. | Johnson & Johnson NJ | $25.10 | Expertise in surgery, orthopedics, and interventional solutions. |

## TABLE 7.1  *(continued)*

| Rank | Medtech Company | Revenue | Specialization |
|------|-----------------|---------|----------------|
| 3. | GE Healthcare IL | $18.30 | Medtech ranging from drug manufacturing and discovery to medical diagnostics. |
| 4. | Fresenius Medical Care Germany | $18.00 | Providing products and services relating to kidney failure and chronic disease. |
| 5. | Philips Healthcare Netherlands & MA | $16.00 | Specializes in cardiology, oncology, and women's health, in the areas of imaging systems, patient care clinical informatics, and home health. |
| 6. | Siemens Healthineers Germany | $14.10 | Centers around products and services for diagnostic and therapeutic imaging. |
| 7. | Becton Dickinson NJ | $12.42 | BD Medical and BD Life Sciences focused on diagnostics, gene and cancer research, and diagnosis of infectious disease. |
| 8. | Cardinal Health Ohio | $12.15 | Primarily a drug wholesaler, with sales also focused around surgical equipment and gloves. |
| 9. | Stryker Michigan | $11.30 | Provides services and products focused on neurotechnology and spine, medical and surgical, and orthopedics. |
| 10. | Baxter International Illinois | $10.16 | Mainly provides products related to renal systems, as well as dialysis and IV solutions. |

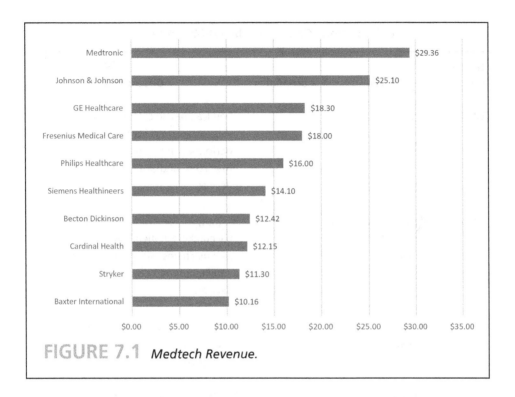

FIGURE 7.1  *Medtech Revenue.*

The U.S. Census Bureau uses seven North American Industry Classification System (NAICS) codes to estimate the size of the medtech industry (Table 7.2).[9] NAICS codes are used by federal statistical agencies to classify business establishments. Of the 6,500 medtech companies in the U.S., more than 80% (5,200) have fewer than 50 employees.[10] The states with the most medtech companies are California, Florida, New York, Pennsylvania, Michigan, Massachusetts, Illinois, Minnesota, and Georgia (Table 7.2).[11]

*Medtech product segments*: The FDA has regulated medical devices since 1976, and it segments medtech products into three classes based on safety, effectiveness, and risk. Products are classified by the risk the device poses to the end-user as well as the intended use of the device. A scalpel may have a low risk use of cutting tissue, but a manufacturer may also market a specialized scalpel specifically designed to make incisions in the cornea. A Class I device has a simple design and poses almost no potential risk; they represent 47% of medical products. Companies must register the device with the FDA, follow labeling and manufacturing guidelines, and alert the FDA prior to marketing. Examples of Class I products are elastic bandages, examination gloves, and hand-held surgical instruments.[12]

Class II devices are more complicated in design and have moderate to high risk. They must have special labeling, meet mandatory performance standards, and have post-market surveillance. Class II products represent 43% of medical

TABLE 7.2 **U.S. Medtech Companies by NAICS Code.**

| NAICS Code | Name | Companies | Description |
|---|---|---|---|
| 325413 | In-vitro diagnostic substances | 167 | Chemical, biological, or radioactive substances used for diagnostic tests performed in test tubes, Petri dishes, machines, and other diagnostic test-type devices. |
| 334510 | Electro-medical and electrotherapeutic apparatus | 2,560 | A variety of powered devices, such as pacemakers, patient-monitoring systems, MRI machines, diagnostic imaging equipment, and ultrasonic scanning devices. |
| 334517 | Irradiation apparatus | 274 | Includes X-ray devices and other diagnostic imaging, as well as computed tomography equipment. |
| 339112 | Surgical and medical instruments | 4,964 | Anesthesia apparatuses, orthopedic instruments, optical diagnostic apparatuses, blood transfusion devices, syringes, hypodermic needles, and catheters. |
| 339113 | Surgical appliances and supplies | 4,189 | Artificial joints and limbs, stents, orthopedic appliances, surgical dressings, disposable surgical drapes, hydrotherapy appliances, surgical kits, rubber medical and surgical gloves, and wheelchairs. |
| 339114 | Dental equipment and supplies | 1,334 | Equipment, instruments, and supplies used by dentists, dental hygienists, and laboratories. Specific products include dental hand instruments, plaster, drills, amalgams, cements, sterilizers, and dental chairs. |
| 339115 | Ophthalmic goods | 984 | Eyeglass frames, lenses, and related optical and magnification products. |

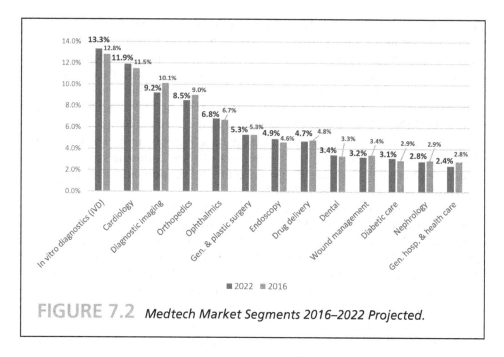

**FIGURE 7.2**  *Medtech Market Segments 2016–2022 Projected.*

products. Examples of Class II devices are powered wheelchairs, acupuncture needles, infusion pumps, X-ray machines, and surgical drapes.

Class III medical products have complex designs and high levels of illness or injury risk. Class III products follow the same guidelines as I and II, but they also require premarket approval by the FDA and a scientific review before marketing. Examples of Class III products are heart valves, implantable pacemakers, and breast implants. These devices are used to sustain or support life, are implanted, or present "potential unreasonable risk."[13] Class III products represent 10% of medtech products regulated by the FDA.

*Medtech market segments*: Medtech is used in a wide range of medical specialties. The four specialties of *in vitro* diagnostics (13%), cardiology (12%), diagnostic imaging (9%), and orthopedics (9%) represent 43% of the total medtech market. Market share for the top 13 medtech medical specialties for 2016 and 2022 (projected) are compared in Figure 7.2.[14]

### Health IT Products and Markets

*Definition*: Health IT is the use of computer hardware and software information processing for collecting, storing, retrieving, sharing, and using health care information, data, and knowledge to support decision-making.[15] The benefits of health IT are improved medical care, better public health, lower health costs, increased efficiency, reduced medical and administrative errors, enhanced customer experience, and optimized reimbursement. Health IT is used to manage hospital departments, medical treatment protocols, clinical trials, claims data, data analytics, electronic health records, and clinical and administrative decision software.[16] It is also essential for population health, customized precision medicine, the development of new clinical therapies, and giving consumers direct access to personal health data.

*Health IT market size*: The health IT market is smaller than the medtech market, but it is also growing rapidly. The size of the global health IT market was $183 billion in 2017, and it is projected to grow at a CAGR of 15.4% and reach $665.36 billion by 2026.[17] The Health IT market is highly fragmented, and there are no NAICS codes that classify health IT companies. The vast majority of health IT companies are privately held, and the number of these companies and their revenues are not publicly available. Figure 7.3 estimates the annual global revenues for the top 10 public companies in 2017.[18]

Another measure of the health IT market size is investment. Nearly $8.1 billion was invested in 2018, and this was 42% more than the $5.7 billion in 2017. There were 368 health IT deals completed in 2018 and the average deal size increased 38% from $15.9 million in 2017 to $21.9 million in 2018 (Figure 7.4).[19] Marketing channels strategies continue to evolve. Of the health IT companies that started with business-to-consumer (B2C) channels, 61% added business-to-business (B2B) and business-to-business-to-consumer (B2B2C) channels strategies. Fitbit had traditionally used a direct-to-consumer channel, but it is now adding an enterprise channel and marketing trackers and smart watches to employers, commercial insurance, and government payers.[20]

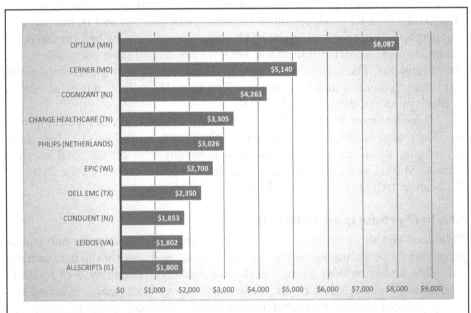

**FIGURE 7.3**  *Top Global Health IT Companies by Revenue, Million $.*

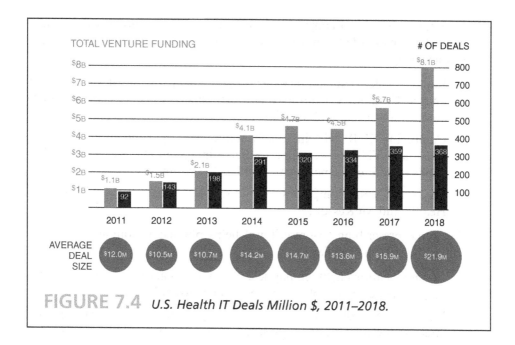

**FIGURE 7.4** *U.S. Health IT Deals Million $, 2011–2018.*

Health IT companies continue to consolidate to expand their portfolio of offerings. Livongo acquired Retrofit and its diabetes prevention program solution to increase its therapeutic offerings. Welltok acquired WellPass, itself a merger between Sense Health and Voxiva, following the acquisitions of health IT companies Mindbloom and Predilytics. ResMed closed out 2018 by acquiring Propeller Health for $225 million with the hopes of becoming "the global leader in digital health for COPD." This was just after ResMed announced a $750 million deal to acquire MatrixCare, an EHR company.

*Health IT product and user segmentations*: The health IT market has a wide range of product segments that are used by clinicians, managers, and consumers:

A. *Health IT Used by Clinicians*

1. The EHR is a central component of health IT infrastructure. Physicians use it to collect, store, and share patient medical information including medical history, test results, and medications:

   - An estimated 87% of physicians have installed an EHR.[21]

   - 35% of physicians reported lack of user-friendliness as the largest problem.[22]

   - EHR market leaders are Epic, Cerner, Meditech, Allscripts, athenahealth, McKesson, and Practice Fusion.

2. Picture archiving and communication systems (PACS) along with vendor-neutral archives (VNA) are widely used to help clinicians store and manage medical images:

- Radiology departments have been the primary repositories of medical images. Cardiology, neurology, and orthopedics are also becoming high volume producers of clinical images.

- Combining EHRs with images from different departments is a problem. PACS and VNAs are starting to merge imaging data stored in imaging banks in different departments and health systems.

- PACS and VNA companies include GE Healthcare, IBM, Carestream Health, and McKesson.

3. Electronic prescribing (E-prescribing) helps physicians communicate electronically with pharmacies:

- Communications between physicians and pharmacies have often been by fax, and paper prescriptions can be lost or misread.

- E-prescribing reduces prescribing errors by eliminating handwriting misinterpretations and giving physicians and pharmacists access to up-to-date prescription histories.

- E-prescribing prompts prescribers to completely fill out the dose, strength, and frequency, and it provides dosage checking and duplicate therapy alerts.

- E-prescribing companies include RxNT, CoverMyMeds, MDToolbox, and Surescripts.

4. Telemedicine and telehealth are terms with different meanings but are commonly used interchangeably:[23]

a) Telemedicine: According to the Center for Connected Health Policy, telemedicine refers to traditional clinical diagnosis, professional consultation, and remote monitoring that is delivered by technology. It can be accessed by consumers through phone, video, kiosks, web, and Bluetooth-enabled technology. Telemedicine services are divided into three categories:

- *Live video* uses teleconferencing technology in real-time for remote medical diagnosis and treatment. The benefit to consumers is convenient, on-demand access to primary and specialty care. Live video also supports remote tele-stroke video diagnosis, primary care consultations with specialists, behavioral health assessments of emergency department patients, and it is especially helpful in rural areas with physician shortages.

- *Store and forward* refers to a secure electronic communications system used to communicate information that has been previously collected. Common examples include emails sent through a patient portal, radiologic images sent from a rural hospital to a radiologist at an academic medical center, or an EKG sent from a primary care physician office to be interpreted by a cardiologist in another practice.

▪ *Remote patient monitoring* transmits patient medical data in real-time to a provider in a different location. It can track patient data or electronically remind patients to take readings when a patient is home or in another care facility. A study of 120,000 adult patients at 32 hospitals found that ICU telemedicine improved best practices, reduced response times, and encouraged usage of performance data.

b) Telehealth: This is a broader term that includes diagnosis and patient management applications, education, and other health care communications supported by technology. It is used in medicine, dentistry, counseling, physical and occupational therapy, home health, chronic disease monitoring and management, disaster management, as well as consumer and professional education.

Telemedicine and telehealth companies include American Well, CareClix, Doctor on Demand, Amwell, and Teledoc.

B. *Health IT Used by Both Clinicians and Managers*
Business intelligence (BI), big data, and analytics are interrelated processes and technologies used to support clinical and business decisions. BI can help health care organizations leverage market trends such as population health management, consumer needs, and risk-based contracting:

a) BI can supply data to answer questions such as which patients will respond to a particular treatment, how can hospital infections be detected earlier, how could the performance of a specific department be improved? If U.S. health care organizations collectively applied BI, a McKinsey & Company analysis indicated that savings would be between $300 and $450 billion annually.[24]

b) BI relies on "big data" from EHRs, consumer mobile devices, and clinical biometric sensors and other sources. For big data to deliver value, it needs to have three characteristics: high volume, high velocity, and a wide variety of data types. The data include structured and unstructured text, images, audio, video, and sensor traces. Artificial intelligence (AI) has the potential to use big data to predict the course of a disease and prescribe the best treatment, but this capability is not yet available.

c) BI is also used in operational analysis, predictive modeling, and clinical research. Examples are forecasting demand for hospital EDs, likelihood of strokes, and genetic and behavioral causes of disease.[25]

d) Companies that supply health care BI software include Qlik, IBM, SAS, SAP, Tableau Software, and MicroStrategy.

### C. *Health IT Used by Managers*

1. Revenue cycle and practice management are the processes that hospitals and physician practices use to manage claims processing, payment, revenue generation, and other functions.[26]

   a) When a patient schedules an appointment, management uses the system to confirm the appointment, verify insurance eligibility, and establish a patient account. Following the appointment, the system electronically transmits an insurance claim to the patient's insurance carrier that includes visit documentation, an ICD-10 diagnosis code, and a CPT procedure code.

   b) The claim is adjudicated by the payer and payment is sent to the provider. Commercial patients are then balance billed for the remaining amount approved by the payer (Medicare, Medicaid, and other government plans do not allow patient balance billing). The system manages claim denials, patient statement processing, and patient collections.

   c) Leading revenue cycle and practice management companies are athenahealth, Change Healthcare, Optum360, and NextGen Healthcare. Investments in these types of systems are predicted to grow by 16% annually with total spending projected to reach $7.09 billion by 2020.[27]

2. Electronic health information exchange (HIE) is the secure transmission of electronic health data among health care providers, payers, government agencies, and other health care organizations.

   a) The HIE market can be segregated into public and private exchanges.

   b) These organizations form a health data clearinghouse, enter an interoperability pact, and agree to share data among their systems. As an example, the State of Maine HIE has data for 98% of consumers and 90% of physicians.

   c) HIEs use a diversified set of health data, a master patient index, and sophisticated algorithms to build predictive analytics for precision medicine. A group of 20 behavioral health centers used HIE data to identify a high co-morbidity between mental health and chronic disease with a sample of 435 patients. Case managers used this information to reduce hospital mental health emergency department visits and reduced annual costs by $6 million.[28]

   d) Epic Systems, Medicity, RelayHealth, InterSystems, and ICA are companies that offer HIE services.

### D. *Health IT Used by Consumers*

1. Consumers frequently rely on the web for health reviews and personal health information. A sample of consumers were asked about health-related reasons for using the web, and the majority of consumers used the web frequently for researching personal health, paying insurance bills, and ordering prescription drugs (Figure 7.5).[29]

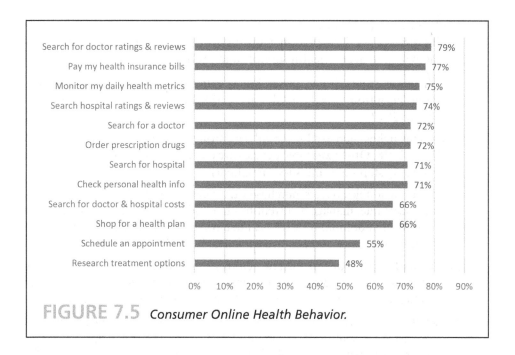

**FIGURE 7.5** *Consumer Online Health Behavior.*

2. A personal health record (PHR) is a consumer's self-maintained electronic health record, and PHRs have the potential to be as important as EHRs.

   a) PHRs help consumers improve their health by updating and sharing immunization records, lab results, screening due dates, blood type, and other health data.

   b) PHRs can be used with provider health portals to securely communicate with clinicians, pay bills, check service costs against insurance allowed amounts, download full medical records, order prescriptions, and schedule appointments.

   c) The Apple Health Record PHR program is integrated with the iPhone and patient portals at NYU Langone Health, Stanford Medicine, and 27 other health systems. Users can view all their medical records from their iPhone using encrypted Fast Healthcare Interoperability Resources (FHIR), a standard for transferring electronic medical records.[30]

   d) The CMS Medicare Blue Button 2.0 program is designed to help 53 million Medicare members securely share their personal health data with providers, clinical researchers, and digital health services. This includes drug prescriptions, primary care treatment and cost, and Medicare coverage. The program also allows research organizations to pre-populate medication lists as part of clinical trial enrollment, and it can help pharmacies assess medication adherence.[31]

3. Mobile health (mHealth) uses mobile phones and other devices to provide health services and information. Consumers track personal health and physical activity and access health services and products.

a) Consumer smartphone ownership is estimated to be 77%, and smartphone adoption among adults aged 65+ in the U.S. quadrupled from 2012 to 2017.[32]

b) Smartwatches increased in popularity from 32% of consumers in 2016 to 53% in 2018. Other wearable devices are earwear, wristbands, and clothing (primarily step-counting shoes in China).

c) 65% of wearables buyers purchased the devices to monitor general health, track heart rate, manage a current health condition, or prevent future health problems. In addition, 67% of wearable owners believe that their device has increased awareness and positively impacted their health and activity.[33]

d) Atrium Health is one of the few health systems to use smart speaker voice recognition in their digital innovation strategy. It created a Google Alexa skill that tells consumers the closest Atrium urgent care and its wait time.[34]

e) Cedars-Sinai in Los Angeles launched an Apple Watch app giving patients access to their health information and care team. The watch app pairs with Cedars-Sinai's patient app and allows users to contact their doctor, search for care locations, and track various elements of their health. The data is then shared with their care provider on their next visit. Importantly, this technology will increase Cedars-Sinai's customer engagement, loyalty, and brand equity by being an active partner in the user's daily wellness routine.[35]

f) Notable mobile health companies include Fitbit and Apple in the U.S. and Xiaomi and Huwai globally.

## FOUR ENVIRONMENTAL FORCES AFFECTING HEALTH TECHNOLOGY COMPANIES

Advancements in health technology are converging people, information, technology, and connectivity that are improving health care and outcomes. Four environmental forces, however, are responsible for trends that marketers need to understand and manage. These forces are social-cultural, economic, political-legal, and technological.

### *Social-Cultural Force:* Trend 1—Consumer Demand for Health IT is Increasing, but Data Security is a Growing Market Threat

Increased financial accountability has resulted in consumers becoming more engaged in their health. This interest in personal health data and information has been aided by advances in technology. Health IT companies are experiencing increased consumer engagement with their products and services.

A 2019 consumer survey found that 76% of consumers searched online for a diagnosis based on their symptoms, treatment options, prescription drugs side effects, or other personal health information. Almost half (44%) of respondents used health IT to track at least one health condition, and 75% shared this data with their physicians. Overall, 18% of consumers participated in online communities based on their particular acute or chronic condition. A quarter (23%) of respondents with a chronic condition joined the corresponding group on PatientsLikeMe, Mayo Clinic Connect, Facebook, or another community platform to exchange information on treatment and management of their conditions with fellow patients.

Nearly two-thirds (64%) searched for physicians and hospitals online. Of the consumers who searched for providers online, 43% selected a hospital and 58% chose physicians or nurse practitioners based on online reviews. Consumers indicated that they are increasingly using information found online to inform their provider choices and what they share in the exam room. This consumer behavior change is also affecting how they make health decisions, and it may conflict with the traditional paternalistic doctor-patient relationship (Figure 7.6).[36]

The *wearables* market continues to grow from 84 million sold in 2015 to 245 million projected in 2019.[37] A third of consumers now track their health using a smartwatch or other wearable device. Weight and blood sugar are the two most tracked measures primarily among consumers with obesity, diabetes, or heart disease. Consumer research indicates wearable technology is most often used for activity and fitness tracking, and consumers are increasingly using these devices to manage sleep and clinical diagnoses. The percentage mentioning sleep management has steadily grown from 22% in 2016 to 31% in 2018, and those using wearables for managing a diagnosis increased from 20% in 2017 to 30% in 2018.[38]

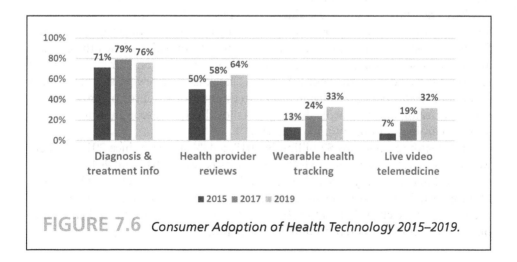

**FIGURE 7.6** *Consumer Adoption of Health Technology 2015–2019.*

A survey of hospital executives found that 47% of hospitals are providing wearables to consumers to manage chronic conditions and to remotely monitor in-home medical devices and smartphone apps. Consumers with diabetes and hypertension who use health trackers such as Fitbit or Apple Watch have been found to be more likely to take their medications as prescribed. Health plans are also offering members discounts on wearable devices or premiums. UnitedHealthcare has partnered with Fitbit and Apple Watch to launch its Motion program that offers monetary rewards. Aetna is collaborating with Apple to allow its members to purchase an Apple Watch and then "earn it back" through healthy behavior.

Wearables only improve health if consumers continue to use them. The percentage of consumers that reported they had stopped using their wearable increased from 27% in 2017 to 39% in 2018, and the number of consumers who stopped using a wearable in 2018 was higher than the number of consumers who began using one. The top reasons consumers reported for discontinuing use were that their health goals were achieved (39%) or that their wearable was not effective in achieving their goals (25%).[39]

Additionally, 64% of consumers indicated that they would continue to use a wearable if it could reduce the number of in-person doctor or hospital visits. Just over half of the surveyed patients (55%) visit a physician or specialist more than once per year. The three reasons consumers gave for wanting to reduce in-person visits were costs, distance traveled, and an overall dislike of health care facilities. This evidence shows that understanding consumer attitudes, motivations, and behavior is important to marketing wearables that improve health.[40]

Like online health search and wearables, *telehealth* is also growing, but consumer use has been relatively low. The Covid-19 pandemic, however, has increased the use of telehealth (see Political-legal force: Trend 3.3 Marketers can take advantage of changing reimbursement to increase use of telehealth, p. 265). Telehealth product segments are live phone, picture or video sent, email, live video, and text. Live video involves a real-time consumer-provider virtual meeting to diagnose illness or disease and to prescribe treatment. Examples of companies that provide live video are Doctor on Demand and American Well. Provider-to-provider telehealth products are remote patient monitoring and asynchronous information store and forward services. Store and forward telehealth allows clinicians to review patient health data and images prior to a patient evaluation. An estimated two-thirds of providers are using telehealth, and the medical specialties most likely to use it are primary care, stroke, neurology, radiology, and pediatrics.[41]

Telehealth revenue was $2 billion in 2018, a 44% increase since 2013.[42] There was a 39% increase in Medicare telehealth visits between 2016 and 2017, but consumer volume was only 334,140 and 465,515, respectively.[43] The Rock Health/Stanford Medicine 2019 consumer survey found that 32% of respondents had used live video telehealth, and the 2019 JD Powers' telehealth study indicated that only 10% of consumers reported using telehealth.[44]

Early adopters of telehealth are typically young, urban, wealthier, and privately insured. Of consumers aged 30 to 49, 34% used a virtual visit at least once, 63% of urban consumers used a visit for their child, and 51% of those with incomes greater than $71,000 have used telehealth. Between 14% and 18% of consumers with private insurance are users compared to only 4% with Medicare, Medicaid, or no insurance.[45] Consumers who had a prior, in-person visit with a provider, followed by a telehealth interaction with the same provider, were more likely to be satisfied (92%) with their telehealth visit than those without a prior personal visit (53%).[46] Consumers report that the types of virtual visits most appealing are a prescription question or refill, receiving results from an oncologist, a pre-surgery appointment, and ongoing care for a chronic condition.

An Advisory Board Company survey found that 77% of consumers reported a willingness to try a telehealth virtual visit, but repeat purchase was very low (Table 7.3). Research has also found that marketing can improve the telehealth customer experience and increase repeat purchases.[47] Saving consumers time is one of the advantages of telehealth services, but a telehealth visit often takes more time than consumers expect. The average experience lasted 44 minutes. This included 17 minutes to complete the enrollment process, nine minutes to wait for a physician or nurse practitioner, and 18 minutes for the actual consultation.[48] Consumers are willing to try a virtual visit if the cost is less than an in-person visit, the visit comes with a satisfaction guarantee, they have discussed a virtual visit in-person with their physician, and if a friend or family member recommends a virtual visit. Using the NPS analysis will help telehealth providers better understand the customer experience and improve customer loyalty.

TABLE 7.3  **Telehealth Consumer Visits.**

| Number of telehealth visits | Percent |
| --- | --- |
| 1 | 81% |
| 2 | 13% |
| 3 | 4% |
| 4 | 1% |
| 5+ | 1% |

Industry demand for personal health data is continuing to increase to support AI diagnostics and precision medicine, but consumer trust in *data security* is continuing to erode. Recent data security questions have been raised about access to personal genetic screening data (Veritas Genetics, 23andMe, and Ancestry), law enforcement, and the federal government. The *Wall Street Journal* reported that Facebook was collecting a range of health data from apps without user knowledge or permission.

The Health Insurance Portability and Accountability Act (HIPAA) requires hospitals, physicians, health plans, pharmaceutical companies and all their respective "business associates" to have safeguards that ensure the confidentiality of personal health data. Interestingly, data from health apps, direct-to-consumer genetic tests, and other consumer-focused health technologies are not covered by HIPAA. The reality is that consumers do not necessarily know where their data are located.

According to a consumer survey, most respondents were willing to share data with their physicians, but the percentage dropped to 73% in 2019 from 86% in 2017. Consumers were less likely to share with insurers, pharmacies, research institutions, tech companies, pharmaceutical companies, and the government (Figure 7.7).[49]

The survey also found several generational patterns concerning data sharing attitudes and behavior. Compared to consumers age 18 to 24, those age 45 to 54 were three times more likely to share data and information with their physician. This trend

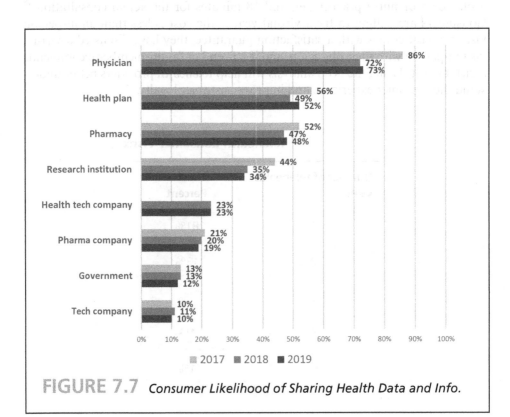

**FIGURE 7.7**  *Consumer Likelihood of Sharing Health Data and Info.*

increased further with those between 55 and 64 being eight times more likely to share, and those age 65 and older were 12 times more likely to share with their physician. Another association was that respondents who frequently interacted with their physician were substantially more willing to share with their physician. Respondents over the age of 45 were three to five times as likely to want to know what health data has been collected compared to the younger 18 to 24 age group.

Consumers who downloaded and used health apps are four times *less* likely to share data with their physician compared to consumers who did not download an app. These respondents were also twice as likely to share their health data with technology companies—the entities with the lowest overall level of consumer trust—compared to those who did not download an app. Consumers who use health care apps are three times less interested in being notified about the data collected about them compared to those not using apps.

Health IT companies have the opportunity to incorporate and communicate data security practices when targeting markets based on their age and data sharing preferences. Further, research can be done to analyze engaged early-adopters of health IT products and services who may be shifting away from traditional health care sources and toward sharing data with technology companies to meet their health needs. It will be important to understand the basis of these attitudes and behavior, measure the size of this market segment, and accurately forecast sales revenue and market share.

### *Economic Force*: Trend 2—Value-Based Care is Changing Medtech Buyer Attitudes and Behavior

Medtech customers have primarily been physicians and hospital approval committees. The rise of value-based payment has now added centralized health system procurement managers, clinical end-users, joint committees on patient outcomes, payers, and other participants in the continuity of care. These buyers are using systematic processes to evaluate medtech technical, implementation, and brand value along with additional focus on price bargaining strategies.[50] Health systems also want partners who will provide value-added services after product delivery. The frameworks below are being used by hospitals to evaluate medtech technical and implementation capabilities.

1. *How health systems are evaluating medtech technical and implementation capabilities.*

Health system managers first rate the importance of different medtech technical capabilities to the organization such as customization, automation, and server management by using a rating scale of high, medium, or low importance. They then rate each medtech offering for these capabilities using a scale of 1 = low to 5 = high (Table 7.4).[51]

Health systems are also evaluating medtech implementation capabilities. Health system managers determine the importance of different implementation capabilities including product testing, support, liability, and achieving financial expectations. Each medtech company is then rated using the 1 to 5 scale for implementation (Table 7.5).[52]

**TABLE 7.4** Medtech Technical Capabilities.

| Capability | | Health System Importance Ratings | | |
| --- | --- | --- | --- | --- |
| | | Medtech Co. #1 | Medtech Co. #2 | Medtech Co. #3 |
| **Customization** | How can the medtech product be customized? | | | |
| | Are peripheral measurement devices provided? | | | |
| | Can multiple devices be used simultaneously? | | | |
| | Is device communication Bluetooth, VPN, or cable? | | | |
| | Does the product include e-messaging, video, artificial intelligence, behavior tracking, group chat, blockchain, integration with other technologies? | | | |

**Automation**

Does the medtech product automatically map patient data to the hospital's EHR?

How reliable are the automatic data updates to the EHR?

Are cloud-based updates available 24/7?

**Server Management**

Are the medtech applications hosted in the cloud (virtual machines), on the medtech company servers, or on the hospital servers?

Will the medtech company monitor the servers 24/7?

Will hospital employees have any responsibility for maintaining the servers?

**TABLE 7.5  Medtech Implementation Capabilities.**

| | Capability | Health System Importance Ratings | | |
| | | Medtech Co. #1 | Medtech Co. #2 | Medtech Co. #3 |
|---|---|---|---|---|
| **Testing** | Will the medtech company lead testing of the offering? | | | |
| | What are the beta product testing procedures, metrics, and schedules? | | | |
| | Is there a user experience (UX/UI) specialist on the implementation team? | | | |
| **Support** | How will the company respond to potential equipment malfunctions and data breaches? | | | |
| | What is specifically included in the plan for employee training and ongoing IT support? | | | |

How does the medtech company meet customer service needs for clinical end-user consumers?

What types of consumer promotion and communications materials are available?

What are the product warranty and liability limitations and the clinical user credentialing requirements?

## Liability

What are the HIPAA compliance and security requirements, and how are they being met?

What has been the product's documented effect on outcomes and ROI?

## Financial

What are the upfront costs and annual maintenance fees?

2. *Market-driven medtech companies are proactively using value-based sales strategies.*

AdvaMed, the medtech trade association, developed a Strategic Value Initiative that supports medtech value-based marketing. AdvaMed conducted marketing research with hospitals and physicians to understand their perceptions and expectations of medtech value. This research led to the development of value frameworks that can be used by medtech companies that begin in product development. The frameworks identify and analyze end-user consumer needs, the needs of providers and other stakeholders, and also other health services and health IT solutions used in conjunction with the medtech product.

The four components of the AdvaMed framework analyze a product's (1) clinical impact, (2) non-clinical impact (e.g., customer experience and out-of-pocket costs), (3) care delivery revenue and cost impact, and (4) public and population health impact on the health care system, employers, and consumers (Figure 7.8).[53]

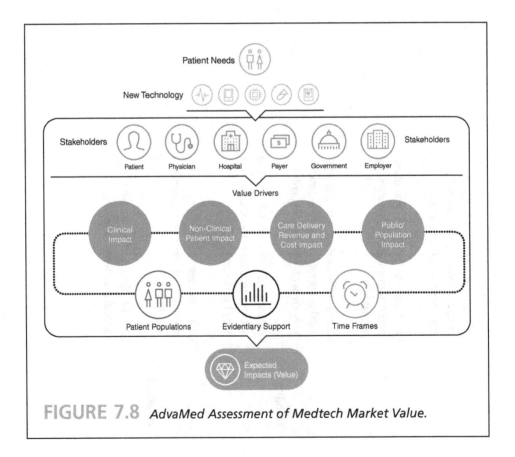

FIGURE 7.8  *AdvaMed Assessment of Medtech Market Value.*

Medtech product value is analyzed using quantitative and qualitative data such as the time and cost of acquiring and implementing the product, changes to customer clinical and operational protocols, and customer staff training needs (Table 7.6). Stryker's JointCOACH product offers joint replacement as well as a user-centered engagement and education platform. The product includes pre-operative preparation, medication information, and recovery information to help ensure a more effective procedure. Patients can use the platform to talk with their care team before surgery and up to 90 days post-discharge.[54]

## TABLE 7.6  AdvaMed Medtech Market Value Analysis Key Questions.

| Clinical Impact <br> *How does this technology...* | Non-Clinical Impact <br> *How does this technology...* | Care Delivery Revenue & Cost Impact <br> *How does this technology...* | Public & Population Impact <br> *How does this technology...* |
|---|---|---|---|
| Affect clinical outcomes compared to other treatment options? | Create more or less preferable options for the patient such as more accessible care settings or less intensive care settings? | Enable the most effective treatment, for a specific patient, at the best time, in the most appropriate location? | Impact life expectancy free of disability and other public and population health measures? |
| Impact patient safety to lower the risk of complications, be less invasive, compared to alternatives? | Enable patients, families, and caregivers to navigate, coordinate, and manage care effectively? | Affect costs to system workflows, care efficiency, site of care, and staff? | Lower unnecessary private and public spending? |
| Impact quality of life in the short and long term? | Impact affordability of treatment expense for different patients? | Help reduce costs associated with variance in clinical outcomes? | Improve provision of care, productivity, and attendance? |

Stakeholders are placing higher priority on using outcome-based payment models where manufacturer payment is linked to specific outcomes.[55] The value-based partnership between Johnson & Johnson's Animas Division and Aetna insurance for the J&J OneTouch Vibe and Ping insulin pumps has payments tied to the improvement of diabetic patient A1c tests. A1c measures blood glucose levels for a three-month period. UnitedHealthcare has a pricing agreement with Myriad Genetics, a molecular diagnostics company, for genetic tests in multiple therapeutic areas including breast cancer, prostate cancer, rheumatoid arthritis, and neuropsychiatry. The agreement provides UnitedHealthcare members with access to BRCA testing using the Myriad myRisk Hereditary Cancer test if they meet hereditary cancer testing eligibility criteria.[56]

Medtech value-based marketing reflects the marketing imperative because it builds ongoing relationships. Relationships are developed with providers, payers, and end-user customers to better understand and meet their respective needs. These new partnerships are fundamentally different from the traditional transaction-based medtech contractual relationships. The majority of surgeons surveyed (62%) indicate that the "strongest existing relationship" with a medtech company is an important purchasing consideration. Examples of a "strong relationship" were best value for price paid inclusive of wrap-around services and training. Ongoing training support was the most important value-added service for 54% of surgeons. In contrast, surgeons rank the traditional medtech sales role of communicating medical device benefits and attributes as only fifth in importance.[57]

Health systems also want a central point of contact for both sales and technical product information. Market-driven medtech companies have responded by replacing product-oriented sales people with strategic problem-solvers who can connect prospective customers with a range of medtech technical experts.[58] This organizational change is expected to financially payout according to a Bain Consulting NPS research study. The study found that medtech companies that implemented market-driven strategies had an average NPS of 30 compared to more traditional product-driven medtech companies that had an average NPS of 6.[59]

3. *Marketing research and strategic positioning can increase medtech market share.*

Most medtech companies are struggling to adapt to the new value-based buying model used by health system purchasers. Secondary and primary marketing research tools can be used to help understand how medtech customers are defining value, demand for different types of value, and the wants and needs of the individuals now participating in the customer buying process. This research supports the development of an effective medtech product positioning strategy using the standard positioning format. An effective positioning will improve the alignment between market needs and product benefits and give medtech companies a competitive advantage.

### *Standard Product Positioning Format*

*To (the target market), the (product) is the brand (frame of reference) that (primary benefit) because (attributes).*

A national marketing research study was conducted with 9,000 medtech health systems buyers to understand the most important medtech product benefits. The study identified the top 10 benefits based on total respondent mentions. Researchers calculated that the average benefit was mentioned by 81% of respondents. Researchers then ranked the five benefits above this average as primary benefits and the five benefits below this average as secondary benefits (Figure 7.9).[60]

The benefits were then analyzed to identify the product attributes that support each benefit (Table 7.7).[61]

The research also examined buyer perceptions of product benefits that were considered strong or weak points of differentiation. A differentiator was considered to be an unmet market need if the benefit performance score was below 60%. There was more differentiation opportunity for medtech products that focused on lower product risk, higher efficacy, consistent outcomes, patient outcomes, and being a proven and trustworthy brand. Supporting product attributes for these benefits are investments in clinical quality and proof of performance studies.

Weak points of differentiation included communicating a high-performing product feature, recommendation by an opinion leader, claiming the product will attract or retain patients, a comprehensive company product portfolio, and focus on a basic undifferentiated product benefit. Since most buyers think that medtech products perform similarly on these functions, promotional spending in these areas was not recommended.[62]

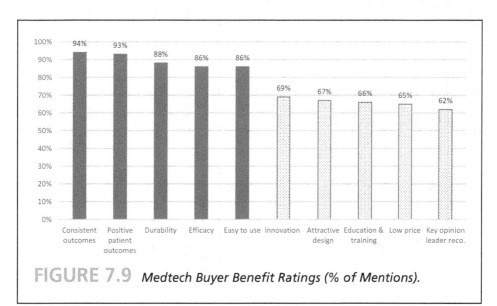

**FIGURE 7.9**  *Medtech Buyer Benefit Ratings (% of Mentions).*

TABLE 7.7  **Medtech Buyer Benefits Supporting Product Attributes.**

| Benefits—Above Average | Consistent Outcomes | Positive Patient Outcomes | Durability | Efficacy | Easy to Use |
|---|---|---|---|---|---|
| Product Attributes | Ensures consistent outcomes | Low patient discomfort | High wear resistence | Product performs as expected | Highly intuitive |
| | Confidence in quality outcomes | Improved patient experience | High-quality components | Short time to results | Simple to operate |
| | Predictable outcomes | High patient compliance | | Long-lasting performance | |

| Benefits—Below Average | Innovation | Attractive Design | Education & Training | Low Price | Recommended By Key Opinion Leader |
|---|---|---|---|---|---|
| Product Attributes | Cutting-edge materials | Appealing look & style | Offsite team training with other customers | Low cost to organization | Colleagues recommend |
| | Advanced technology | Contemporary design features | Certified trainers | Low cost to patients | Distributor recommends |
| | Product development focus | Sleek design | Custom training | Offers price promotions | Peers recommend |

The research also compared perceptions of benefit importance with product performance. All benefits were analyzed based on perceptions of importance and performance. If the average benefit performance score was lower than 60%, then the benefit was considered to satisfy an unmet need. The top six benefits with high importance and low performance gaps were patient outcomes, familiar procedure, efficacy, customer service, basic product features, and flexible contract options (Figure 7.10). By understanding the most important product benefits and the best opportunities for differentiation, marketers can effectively position medtech products to increase revenue.[63]

### *Political-Legal Force*: Trend 3—Regulation is Adapting to Better Support Health Technology Innovation

Medtech and health information technology customers want increased access to data and algorithms to improve clinical outcomes and to lower costs. Customers need health technology companies to be more market-driven and innovative to increase product value.

GE Healthcare has responded to this need by developing an AI app to help clinicians find the cause of rejected X-ray images and reduce the need for re-scans. Researchers are now using machine learning to extract large data sets from MRI, CT, and PET images to improve cancer diagnosis and better predict responses to treatment. The next step is to automate workflows that seamlessly integrate data output with other customer clinical applications.

1. *The medtech industry needs to further increase innovation and value.*

The medtech industry has been criticized by some as not sufficiently responding to customer needs for increased innovation. The EY *2018 Pulse of the Industry*

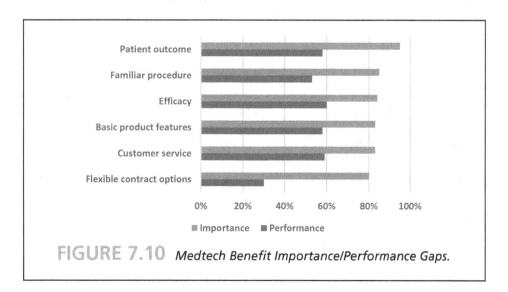

FIGURE 7.10 *Medtech Benefit Importance/Performance Gaps.*

reported that only 16 of the 43 therapeutic devices receiving FDA premarket approval between January 2017 and June 2018 had a health information component or made use of data analytics. Medtech capital investment was dominated by short-term growth strategies focused on returning cash to shareholders.

Some medtech companies have responded to this criticism by arguing that government regulation is responsible for their lack of innovation. The FDA requires that medtech products with the highest levels of risk—due to insufficient product safety data, and the absence of comparable products—must apply for approval as Class III devices. These products are required to follow the more time-consuming and expensive Premarket Approval (PMA) pathway for approval. FDA review of an application for premarket approval is supposed to take six months—twice as long as the 510(k) for Class I and Class II products—but it usually takes longer. A 510(k) is a premarket submission made to the FDA to demonstrate that the device to be marketed is as safe and effective and is substantially equivalent to a legally marketed device. It costs a manufacturer an average of about $94 million to bring a medical device onto the market through PMA, compared to $31 million for the much less stringent 510(k) process.[64]

A fast track process for Class III devices, known as De Novo, was initially added to the Food and Drug Administration Modernization Act (FDAMA) in 1997, but regulations for this process had not been developed. FDA databases from 2015 to 2017 show that 98% of all medtech product submissions were for 510(k), 1% were PMA, and 1% were De Novo (Table 7.8).[65] The EY report concluded that medtech companies that do not give priority to data-based innovation supported by R&D investment from the beginning of the product lifecycle may become irrelevant.[66]

The FDA added regulations to the De Novo submission process in 2018. New Class III medtech products with relatively low to moderate risk may now apply for the De Novo process by using the 501(k) submission form that is also used for

TABLE 7.8 **Medical Device FDA Submissions 2015–2017.**

|  | 510 (k) | | PMA | | De Novo | | Total |
|---|---|---|---|---|---|---|---|
| **2015** | 3,039 | 98.0% | 43 | 1.4% | 18 | 0.6% | 3,100 |
| **2016** | 2,941 | 97.8% | 39 | 1.3% | 26 | 0.9% | 3,006 |
| **2017** | 3,117 | 97.7% | 45 | 1.4% | 30 | 0.9% | 3,252 |
| **Total** | 9,097 | 97.9% | 127 | 1.4% | 74 | 0.8% | 9,358 |

Class I and Class II products.[67] Once a product is submitted to the FDA under De Novo, the FDA will decide within 120 days if the device is "novel" and if there is no existing classification or a predicate device already on the market.[68] This regulatory change is expected to improve the approval of innovative medtech products and change the percentage of product submissions.

2. *The FDA has developed an innovative approach to regulating health technology software.*

In 2016, Congress passed the 21st Century Cures Act (Cures Act) and authorized $6.3 billion to fund processes that accelerate and streamline medtech and health information technology development. The FDA developed a Digital Health Innovation Plan in 2017 to implement this legislation, and the plan has four important sections:[69]

a) *Implementation of the digital health provisions of the 21st Century Cures Act.* An important element of the plan specifies the types of products that are not regulated by the FDA. The following five product groups are not considered to be regulated: (1) administrative support software, (2) wellness software, (3) electronic health records, (4) certain device or laboratory data transfer software, and (5) certain clinical decision support software.

b) *Guidance on low-risk digital health products.* The FDA will issue guidance on products that meet the technical definition of a medical device but have low enough risks that the FDA will not require premarket regulation. This supplements previously released guidance on general wellness products, mobile medical apps, medical device data systems, medical device accessories, and other low-risk digital health products,

c) *A third-party certification pilot program.* The Software Precertification (Pre-Cert) Pilot Program aims to look first at the software developer or digital health technology developer rather than primarily at the product, which is how the FDA currently evaluates traditional medical devices. The Pre-Cert program's goal is to reduce the amount of submission materials required from manufacturers of software-based medical devices and expedite the review process for companies that demonstrate a "robust culture of quality and organizational excellence, and who are committed to monitoring real-world performance," according to the FDA.[70] Since most software companies are able to quickly respond to glitches, adverse events, and other safety concerns, the FDA is working to establish an equally responsive regulatory framework.

The voluntary Pre-Cert program began in 2019 and is pilot testing manufacturers of software *as* a medical device (SaMD) and will be expanded to manufacturers of software *in* a medical device (SiMD) and software integrated with medical device hardware. The marketing benefit of pre-certification is access to a streamlined FDA premarket review and opportunities to collect and leverage real-world post-market data. In return, the FDA expects companies to ensure high-quality software products throughout the life of the medtech product by enabling companies to demonstrate their cultural capabilities related to quality and excellence.

The FDA is using the Total Product Lifecycle (TPLC) process to evaluate and monitor a medical device with software from its premarket development to post-market performance. The model's five criteria are patient safety, product quality, clinical responsibility, cybersecurity responsibility, and proactive culture (Figure 7.11).[71] The initial nine companies selected for the Software Pre-Cert pilot program in September 2017 from over 100 applicants were Apple, Fitbit, Johnson & Johnson, Pear Therapeutics, Phosphorus, Roche, Samsung, Tidepool, and Verily (Google).

d)  *Use of real-world evidence to support the development of digital health products.* The FDA allows developers to leverage real-world data gathered through external data sources to expedite market entry and subsequent expansion of indications. An example source of real-world data is the National Evaluation System for Health Technology (NEST). NEST is a virtual system for evidence generation based on strategic alliances among data sources including medical registries, electronic health records, payer claims, and other sources. The FDA is a member of the Medical Device Innovation Consortium (MDIC), the public-private partnership that operates NEST.

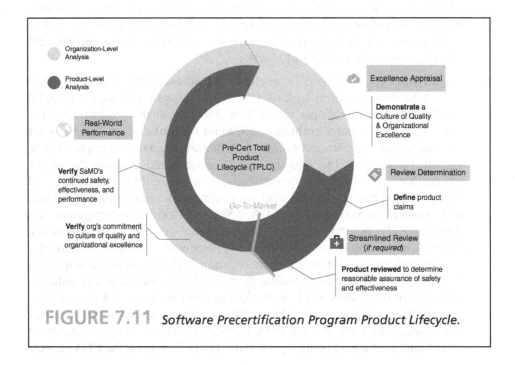

**FIGURE 7.11**  *Software Precertification Program Product Lifecycle.*

Current Health, a health technology company based in Edinburgh, Scotland, has developed an upper arm wearable, remote monitoring device and has received FDA clearance. Current Health is responding to the problem of tracking consumers with chronic conditions and high rates of hospitalization, readmissions, and costs. Focusing on heart failure and chronic obstructive pulmonary disease (COPD), the Current Health product monitors respiration, pulse, oxygen saturation, temperature, and mobility. It uses Bluetooth to collect ICU-level quality data, continually update physicians on their patient's condition, and alerts physicians to take action if the data signal an emerging problem. Current Health received Class II FDA clearance for in-hospital use in February 2019 and began working for Mount Sinai Hospital in Brooklyn, the Banner Health system in Phoenix, along with several NHS Trusts in the UK. The company has demonstrated reduced readmissions and pressure on clinical staff. A second FDA clearance followed in April for in-home remote patient monitoring.[72]

3. *Marketers can take advantage of changing reimbursement to increase use of telehealth.*

CMS has regulated telehealth in the past by narrowly restricting reimbursement for live video, remote patient monitoring, mobile health, and store-and-forward. Medicare was limited to providing telehealth reimbursement to rural sites that must be in Health Professional Shortage Areas and outside Metropolitan Statistical Areas, among other restrictions. Congress passed the Creating High-Quality Results and Outcomes Necessary to Improve Chronic Care Act of 2017 (CHRONIC Act) to improve health outcomes, access, and reimbursement for telehealth services for consumers in Medicare Advantage plans. It benefits rural consumers because it removes the restriction that telehealth services are only available at selected clinical sites. The CHRONIC Act also eliminates geographic restrictions that did not allow Original Medicare consumers residing in urban and suburban areas to use telehealth and telestroke services. The Veterans Administration alone is already projecting savings of $1 billion over the next 10 years from their partial roll out of telehealth services. Larger scale implementation, according to a CBO report, is projected to save just as much over the 2020s.

In 2019, CMS further proposed a set of "new virtual telehealth services" that are explicitly designed to not be considered traditional Medicare telehealth services. These new regulations would increase Medicare beneficiary access and provider reimbursement. New procedure codes would be established for store-and-forward and remote patient monitoring, provider-to-provider consults, new "brief virtual check-ins" for patients to consult with their provider about whether they need an in-person visit, and the elimination of geographic restrictions for stroke and diabetes.

The Independence at Home (IAH) section of the CHRONIC Act helps keep seniors in their homes longer where they are more comfortable and have more control over their lives. Staying at home allows family and friends to offer support and improve adherence to medication and therapy regimens.[73] This regulation also supports the use of telehealth in the home. Synzi is a telehealth platform that uses a combination of video, email, and secure messaging tools to help home health providers stay in touch with patients. According to Synzi, the platform can result in a 40% increase in home health referrals, better quality care, and higher financial margins.[74] Another telehealth home health pilot program in Colorado reported a 62% reduction in 30-day re-hospitalizations for congestive heart failure, chronic obstructive pulmonary failure, and diabetes. ED use, nurse home visits, and costs of care also fell over a 60-day episode of care.[75]

Marketing research can be effective in supporting telehealth technology effectiveness. In 2014, UK health tech company 3Rings launched a plug adapter to monitor the use of electrical appliances such as kettles to prevent accidents and fires in the homes of seniors. Adult children caregivers could set alarms using a phone app to alert them if appliance usage was unusual. Unfortunately, a number of seniors thought the adaptors were wasting electricity and unplugged them.

The people caring for the seniors were themselves likely to be older, and they were nearly as unsavvy about properly using the technology as the ailing seniors. Unfortunately, 3Rings went out of business in 2019. 3Rings may have been saved if they had used ethnographic marketing research. This research would have observed exactly how caregivers and end-users actually used the plug adaptors. The device disconnection behavior could likely have been prevented by applying user-centered product design and more effectively educating buyers.[76]

In March 2019, only about 33% of inpatient hospitals and 45% of outpatient facilities offered telehealth services to their patients. Medicare limited telehealth reimbursement to services such as routine visits in certain circumstances. Patients were required to reside in a rural area, had to travel to a local medical facility that offered telehealth, and were generally not allowed to receive telehealth services in their home.

The Covid-19 pandemic immediately led to increased demand for telemedicine and telehealth services in March 2020. CMS reacted by waiving limitations on the types of care providers eligible for Medicare telehealth reimbursement. Physical and occupational therapists, licensed clinical social workers, and speech language pathologists became eligible. Hospitals were allowed to bill for outpatient services furnished remotely by hospital-based practitioners to patients in their homes. CMS also expanded the use of audio-only phone service reimbursement to include many behavioral health and patient education services. Telehealth reimbursement levels became equivalent to office or outpatient services reimbursement.[77]

The percentage of hospitals using telehealth and telemedicine systems also increased from 33% in March 2019 to 75% in March 2020. Total telehealth claims increased by 1,480% year-over-year from this same time period. Claims further jumped 4,545% from April 2019 to April 2020. Zoom video conferencing was the telemedicine and telehealth software market leader among health care providers, with 26% market share in June 2020.[78] It is unclear if telehealth changes will continue following the pandemic. Congress is under particular pressure, however, to pass laws to make expansion of telehealth coverage permanent, and CMS has signaled a willingness to review and likely revise its pre-pandemic guidelines for Medicare and Medicaid coverage.

### *Technological Force*: Trend 4—The "Big 5" Tech Companies View Health Care as a Market Opportunity

The Big 5 tech companies—Apple, Google, Amazon, Microsoft, and Facebook—are increasing their penetration of the health care market. Their ability to engage consumers could disrupt other smaller health technology companies as well as health systems. A survey found that 80% of health system executives are very or somewhat concerned that Big 5 products could be a competitive threat.[79]

1. *The Big 5 have access to billions of consumers and investment revenue, but they have a problem with data security.*

The primary strengths of the Big 5 include billions in annual revenues and relationships with billions of consumers (Table 7.9).[80] Apple has 1.4 billion devices in use, 95 million consumers have Amazon Prime memberships, and Google has over 1 billion consumers using each of its seven unique products every month. Another important strength is collecting and managing customer data, and this competitive advantage could be applied to the health care market. Medical diagnosis would improve if a consumer with a heart problem uses a watch with a medical grade monitor to detect arrhythmias.

A Rock Health/Stanford Medicine consumer survey, however, found that only 10% of consumers were willing to share health care information with any technology company. Of those consumers, 56% were willing to share with Google

**TABLE 7.9  Big 5 Tech FY18 Annual Revenue in Billions.**

| Big Tech Companies | Annual Revenues—billions |
|---|---|
| Apple | $265.6 |
| Amazon | $232.9 |
| Alphabet/Google | $136.8 |
| Microsoft | $110.4 |
| Facebook | $55.9 |

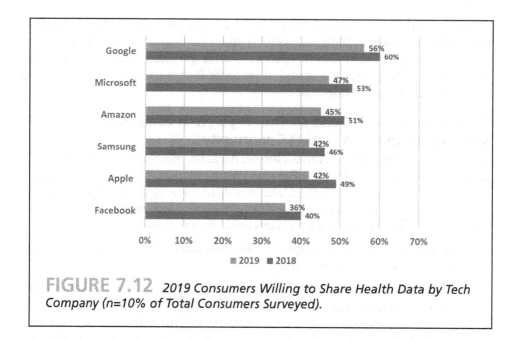

**FIGURE 7.12**  *2019 Consumers Willing to Share Health Data by Tech Company (n=10% of Total Consumers Surveyed).*

followed by Microsoft (47%) and Amazon (45%). Willingness to share health data dropped from 2018 to 2019 for each tech company (Figure 7.12).[81]

Data security may be the Big 5's greatest weakness in entering the health care market. Nearly a quarter of all data breaches happen in health care. As more consumer data are analyzed in the cloud and shared, the greater the potential risk for hacking or misuse. The *Financial Times* (FT) researched a range of 10 health care sites to understand how they were sharing consumer data. This analysis excluded data sent to analytics companies to improve the performance of a website, and consent was given for cookies on all websites that requested it. The privacy policies, however, did not adequately outline that sensitive data would be shared with third parties. Neither did they spell out how any data that were shared would be used.

The FT found that drug names entered into the Drugs.com website were sent to Google's DoubleClick ad unit. Questions related to disease symptoms and diagnoses typed into the WebMD search box were shared with Facebook including symptoms for "drug overdose." Ovulation cycle data from BabyCenter was sent to Amazon Marketing and others. Keywords such as "heart disease" and "considering abortion" entered into the British Heart Foundation, Bupa, and Healthline sites were shared with data collection firms Scorecard Research and BlueKai.[82] Big 5 tech companies could use marketing research to clearly understand consumer data-sharing preferences and then implement them if they were really interested in rebuilding consumer trust.

The Big 5 tech companies are primarily using two health marketing channels strategies.[83] The first is to collaborate with health systems, payers, and other health technology companies. The second is to use their tech platforms to create new direct-to-business or direct-to-consumer channels. Apple and Alphabet (Google's parent company) are expected to have the most impact on the health care market in the near term. Amazon's health care venture with JPMorgan Chase and Berkshire-Hathaway will cover roughly 1 million employees, but Apple and Alphabet have the potential to generate or enable valuable health insights for billions of users (Table 7.10).

TABLE 7.10  **Big 5 Tech Health Product Lines.**

| Apple | Google | amazon | f | Microsoft |
|---|---|---|---|---|
| Health | Verily: Sensors, precision medicine, interventions, pop. Health tools | Berkshire Hathaway-Chase partnership | Behavioral health detection | AI-powered virtual health assistants |
| CareKit | Cityblock Health | Alexa virtual assistant | Clinical trials | HoloLens |
| ResearchKit | DeepMind Health (AI) | PillPack | | Walgreens partnership |
| Apple Watch ECG | Calico (extended lifespans) | Rx licenses | | Enabling team huddles |
| Early detection | | Over-the-counter product line | | |
| Medical clinics | | Amazon Care employee health services | | |

2.   *Apple launched its Health app in 2014 and by 2018 it was downloaded by 140 million U.S. consumers.*

The app tracks activity, monitors sleep, and offers mindfulness stress reduction. Apple also offers three kits for developers to build health-related apps for iPhone and Apple Watch. HealthKit is a developer framework to send and receive information, ResearchKit is used to create apps for medical research and clinical trials, and CareKit connects consumers and their care providers. Apple is pursuing the following six health technology strategies.

a)   *Connect consumers to their electronic health records*: Starting in January 2019, iPhone users could use the Health app to download, store, and share parts of their EHR. Providers can also send lab test results, medication instructions, and other data directly to consumers. More than 300 providers using Epic, Cerner, athenahealth, or CPSI EHRs are participating.

b)   *Help providers more closely monitor consumer health*: HealthKit is being used by Duke Health and Stanford Medicine to enable chronically ill consumers to track and report management of their symptoms. Providers are also using CareKit tools to manage population health interventions. Examples are promoting large scale behavioral changes like improving diet and medication adherence.

c)   *Increase efficiency of clinical trials participant recruitment*: Duke Health completed a study using the iPhone's facial recognition technology to screen young children for autism and other neurodevelopmental disorders. The app was downloaded 10,000 times, and usable data was collected on 88% of the videos the parents uploaded.

d)   *Use channels marketing to target health plans*: Apple entered agreements with UnitedHealth Group and with Aetna to provide discounted Apple Watches to health plan members who walk more than 10,000 steps per day. Apple is also in talks with at least three Medicare Advantage plans about providing subsidized watches for early detection of atrial fibrillation, an irregular heart beat condition, among consumers over age 65.

e)   *Directly provide consumer primary care*: AC Wellness is a primary care physician group that is also an Apple subsidiary. The practice offers care to Apple employees in Santa Clara County, California. Many of the AC Wellness physicians have backgrounds in alternative medicine and wellness, and the practice also employs a number of health coaches to help coordinate care and guide consumers. The AC Wellness clinics can also be used as a laboratory to test and modify new Apple health technology products.

f)   *Apple Heart Study shows a lot of promise but cardiologists still have questions*: The results of the Apple Heart Study were published in the *New England Journal of Medicine* in November 2019. More than 400,000 people signed up for the Apple Heart Study making it one of the largest research efforts to rely on a wearable, the Apple Watch. About 0.5% of participants received notification from the watch's electrocardiogram sensor of atrial fibrillation. These tools for monitoring heart health are evidently developing faster than the medical community can respond to them. Physicians are unsure that they should be used on a general population because clear treatment protocols have not been established. This is especially true for young people who are found to have atrial fibrillation in the earliest stages without any other risk factors.

3. *Google, and its holding company Alphabet, wants to build "smart" health products with or without industry partners.*

Four Alphabet subsidiaries are currently investing heavily in the development of a wide range of health technology projects: Google, Verily, DeepMind Health, and Cityblock Health.

Google has offered big data storage and management services to hospitals for years, and its machine learning, G-suite apps, and other data services are all HIPAA compliant. Google Cloud—much like its consumer personal health information product Google Health that failed due to low market demand in 2011—is now targeting hospital customers to collect and organize a variety of medical data from lab results to medical records to X-ray images in a single location. This product meets a need because patient data is often inaccessible and spread throughout hospitals and clinics resulting in expensive duplicate tests and procedures. Stanford School of Medicine is one of the first program participants.

Another Google Cloud product is Big Query, a serverless data warehouse that combines and analyzes patient records with other massive data sets. The Colorado Center for Personalized Medicine at the University of Colorado is using Big Query to build a 6-million record genomics database. Data are being combined from EHR data from the health system, external health insurance claims, public health data, and environmental data to devise personalized patient therapies.

Verily Life Sciences has a range of direct-to-consumer health products to treat diabetes and other chronic conditions. Liftware Steady is an electronic stabilizing handle and a selection of attachments that include a soup spoon, everyday spoon, fork, and spork. This tool was designed to help people with hand tremor caused by Parkinson's disease or essential tremor to eat more easily. Verily is partnering with the Gilead Immune Profiler platform to better understand the immune system. This product combines genomic and immunologic laboratory technologies with Verily's health data analysis to build maps of inflammatory disease, and others. Verily is collaborating with medtech company Dexcom to offer a continuously reporting glucose meter and a disposable glucose sensor worn like a bandage for up to 14 days. Verily is working with Stanford Medicine and Duke Health on its answer to the Apple Watch, the Study Watch, to detect heart disease.

Verily has also teamed with Fitbit to connect consumer health data with consumer EHRs. Google announced in November 2019 that it was acquiring Fitbit.

The DeepMind Health subsidiary based in London is focused on AI. It has been providing the Streams AI app to the UK National Health Service and U.S. Department of Veterans Affairs. Streams uses hospital data and AI to give clinical staff early alerts for patients experiencing severely deteriorating health. It can now predict acute kidney injury up to two days before it happens. DeepMind Health FY19 losses were $571 million and cumulative debt was over $1 billion. Cityblock Health is piloting a program in Brooklyn, New York, that offers primary care to low-income consumers in their own homes. It uses big data to identify where care is needed and does not rely on existing health infrastructure. Cityblock sends its own clinical employees to the homes of people needing care and visits are usually reimbursed by Medicaid.

4.   *Amazon announced a joint venture with Berkshire-Hathaway and JP Morgan Chase in January 2018.*

When Amazon made this announcement, the market value of the 10 largest health insurance and pharmacy stocks dropped by a combined $30 billion in the first two hours of trading.[84] The goal of this nonprofit organization named Haven is to use innovation to lower health care costs, beginning with the three companies' 1.2 million employees. The overall strategy is to leverage data and technology to change incentives, improve the patient experience, and create a better system.

Specific strategies announced by Haven are communicating health pricing to employees, helping employees better understand and use health insurance benefits, reducing prescription drug pricing, integrating technology to improve the consumer experience, and incentivizing employees to be more engaged and accountable for their health. Using employee marketing research to understand how best to change employee health attitudes and behavior will improve strategy effectiveness. Haven is expected to market these innovative solutions to other employers.

Also, in 2018, Amazon acquired the company PillPack and its "Basic Care" product line of over-the-counter health and medical products, to potentially disrupt the retail pharmacy market through its customer-driven strategy. PillPack targets high-cost, chronically ill consumers and the growing number of self-pay consumers with high deductible health plans. Their website lists drug prices online, centralizes all consumer prescriptions, and is responsible for coordinating all insurance administrative requirements. It uses same-day or one-day free shipping to consumers' homes. Shipments include customized daily packets containing all drugs needed for a particular day and a monthly medications list with photos of all drugs prescribed, and consumers have 24/7 access to PillPack pharmacy support.[85]

Amazon has used its data processing capabilities to build a tool to monitor and care for employees away from hospitals and physician offices called Amazon Care. Launched in September 2019, Amazon Care is an app-based medical service for its employees in Seattle that is expected to cut costs and improve the customer experience. Separate from Haven, this service combines an app for video calls and text chats with doctors or nurses and visits from "mobile care nurses" at employees' homes and offices. Amazon said it was piloting the benefit for employees to help them get fast access to health care without an appointment.[86]

Additionally, Amazon is offering its Alexa voice assistant to health systems. The UK's National Health Service is partnering with Amazon's Alexa for health advice supplied by the National Health Service. In the U.S., six health systems are working with a HIPAA-compliant version of Alexa that can share and receive protected health information.[87]

5. *Microsoft and Facebook are targeting the health care market with their core businesses of software and social networking.*

Microsoft is interested in being the cloud provider of choice for the health provider market, and it has developed an effective strategic positioning. This positioning can be summarized as "We are not a health care company.", and it communicates a valuable benefit and differentiates Microsoft from its competitors. Providers have felt threatened by other Big Tech companies that have diversified into directly providing health services. Examples include Apple's launch of health clinics for its employees and Amazon's acquisition of PillPack.

This positioning, according to the CEO of Providence St. Joseph Health, was the primary reason why Microsoft was selected over Google, Apple, and Amazon for a multi-year strategic alliance to move data and applications from the health system to Azure, the Microsoft cloud service. Providence is a 51-hospital Catholic, not-for-profit health organization operating in seven states. Microsoft will also provide their 119,000 physicians with access to the Microsoft Office productivity software and collaboration tools. In addition, Microsoft will work with Providence to turn an existing Seattle facility into a "hospital of the future" by retrofitting it with technology such as natural language processing (NLP) and machine learning tools.[88]

Microsoft is collaborating with other tech companies to improve health care value. Examples are AI, pharmaceuticals, EHR documentation, and behavior health.

a) UCLA Health will use Azure and Microsoft's AI tools to store its data from different sources, analyze and customize it to the individual, and use it for disease prevention. They will build algorithms to predict when a hospitalized patient's condition is at risk of deteriorating by using structured data (lab results and medication information) with unstructured data (chart documentation, genomics, and medical images).

b) Pharmaceutical company Novartis is also working with Microsoft AI tools to uncover new insights through mining 2 million patient years of clinical data from hundreds of studies completed over the past 20 years.

Novartis will also use Microsoft AI and machine learning to shorten the drug discovery process that currently requires an average of 14 years and up to $2.5 billion.

c) Microsoft is working with the software company Nuance Communications to add AI and NLP to hospital exam rooms. This system will listen in on patients' visits and automatically create a document in the EHR. Microsoft is also collaborating with SilverCloud Health, a behavioral health support platform, to use Microsoft AI to improve the delivery of more personalized mental health care. This collaboration is expected to result in earlier interventions and improve mental health clinical outcomes.[89]

Facebook health care initiatives are also focusing on mental health in addition to clinical trials and heart and cancer preventive health. Facebook uses AI to monitor user online behavior for patterns that may indicate depression or result in suicide. The photos a user posts on Instagram may signal depression depending on the colors they contain, the times they are posted, and whether they show faces. Facebook is monitoring and managing consumer groups that discuss different health symptoms to help drug companies improve recruitment for clinical trials.[90]

Facebook is collaborating with the American Cancer Society, the American College of Cardiology, the AHA, and the CDC to motivate consumers to get cholesterol, blood pressure, and breast cancer screenings and seasonal flu vaccines. Their preventive health tool will also direct consumers to Federally Qualified Health Centers (FQHCs) near them for health services that are either at no cost or available at a sliding scale depending upon their income.[91]

## HEALTH TECHNOLOGY PROBLEMS AND STRATEGIC MARKETING SOLUTIONS

Health technology companies are facing rapidly changing market opportunities and threats. Health system, physician, payer, and employer customers are searching for value through and evidence-based care. Consumers are adopting select health tech tools but are increasingly distrustful about sharing health data. New regulations and competitive moves are reported daily. This section explores how strategic marketing can help health tech companies respond to these challenges.

### 1. *Marketing Problem—Health System Customers are Buying Health Technology Based on Value.*

Rather than selecting products and services based primarily on the lowest price, health tech customers are demanding outcome and quality data to forecast ROI. Marketing research indicates that only 10% of executives believe that new health tech products are aligned with health system needs. Additionally, 90% are convinced that health tech companies cannot provide the evidence needed to support product value and competitive differentiation.[92]

### *Marketing Solution*—Develop Sales and Marketing Strategies Based on the Marketing Imperative.

The marketing imperative targets and builds relationships with the right customer, offers solutions that meet their specific needs, and defines differentiated quality packages that have a competitive advantage. Some health tech companies have developed an effective four-step sales strategy based on this fundamental marketing strategy.[93] ProFlow uses this sales strategy to market their smart infusion pump.[94] Infusion pumps are medical devices that deliver fluids to patients such as insulin or other hormones, antibiotics, chemotherapy drugs, and pain relievers.

"Smart" infusion pumps use a combination of computer technology and drug libraries to reduce errors such as an incorrect dose, rate of administration, solution concentration, or human failures in pump programming. If a bedside clinician tries to administer a medication either above or below a "soft" limit, the smart pump will warn the user to recheck the settings. Entering a value outside of a "hard" limit will prevent the initiation of the infusion and will prompt the clinician to reprogram the pump or cancel the procedure.

*Step 1*: *Determine how target customers define product value*

Step 1 begins with understanding how different customers define value. Secondary marketing research was conducted to analyze the environmental forces affecting health systems and identify problems they were facing. ProFlow learned that product safety was a high priority for health system purchasing, and there was a strong financial relationship between safety and superior quality and improved incomes. In the case of infusion pumps, adverse drug events (ADEs) were increasing, and IV pump programming errors were responsible for a significant number of deaths. Additional market intelligence also found that health system chief information officers expected health technology products and companies to be accountable for reducing medical errors.

*Step 2*: *Map product benefits to buyer definitions of value*

In Step 2, health technology companies map the customer information from Step 1 to the benefits provided by their products. This analysis may find that product design modifications are needed to better align product benefits with customer needs. ProFlow found that medication administration errors were responsible for 38% of pump errors. They used smart pump industry data to evaluate computerized practitioner order entry (CPOE), bar coding, drug-dispensing robots and cabinets, integrated pharmacy systems, and clinical decision support. There were 125 annual overdose ADEs and 15 underdose ADEs *prevented* by smart pumps at the average 300-bed hospital. These ADEs would not have been prevented by CPOE-driven decision support software, bar coding, or other health technology.

***Step 3***: *Validate product value*

Step 3 reviews product performance and company reputation. This quantitative evaluation compares actual performance to marketing claims, customer expectations, and to competitors. This analysis may show that performance needs to be improved or changed to meet customer needs and overcome competitor threats.

ProFlow worked with its customers to quantify its smart pump impact on medication errors and ADEs. Comparative models were developed to accurately project the number of ADEs that could be prevented with its smart pump compared to bar code and CPOE technologies. ProFlow smart infusion pumps prevented between 9 and 10 ADEs over a seven-year period per $10,000 invested by a 300-bed hospital. This investment compares to bar code technology that prevented 3 to 5 ADEs, and CPOE that prevented 1 to 2. Importantly, the evidence found that ProFlow smart pumps had the highest cost-benefit and ROI among these three technologies.

***Step 4***: *Communicate with prospective customers*

Finally, Step 4 identifies the product and company information content and information services preferred by particular customers. Health system decision-makers have different information needs and communications channels depending on the product. For example, preferred information channels have ranged from key opinion leaders, to attending professional meetings, or to word-of-mouth from colleagues.

ProFlow research found that their target customers preferred to receive written communications about how ProFlow solved specific client problems. Executives also wanted to see client problem/solution cases summarized on the ProFlow website. If the decision-makers were interested in learning more, they wanted quantitative performance analyses—including tables and figures—discussed in a slide presentation. ProFlow created these communications using the preferred content and media channels.

## 2.   *Marketing Problem*—Complete Drug Availability and Pricing Information is Not Available.

More than 3,400 drugs increased in price in the first six months of 2019, representing a 17% jump over the same period in 2018. The average price went up 10.5%, five times the rate of inflation, and the number of consumers not able to afford the medicines they needed is growing. At the time of prescribing, physicians do not have information on the drugs covered by a consumer's insurance, drug prices and possible substitutes, or information on the prescriptions that require a prior authorization (PA) in order to be filled by the pharmacy.[95] Consumers not following medication recommendations and abandoning their prescriptions at pharmacies costs the U.S. health care system an estimated $280 billion annually.[96]

### Marketing Solution—Improve the Customer Experience to Increase Brand Equity.

CoverMyMeds is a health IT company (Columbus, Ohio) that wanted to help consumers obtain the medicine needed by giving physicians the information they needed. CoverMyMeds understood that improving the customer experience would lead to increased value and brand equity. The company believed that automating the prescribing process would give physicians the information they needed to improve medical outcomes.

CoverMyMeds began the new product development process with consumer and physician marketing research. The first research phase was to conduct two quantitative studies to understand consumer and physician attitudes and behavior. The consumer survey (N=1,000) found:

a) 75% of consumers received a prescription that cost more than they had expected.

b) 50% could not pay for the drug at the pharmacy because the cost was too high.

c) 37% stopped taking a drug because it was too expensive.

d) 87% wanted their physician to give them drug cost information before it was prescribed.

Additionally, 42% of consumers with high deductible health plans used apps such as GoodRx and Blink Health to track prescription drug prices, find drug coupons, and use pre-negotiated prices. Unfortunately, this information was insufficient for most consumers.

The CoverMyMeds physician survey (N=1,300) found that:

a) 70% of physicians were interested in talking with consumers about drug options and affordability.

b) Only 52% of physicians had access to drug formulary and benefit data in their EHR at the point of prescribing. These physicians, however, had a low level of trust in this data, giving it a 5.7 trust rating on a scale of 1-low and 10-high.

c) The prescribing information needed by physicians included patient drug benefit coverage, drug prices negotiated between the health plan and pharmacy, and the pharmacy cash prices.

d) Physicians also wanted to have discussions with patients concerning their out-of-pocket spending limits, alternative drug options, and patient assistance payment programs.

The second phase of the physician research used ethnographic observation to shadow physicians and document each step of their manual prescribing workflow. This research was used to develop an automated workflow that delivered the needed information and used a sequence of steps familiar to physicians. This new product, named RxBenefit Clarity, provided real-time benefit check information. Through a collaboration with the health web communications firm RelayHealth, RxBenefit Clarity gave physicians access to medication-specific prescription cost information in real-time and at the point of care.

Physicians now had the same benefit coverage and pricing information as a pharmacist. Physicians can determine if patients will need to pay a $20 drug co-payment, if a drug is covered under the patient's benefit plan, and if an insurance PA is required—all through the patient's EHR at the time of prescribing. If a PA is required, it is submitted electronically directly through the EHR, and this stream-lined process eliminates administrative costs and reduces consumer waiting times. Physicians can also identify clinically-approved therapeutic alternatives and pharmacy mail order availability. Pharmacies can access RxBenefit Clarity to verify benefit eligibility lookups, a capability pharmacists only currently have 35% of the time. Pharmacies use these lookups to find and fix benefit eligibility data using historic claims and to find the lowest drug prices by analyzing drug claims databases using machine learning. RxBenefit Clarity supports improved medication adherence by helping physicians, pharmacies, and consumers make more informed health care decisions.

The physician research conducted by CoverMyMeds also informed the RxBenefit Clarity promotion strategy. CoverMyMeds focused on education and word-of-mouth communications, and the CoverMyMeds sales team built relationships with both medical and health system key opinion leaders. Personal marketing communications was used at tradeshows and industry events; and personalized email was used to generate leads and attendance for online webinars that explained the benefits of RxBenefit Clarity.

### 3. *Marketing Problem*—An Innovative Drug Inhaler Company Needed to Develop a Supply Chain Strategy to Exploit a Market Opportunity.

Handheld inhalers are used by consumers suffering from lung conditions such as asthma and COPD. These devices were designed to spray albuterol and other drugs into the lungs using chlorofluorocarbons (CFCs) gases. Albuterol was a $1 billion global market when the FDA banned CFCs because it was shown to delete ozone in the atmosphere.[97] The gas hydrofluoroalkane (HFA) was recommended as a substitute, but HFA tripled the cost of CFC inhalers.

Respirics, a start-up medtech company, responded to this market threat by creating an innovative dry powder inhaler that propelled albuterol using breath instead of a gas. The product was named Acu-Breathe, and the primary benefit was improving the customer "inhaler technique" experience and more efficient and consistent dosing. Respirics had first-mover advantage and its intellectual property was protected by nine patents through 2021, but it desperately needed to create marketing supply chain strategies for Acu-Breathe manufacturing and distribution.

*Marketing Solution*—Evaluate and Contract with High-Performing Channel Partners that Match the Respirics Market-Driven Culture.

A company should initially consider the needs of the target market and then design the supply chain backward. Channels partner examples include manufacturers, suppliers, wholesalers, retailers, and other intermediaries. The channels a company chooses affect all other marketing decisions, and Respirics needed to contract with partners that were market-driven and fit their cost model. Channels decisions involve relatively long-term commitments as well as policies and procedures to specify mutual goals and responsibilities. Product pricing is influenced by the types and costs of distribution. Costs are often higher for products that require many channel partners because each member of the distribution chain needs to be compensated.

Respirics began searching for a manufacturing partner for Acu-Breathe by evaluating 165 applicants from all over the world, and Computime headquartered in Hong Kong was selected. This decision was based on Computime's corporate culture of "put the customer first" and on price. The cost of producing Acu-Breathe in the U.S. was double the cost of producing it in Chinese factories. The Computime culture was quickly put to the test when the initial manufactured lots had a failure rate of 7.5%. After Respirics explained that this rate was unacceptable, Computime's management enhanced the quality assurance process by testing 100% of the units produced. The result was a reduction to a 1% initial failure rate, and volume was then increased to 300,000 units annually.

Another key channel characteristic is how well an intermediary can support the company's sales forecast and growth. Respirics entered into a sales arrangement with a U.S. biopharmaceutical company with sales experience with late-stage respiratory disease products. This sales distribution partner agreed to contact national pharmacy companies and their retail outlets, and high-prescribing physicians such as allergists and pulmonologists. This channels partner also agreed to secure Acu-Breathe reimbursement with health plans and other third-party payers. Unfortunately, this partner did not reach these objectives because it was unable to increase its sales force in the allotted time. Respirics attempted to collaborate with the channels partner to solve this problem, but it was insurmountable. Respirics began to miss revenue objectives, the search for a another distribution partner was unsuccessful, and Respirics was forced to close.

### 4. *Marketing Problem*—A Medtech Company Wanted to Increase its Hyperbaric Oxygen Chamber Market Share, but Market Demand was a Concern.

Técnico is an industrial fabrication, repair, and installation company, located in the Southeast, that had acquired a multiplace hyperbaric oxygen chamber (HBOC) business. Hyperbaric chambers increase air pressure up to three times higher than normal. This pressurized air allows the lungs to absorb more oxygen than would be possible by breathing pure oxygen at normal air pressure. This enriched oxygen is carried by the circulatory system throughout body.

Multiplace HBOCs are large, specially-built steel rooms that can treat up to 15 patients at a time for various medical conditions. Patients are seated or placed on a bed in the chamber and wear oxygen masks. The duration of a session, or dive cycle, is usually two hours. Multiplace chambers can cost several million dollars. A monoplace hyperbaric chamber holds a single person at one time, and they are typically about 8 feet long. The price of a new monoplace chamber ranges from $80,000 to $150,000. Técnico's one multiplace chamber customer was the U.S. Navy, and  Técnico's goal was to penetrate the HBOC market and increase market share.

### Marketing Solution—*Analyze the HBOC Market to Identify Opportunities and Threats and Determine if a Market Penetration Strategy Would Have a Positive ROI.*

Técnico decided to use a market-driven growth strategy, and they began with *secondary marketing research*. Técnico needed secondary research to answer three questions:

1.  What was the size of the hyperbaric oxygen chamber market in the U.S.?

2.  What were characteristics of a successful hyperbaric oxygen therapy (HBOT) hospital program?

3.  What were the strengths and weaknesses of competing companies?

*Market size*: There were 790 total chambers in North and Central America, and 80% were monoplace and 20% were multiplace chambers. More than two-thirds of monoplace chambers (78%) were installed in hospitals, and nearly half (46%) of multiplace chambers were in hospitals. The most common medical conditions treated by HBOT were nonhealing wounds like diabetic foot ulcers, oncology, sports medicine, cerebral palsy, severe anemia, brain abscesses, burns, gangrene, carbon monoxide poisoning, and decompression sickness (the bends). The coastal states of Texas, Florida, and California had 40% of all monoplace installations and 42% of multiplace chambers.

*Target markets*: Hospitals needed sufficient patient volume and financial strength to profitably offer HBOT. Industry standards were that hospitals should have a minimum of 200 beds to make monoplace chambers profitable and at least 500 beds for multiplace chambers. Hospitals needed a "physician champion" to support the HBOT program at the hospital. Hospitals also benefited from being the hub of a regional referral network to generate the patient volume needed for HBOT profitability. A second HBOC target market was resellers that purchased hyperbaric chambers and resold or leased them to hospitals as part of a turnkey wound management service line.

*Competitors*: There were three primary HBOC competitors. Sechrist Industries (California) was the market leader selling both multiplace and monoplace hyperbaric chambers with an installed global client base of nearly 900 units. Perry

Baromedical Corporation (Florida) was a smaller company that began building submarines but had moved into multiplace chambers in a range of sizes. Environmental Tectonics Corporation (Pennsylvania) was the third largest competitor selling both monoplace and multiplace product lines.

A critical conclusion drawn from the secondary research was that hyperbaric medicine physicians played a critical role in HBOT program direction and chamber selection. Técnico then decided to use *qualitative primary research* to interview a sample of U.S. hyperbaric medicine physician key opinion leaders to understand their HBOC attitudes and buying behavior. The interviews found that key HBOT physician leaders wanted an innovative, multiplace chamber that was designed to be modular and could be staged.

The modular design would allow a hospital to enter the HBOT market cost-effectively by buying a single compact multiplace chamber with a capacity of three to four patients. Assuming volume growth, the hospital could expand the service by adding a second stage to the first chamber. The physicians indicated that the most important factors for selecting a chamber manufacturer were proven product quality, personnel competence, company financial stability, and a strong customer reputation. The importance of this conclusion would later prove to be critical.

A *product concept test* of the innovative modular chamber followed with two target markets. Six in-depth interviews were conducted with HBOT buyers at hospitals, and four were conducted with executives at national wound care companies. While market demand for traditional multiplace chamber was very low, the hospital respondents confirmed interest in potentially buying the cost-effective module chambers. The best hospital prospects currently had an HBOT service line experiencing increasing volume, and they had three or four monoplace chambers already in place. There was no demand among wound care service respondents for modular or traditional multiplace chambers.

*Results*: Técnico decided not to pursue the development of the innovative modular multiplace product line. Several months later, one of the key opinion leader survey respondents called about a potential market opportunity. The Khrunichev State Research and Production Space Centre in Moscow, Russia, was searching for a U.S. distribution partner for their monoplace chambers. Representatives of Técnico traveled to Moscow, and they successfully negotiated a memorandum-of-understanding to sell, distribute, and service the Khrunichev chambers.

The relationship with Khrunichev was good, but hospitals had sales objections. Técnico priced the Russian chambers in line with comparable U.S. built chambers. Hospital perceptions of the Russian chambers, however, did not align with their needs for product quality, personnel competence, company financial stability, and a strong customer reputation, as identified in the research. Unfortunately, Técnico was not able to lower its pricing to profitably sell the monoplace chambers.

### 5. *Marketing Problem*—A Health IT Start-Up Had Customers but was Uncertain About how Best to Scale its Business.

Health plans typically auto-adjudicate 85% of submitted claims, but the remaining 15% require manual review. Healthcare Productivity Automation (Nashville, TN) custom-built software robots to lower health plan costs by automating manual claims review processes and other administrative tasks. The product, Health Mason, was software-as-a-service (SaaS) that had been sold to three health plans with more than 100,000 members each.

The Healthcare Productivity Automation average customer had 34,000 transactions per month. The Health Mason price ranged from $.50 to $1.50 per transaction, depending on the level of complexity. Each client generated an estimated $408,000 in revenue. Healthcare Productivity Automation was interested in adding customers and increasing revenue, but they believed that a market-based sales forecast analysis and a strategic marketing plan would best support expansion.

### *Marketing Solution*—Use a Sales Funnel to Estimate the Number of Prospects Needed to Reach the New Business Revenue Objective.

A strategic marketing plan analyzed the Healthcare Productivity Automation market, set goals and objectives, and developed marketing strategies. The 12-month new business revenue objective was $2,000,000. This revenue assumed each new customer would generate $400,000, and a minimum of five new customers were needed in the next 12 months (Table 7.11).

A sales funnel analysis was used to identify and quantify the sales stages. A sales funnel evaluates the stages that are required for customers to buy a company's product. The funnel quantifies each stage beginning with the number of prospects needed at the top of the funnel to reach the sale objectives at the bottom of the funnel.

An evaluation of the sales process for the three Healthcare Productivity Automation customers found they had passed through four sales stages in becoming customers: (1) qualified prospect, (2) active prospect, (3) proposal prospect, and (4) contract prospect (Table 7.12).

Each stage included a projection for the number of prospects that would move successively through to the next stage. The time from qualified prospect to customer was 10 weeks (Figure 7.13). Healthcare Productivity Automation found that in order to close five customers they needed 60 qualified prospects, or five per month.

**TABLE 7.11**  **Annual Revenue and Customer Assumptions.**

| | |
|---|---|
| 1. Annual revenue objective | 2. $2,000,000 |
| 3. Average deal size | 4. $400,000 |
| 5. Number of closed sales | 6. 5 |

TABLE 7.12  **Sales Prospect Funnel Stages.**

| Qualified Prospect | Active Prospect | Proposal Prospect | Contract Prospect |
|---|---|---|---|
| • The particular problem is a priority<br>• Technical access<br>• Budget availability<br>• Will commit to a 30- minute phone discussion | • Prospect meets with HCPA to explain manual workflows<br>• HCPA documents manual workflows<br>• Workflows are mutually confirmed<br>• Technological access to IT is confirmed | • HCPA submits statement-of-work (SOW) to prospect<br>• Prospect agrees to SOW<br>• Prospect is billed and pays confirmation fee | • HCPA automates manual workflows<br>• Workflows are tested and reported to prospect<br>• HCPA contract is submitted and accepted |

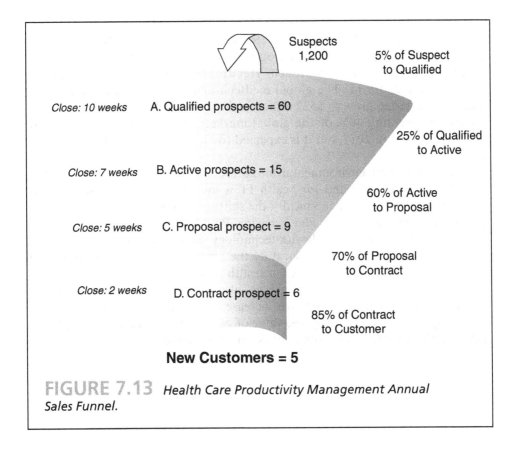

Suspects
1,200

5% of Suspect to Qualified

Close: 10 weeks    A. Qualified prospects = 60

25% of Qualified to Active

Close: 7 weeks    B. Active prospects = 15

60% of Active to Proposal

Close: 5 weeks    C. Proposal prospect = 9

70% of Proposal to Contract

Close: 2 weeks    D. Contract prospect = 6

85% of Contract to Customer

**New Customers = 5**

FIGURE 7.13  *Health Care Productivity Management Annual Sales Funnel.*

Since only 5% of suspects became qualified prospects, 1,200 suspects were needed to start the sales funnel. Suspects are defined as any potential buyer, and for Healthcare Productivity Automation these were health plans with more than 100,000 members. Suspect names, titles, companies, emails, and phone numbers are available from suppliers like Dunn & Bradstreet, professional societies like American Health Insurance Plans, and by attending health plan conferences that publish attendee contact information. Sales tools to build awareness with suspects are "cold calls" using phone with email, trade publication advertising, and exhibiting at industry trade shows.

There were an estimated 800 health plans in the target market, and this sales funnel analysis alerted Healthcare Productivity Management executives that this number of health plans was not large enough to sustain long-term company revenue growth. Management then began developing diversification strategies to automate manual tasks in other health care organizations—such as health systems, physician practices, and reference labs—as well as in banking, hospitality, and other types of insurance.

## CHAPTER SUMMARY

Marketing health technology products and services has traditionally used a product-driven approach, but environmental forces have created incentives to move to a market-driven approach. Health technology can be divided into medtech and health IT. The global medtech market was $387 billion in 2016 and is projected to grow to $522 billion in 2022. The U.S. market is the world's largest representing 40% of the global market. The global health IT market was $183 billion in 2017, but it is expected to also grow rapidly to $665 billion by 2026.

Four important environmental forces are affecting health tech companies. Socially, consumer demand for health IT is increasing, but data security is a growing market threat. Economically, the shift to value-based care is now changing medtech buyer attitudes and behavior. Politically and legally, regulation is adapting to strongly support health technology innovation. Technologically, the "Big 5" tech companies are penetrating the health care market and competing with smaller tech companies as well as health providers.

Medtech and health IT companies are also using strategic marketing tools to implement the marketing imperative, increase brand equity, and improve the customer experience. Additionally, the value of customer-driven channels, sales, and other marketing strategies should not be underestimated.

## DISCUSSION QUESTIONS

1.  Health information technology companies have earned a reputation for marketing new products that do not always perform as promised. Would you classify this perception as new product failure? Why or why not?

2.  Your small orthopedic implant company has traditionally distributed its products through wholesalers and distributors. Your vice president of marketing has recommended adding a direct web-based distribution channel. As the CEO, you are concerned that this change will result in channel conflict. What are the benefits and drawbacks of this strategy? How do you think different types of customers, wholesalers, distributors, and competitors will react if this strategy is implemented?

3.  Medtech and health IT companies spend heavily on trade shows to reach prospective customers. Research a sample of major trade shows for these two market segments. Analyze the target markets, the advantages, the disadvantages, and the best practices for exhibiting at these trade shows.

4.  Compiling consumer names, addresses, phone numbers, and other information in databases is vital for direct marketing. Health care information confidentiality and privacy are protected by regulation, but consumer trust in data security is a major market threat. Explain how health care marketers can ethically and legally gather and use information to build relationships with consumers in this environment?

## HEALTH TECHNOLOGY MARKETING CASE: SLEEPIO

Trading sleep for a few more productive hours of work, fun, or exercise is often tempting. Sleeping less than eight hours a day, however, has been found to be a risk factor for obesity, diabetes, and cardiovascular disease. Major restorative functions in the body such as tissue repair, muscle growth, and protein synthesis occur almost exclusively during sleep. Poor or inadequate sleep can also cause irritability and stress, and can reduce the brain's ability to consolidate factual information and memory.

Only 11% of U.S. college students sleep well, and 40% of students feel well rested only two days per week.[98] The workplace is also a less productive and congenial environment because 65% of U.S. workers experience sleep problems. The U.S. economy is estimated to be losing $411 billion annually through tired or absent employees, and those sleeping less than six hours a night are 13% more likely to die earlier than those getting seven to nine hours sleep every night.[99]

Peter Hames had a job working in business development in England when he began suffering from chronic insomnia. He had studied developmental psychology at the University of Oxford, and he asked his National Health Service general practitioner for a referral to a cognitive behavioral therapy (CBT) program. Disappointingly, his doctor only offered sleeping pills. Hames was able to overcome his sleep problems, however, through a book on CBT written by sleep scientist Colin Espie at the University of Glasgow. Hames contacted Espie in 2010 and invited him to be a co-founder of a CBT sleep-based start-up called Big Health (www.bighealth.com).

The first product that Big Health developed was Sleepio, a personalized mobile app clinically proven to improve sleep quality. Sleepio helps people fall asleep, stay asleep, and feel better during the day without the need for sleeping pills. While CBT is usually provided in a face-to-face setting, Sleepio uses an online app to combine CBT with online entertainment.

The first step is to complete an in-depth sleep questionnaire used to tailor the product for each user. The questions cover personal goals, thoughts, daily schedule, lifestyle, location, and other standardized clinical measures. Sleepio uses an animated sleep expert, "The Prof" chatbot and his narcoleptic dog "Pavlov" to virtually teach users CBT sleep techniques based on their specific problems and progress. Six 20-minute sessions per week follow with users recording their sleep experience in an online sleep diary. Fitbit and Jawbone customers can also upload their sleep data to Sleepio.

On-demand user support is provided 24/7 by The Prof. If users wake in the night with a sleep problem, they can open the app and The Prof appears in his bed clothes with questions and a relaxation plan. A text message in the morning follows, and the problem is added to the sleep diary. Another support feature is the Sleepio user community. Advice and coaching are available to new users from Sleepio "graduates" through an anonymous and secure online community. Users are in control throughout. They can pace the sessions as they wish and implement the toolbox of techniques that are most helpful to them.

The Sleepio product was clinically tested in a placebo-controlled randomized clinical trial, and the study was published in the peer-reviewed journal *Sleep* in June 2012. It found that Sleepio helped poor sleepers fall asleep up to 50% faster, reduce nighttime awakenings by up to 60%, boost daytime energy and concentration by up to 50%, and achieve a more reliable sleep pattern. *The Lancet* published a commentary on the clinical trial and called it a proven intervention for sleep disorders using the internet.

Direct-to-consumer pricing is not easily found on the Sleepio website, but internet research uncovered a U.S. consumer price of $400. Sleepio is available as a covered health benefit to 12 million people through deals with U.S. employers and the UK's National Health Service. Sleepio distribution appears to be focused on an indirect channels strategy. In June 2019, Big Health announced a partnership with the CVS Caremark pharmacy benefits manager (PBM). CVS Health owns the PBM, retail pharmacy chain CVS Pharmacy, and health insurer

Aetna among many other brands. The CVS Caremark deal increases Sleepio access to an estimated 90 million plan members who have their medications managed by CVS Caremark. Sleepio consumer promotion appears to rely on referrals from employers, physicians, and pharmacists. Other promotional vehicles used are online advertising, public relations, poster and print advertising, as well as word-of-mouth.

## CASE QUESTIONS

1. What are the Sleepio market segments? Select the most important target market among these segments and explain the reason for your choice.

2. Big Health appears to be differentiating Sleepio not only from sleep drugs but also from face-to-face CBT. Identify the most important Sleepio competitors by considering any aid for healthier sleep. Analyze the strengths and weaknesses for the three most important competitors.

3. The Big Health indirect channels strategy is increasing consumer access to Sleepio, but consumers must be convinced to try it. How can Big Health measure and increase consumer word-of-mouth?

4. Write an effective strategic positioning for Sleepio using the standard format. Explain your rationale for the target market, frame of reference, primary benefit, and key differentiators.

### *Standard Product Positioning Format*

To (the target market), the Sleepio is the brand (frame of reference) that (primary benefit) because (key differentiating attributes).

# CHAPTER

# BIOPHARMA MARKETING

## LEARNING OBJECTIVES

In this chapter we will address the following questions:

1. What are the value propositions for the biopharmaceutical industry?

2. How is the biopharmaceutical market structured and how it is evolving, including supply chain arrangements?

3. How can strategic marketing be used for competitive advantage given marketplace challenges?

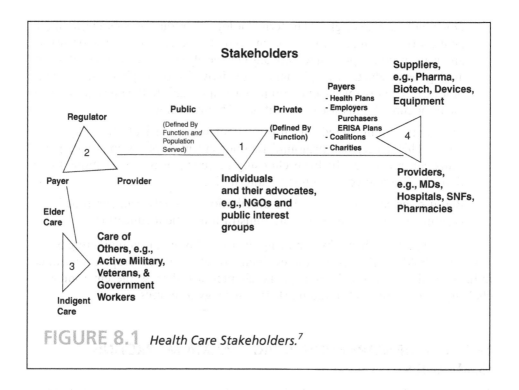

FIGURE 8.1  *Health Care Stakeholders.*[7]

example, in 2013 the U.S. division of Tokyo-based Astellas (which has a focus on neurological products) partnered with Humana, an insurer with a significant Medicare Advantage membership.

- Biopharma companies need clinical data to develop useful products and providers need cutting edge solutions to position themselves as leaders in their field. An example of such cooperative interests is the 2014 agreement between Geisinger Health System in Pennsylvania and Regeneron, a New Jersey-based biopharma company. Geisinger provides patient samples and clinical information; Regeneron sequences DNA and develops therapeutic solutions.

- Since drug development is very costly, pharma companies are looking to reduce discovery time. An example of a cross-category venture to meet this need is Novartis's 2019 announcement that it was partnering with Microsoft to use the latter's AI expertise.

- In an effort to identify more patients for their anticoagulant (blood thinner) products, in 2019 the Bristol-Myers Squibb-Pfizer Alliance announced a collaboration with Fitbit, whose product not only measures pulse but also irregularities such as atrial fibrillation. Shortly after that announcement, Microsoft revealed its intention to buy Fitbit.

- On the retail sales end of the industry, the best-known recent example of cross-category activity was CVS's $69 billion acquisition of insurer Aetna in 2017. (Legal challenges were finally settled in 2019.)

- Additional retail diversification occurred in 2018 when Walgreens and LabCorp announced the opening of 600 in-store testing sites.

As the above examples indicate, cross-category relationships among stakeholders can be complex, but potentially rewarding.

### Stakeholder value propositions

A successful value proposition will satisfy a stakeholder's preferences among product features of *quality, accessibility, and cost.*[12] Since each type of stakeholder will have a different value proposition, these three elements will first be explained. The biopharmaceutical marketer must be familiar with these concepts before crafting a product strategy.

1. Quality: Many stakeholders believe that the *quality* of pharmaceuticals is the responsibility of the FDA, which is supposed to assure they are safe, efficacious,[13] and produced according to good manufacturing practices. Likewise, when something goes wrong (such as an unanticipated side effect or product contamination), stakeholders turn to the FDA for prompt resolution. Given this belief of government assurance, quality is often taken for granted. Products can differentiate themselves on quality by features such as fewer side effects and better achievement of therapeutic goals compared to competitors. However, these comparisons must often be made broadly, since different classes of drugs can treat the same condition. For example, hypertension (high blood pressure) can be treated with diuretics, beta blockers, ACE or ARB inhibitors, or calcium channel blockers, to name a few classes of useful medications.

2. Access: Consideration of product *accessibility* is a bit more complex, since it involves understanding the value chain of this sector. Some factors that influence provision of this feature are:

   a) *Drug development process*: This activity[14] progresses from basic science discoveries, through establishment of proof-of-concept for a potential chemical entity, to rigorous testing, patent application, and submission to the FDA for approval. The time from initial discovery to commercial availability is often about 10 years. This process can often delay promising medication for those who are in immediate need,[15] creating publicity problems for the marketing manager.

   b) *FDA review and approval*: This step[16] can take varying amounts of time depending on the unique nature of the product, balancing potential harm with benefit, the urgency of introduction into the marketplace to meet health care needs, and generic status. Again, during this review, potential patients and their advocates press the FDA for access to promising medications.

c) *Manufacturing*: Given the global nature of the sources or components of health care products, it is difficult for companies to directly own and control the manufacturing process from start to finish. Consider, for example, a pill. The raw ingredients (often originating in India or China) are transformed into a therapeutic chemical entity, after which it is crafted into a form (tablet, capsule, etc.) that can be swallowed. The final product must then be bottled, labeled, and shipped. All of these processes may be done at different sites by different companies. A problem at any stage can cause access difficulties for stakeholders. While usual demand management techniques can help mitigate potential problems, sometimes the marketing manager needs to be skilled in crisis management. Two examples illustrate the need for such a crisis management plan: drug production for many products was delayed by Hurricane Maria hitting Puerto Rico;[17] Pfizer needed to quickly ramp up production of the chemotherapy drug Vincristine when the only other manufacturer (Teva) decided to discontinue production.[18]

d) *Distribution*: Once manufactured, a drug can be sold directly to intermediaries such as pharmacies, hospitals, or physicians. However, other distribution channels are also common. Biopharma companies may sell their products to wholesalers or distributers who then negotiate prices and deliver the product to the previously mentioned customers. The three largest companies in this category are AmerisourceBergen Corporation, Cardinal Health, Inc., and McKesson Corporation, which together control more than 90% of the market. Further, pharmaceutical benefit management companies (PBMs) often act on behalf of insurance companies and other payers to purchase large quantities of medications, negotiate prices on behalf of their clients, and manage sales to patients. Distribution can be either at a physical location, such as a pharmacy, or through the mail.

e) *Formularies*: Payer and provider organizations often develop lists of drugs to which they give preferred status for payment. Decisions about what medications to include and how to prioritize them for payment often come from a Pharmacy and Therapeutics (P&T) Committee, comprised of clinical specialists and those who may regularly prescribe the drugs (such as primary care physicians). Pharma companies often refer to those who influence these decisions (and are influential recommenders of therapeutic options) as Key Opinion Leaders, or KOLs. Payers' formularies may have many categories of preferred drugs, depending on how the underlying insurance product is structured. These levels may include (from least to most costly): generics, branded and preferred, branded on formulary but not preferred, non-formulary, and specialty pharmaceuticals. When filling a prescription, patients usually pay a fixed amount called a co-payment that depends on its category. For specialty pharmaceuticals that are self-administered (for conditions like multiple sclerosis, inflammatory bowel disease, and rheumatoid arthritis) patients frequently pay a percentage of the charge, called co-insurance.

f) *Administration by specialists*: Some drugs can only be prescribed or administered by physicians with certain specialty training. A shortage of such practitioners or scheduling problems can cause product access delays that are out of the control of the manufacturer or supply chain. For examples, oncologists administer chemotherapy in their offices or outpatient facilities. A patient with cystic acne must obtain a prescription from a dermatologist if Accutane (isotretinoin) is needed.

3. Cost: While *quality* and *access* are important product features, all stakeholders (except the biopharma companies themselves) consider *cost* the most important of the three. Figures 8.2 and 8.3 show the rapid spending growth for pharmaceuticals and sources of payment, respectively.

In order to understand the drivers of cost in this field the marketing manager must understand that it is comprised of three elements: price, volume, and intensity. These characteristics are discussed below.

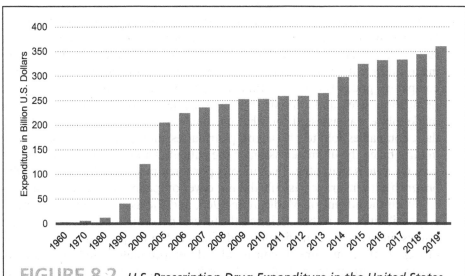

FIGURE 8.2 *U.S. Prescription Drug Expenditure in the United States 1960 to 2019 (in Billion U.S. Dollars).*[19]

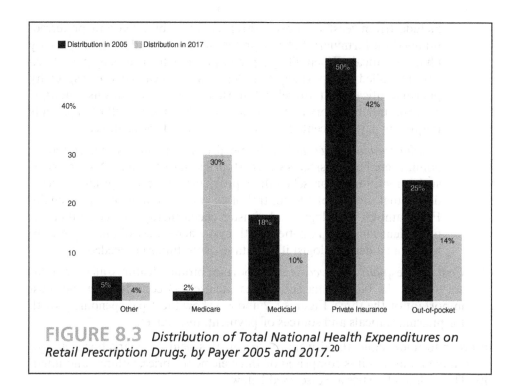

**FIGURE 8.3** *Distribution of Total National Health Expenditures on Retail Prescription Drugs, by Payer 2005 and 2017.*[20]

a) *Price*: This element is the one to which stakeholders pay the most attention. However, many prices can exist for the same product, leading to market confusion. Appreciating this pricing complexity will enable a better understanding of different value propositions. For most of the history of pharma companies, prices were set according to traditional marketing processes: given production, sales, and administration costs, plus a desired profit margin, the marketplace was assessed for what customers were willing to pay. In those days, companies sold to physicians, pharmacies, and hospitals. Those clients, in turn, billed the ultimate customer, the patient, who paid cash for the products. Of note is that, other than union-sponsored programs, before the 1990s *private* health insurance usually did not cover outpatient pharmaceuticals.

With the advent of Medicare in 1966, and the assumption of payment responsibilities for its beneficiaries, the federal government started to have an interest in the cost of medications administered in hospitals and physicians' offices. At the same time, Medicaid also developed state-based programs to pay for outpatient drugs. Instead of developing a national formulary with a fee schedule, federal programs pegged payments to a percentage of the Average Wholesale Price (AWP), a largely arbitrary number that pharma companies set so their immediate customers could maximize *their* profit. The process works in the following way: Biopharma companies set an AWP as high as they can. They then bill customers, like physicians, an actual *sales price* much lower than the AWP. The customers then bill payers a percentage (such as 75%) of AWP. The difference is the provider profit. (Subsequently, private payers also used the AWP methodology to pay providers.) Because of continued losses, federal programs attempted to control payments by reducing the percent of AWP they allowed.

Despite these lowered percentages, continued rising expenses led to passage of the Medicare Modernization Act (MMA) in 2003, which mandated that, starting in 2005, the payment method for these items would be changed to an *Average Sales* Price (ASP), plus 6%, i.e., the federal government would average the national sales prices for individual drugs to all customers (netted for rebates) and add 6% to payments. With this change, the pricing incentive for manufacturers shifted to increasing sales prices, since a larger ASP would result in a more profitable ASP + 6% for customers. As would be expected from this change, physicians use more expensive versions of drugs to treat the same conditions.[21] (This situation is the one that prevails today and is the reason many stakeholders want the federal government to negotiate actual prices directly with pharma companies.)

The market became even more complex when the MMA also created a prescription drug benefit for Medicare beneficiaries, viz. Medicare Part D. Under this plan, individuals purchase a private pharmaceutical plan that covers self-administered medications. Further, the MMA allowed Medicare managed care companies (now called Medicare Advantage, MA, plans) to negotiate prices with manufacturers—as mentioned, something the federal government still does not do.

At present, asking how much a medication costs (or how much will be paid) requires a complicated answer that depends on such factors as the setting where the drug is administered and specifics of the patient's insurance plan. Examples of coverage include:

Medicare inpatient
Medicare Part A pays hospitals under the all-inclusive Diagnosis Related Group (DRG) methodology; medication costs are bundled into the payment. Because the payments are set for *categories of diagnoses*, this method is often called a prospective payment system.

From a biopharma perspective (as well as any other medical product), the problem with such a system is that it cannot easily account for payments required by the constant introduction of new technologies.

If providers want to receive additional payments for these innovations, the *supplier* must petition CMS explaining the reasons for the added amounts.

If successful, this tactic can result in additional revenue if CMS subsequently: (1) pays more for an existing DRG, (2) reclassifies DRG codes to include some with higher payments (as was done in the past with some cardiovascular services), or (3) in the case of Ambulatory Payment Classifications (APCs) for outpatient services, grants what are termed "transitional pass through payments." These latter payments are time-limited additions (for example, three years) to the APCs to which they apply. To qualify, the applicant must demonstrate that the technology is:

- New—that is, generally, that it has been commercially available for no more than two or three years prior to the year for which the additional payment is sought.
- High cost relative to other cases in the relevant DRG category.
- A substantial clinical improvement over existing services or technologies for the Medicare patient population.[22]

### Medicare outpatient

Medicare Part B pays physicians for medications patients cannot self-administer, such as chemotherapy. After an annual deductible, the patient pays 20% of the Medicare-allowed charge. This amount is usually picked up by a supplemental insurance policy. For self-administered medications, such as pills or insulin injections, patients pay out-of-pocket or, if insured by a Part D or MA plan, a set charge for each prescription.

That specified amount can be a fixed payment (co-pay) or a percentage of the charge (co-insurance). The amounts will increase based on the formulary status of the drug, as explained earlier. Medications can be obtained in person at a pharmacy or by mail order (for larger amounts). The latter method costs the same or less than in-person purchase. Outpatient hospital (such as the emergency room or ambulatory care facility) allowed charges are based on Medicare's APCs, which groups services for an episode of illness into one payment. Pharmaceuticals are bundled into these payments. Other sites, like dialysis facilities (covered under Medicare's End Stage Renal Dialysis Program), are paid global rates for most medications delivered during care in those facilities. Likewise, patients in skilled nursing facilities have coverage for medications based on a global payment method.

### Medicaid

It is important to note two general Medicaid payer types—plans run by the state and private plans under state contract, most of which are managed care plans like Health Maintenance Organizations. Under both types of plans, patients either do not pay for drugs or have very small co-payments of several dollars. Medicaid inpatient payment programs vary by state; however, pharmaceuticals are covered as part of the hospital bill. Patients do not pay for these items.

Medicaid physician office payment amounts will also vary by state. Often payers have limited formularies and set prices they will pay physicians for medications. Patients may have a small co-pay for the office visit. For individual consumers, usually the choice of pharmacies or mail order sites is more limited than with either Medicare or private insurance. The patient pays little or nothing for the prescriptions.

Before discussing private insurance, it is important to understand another payment mechanism that affects pharma companies when they deal with providers who care for a large proportion of Medicaid and uninsured patients, the 340B program.

### 340B Program

The current Medicaid outpatient pharmaceutical pricing structure was created by the Omnibus Budget Reconciliation Act of 1990 (OBRA'90), which mandated pharmaceutical companies sell their products at lowest prices to Medicaid programs. In order to compensate for these reductions, drug manufacturers raised prices for the Veterans Administration and certain federally-funded clinics and public hospitals. As a result, Congress passed the Veterans Health Care Act of 1992 (VHCA, P.L. 102–585). The VHCA amended the Public Health Service Act with Section 340B[23] that required drug manufacturers to enter into another pricing agreement with the U.S. Department of Health and Human Services (HHS) called the Section 340B Drug Pricing Program.[24] The outpatient medications covered by this program generally include: FDA-approved prescription drugs, over-the-counter (OTC) drugs written on a prescription, biological products that can be dispensed only by a prescription (other than vaccines), and FDA-approved insulin.[25]

In order to participate in the Federal funding of outpatient drugs dispensed to Medicaid patients, drug manufacturers must enter into pharmaceutical pricing agreements (PPAs) with the Secretary of HHS to sell their products at a discount to certain health care providers, known as "covered entities." A covered entity is statutorily defined and includes various types of health centers, HIV/AIDS program grantees, and specialized clinics, including Federally Qualified Health Centers (FQHC), Federally Qualified Health Center Look-Alikes, Native Hawaiian Health Centers, Tribal/Urban Indian Health Centers, Ryan White HIV/AIDS Program Grantees, Black Lung Clinics, Comprehensive Hemophilia Diagnostic Treatment Centers, Sexually Transmitted Disease Clinics, Tuberculosis Clinics, and Title X Family Planning Clinics.[26] The drug rebate program is administered by CMS's Center for Medicaid and State Operations (CMSO), under the aegis of the Office of Pharmacy Affairs and Information Services (OPAIS) of the Health Resources and Services Administration (HRSA), a unit of HHS.

The purpose of the pricing is to set a maximum drug companies can charge covered entities for their products.[27] According to the OPAIS, "Participation in the Program results in significant savings estimated to be 20% to 50% on the cost of pharmaceuticals for safety-net providers."[28] By October 1, 2017, 12,722 covered entities and 20,000 contracted pharmacies participated in the program. In January 2018, 743 pharmaceutical manufacturers were participating in the program.[29]

Covered entities find this program so attractive, not only because it helps them to afford providing medication to their needy patients but also because they can sell these discounted drugs at market rates for other patients, thus gaining significant profits. The reason for this latter benefit is that the HRSA definition of a patient[30] is not limited to those who are low income, uninsured, or underinsured. Pharmaceutical companies have naturally become angry at this use because it can cut into their profitability. The problem with its resolution is that HRSA does not have regulatory authority to clarify the definition of an eligible patient; therefore, Congress must pass legislation clarifying this meaning. Hospital groups have strongly lobbied to keep the program intact, since they claim its profits subsidize other, underpaid, activities. Until Congress clarifies the role of this program, at least three major problems remain:

(1) The 340B statute does not require covered entities to report the level of charity care provided. As a result, there is a lack of data on how much charity care is provided by covered entities. Further, because there is no universally accepted definition of charity care, drawing a fair comparison of charity care provided across covered entities is difficult, if not impossible. Finally, while charity care spending often exceeds program savings, charity care levels have been on the decline at some hospitals, even as program savings increase.

(2) There is a financial incentive for 340B hospitals to prescribe more, and/or more expensive drugs to Medicare Part B beneficiaries, and prescribing trends indicate that 340B hospitals do prescribe more expensive drugs to Medicare Part B beneficiaries as compared to non-340B hospitals.[31]

(3) Pharmaceutical manufacturers are still fighting this program for two reasons. First, they are required to lower their product prices for covered entities without strict oversight of the recipient of those medications. Second, those reduced prices are figured into the ASP to pay for a much larger population.

### Private insurance

Inpatient payments can be by several methods:

- Charges or discount on charges. The payer will cover a certain amount of the bill and the patient will be responsible for the remainder. Pharmaceuticals are an itemized expense on the patient's bill. The patient may pay a percentage of hospital charges.
- Per diem. Payers pay an all-inclusive charge per day. Under this scheme, drugs are included in the daily payment. The patient usually pays nothing.

- Global fee. If the total fee for the admission is by diagnosis (as with DRGs) or by procedure (such as a joint replacement), the patient usually pays nothing.

    Outpatient physician's office patients may pay a percentage of the cost of non-self-administered medications, such as chemotherapy; or the cost may be included for a required co-payment. Which method applies depends on the insurance plan. In other settings, payments vary widely and can range from a global episode of care, to a daily charge, to a per-item basis.

b) *Volume*: The volume value proposition occurs when a medicine can be administered fewer times per day and/or fewer doses per course of treatment. For example, an antibiotic that can be taken once daily for three days (such as azithromycin) will be more valued than one that needs to be taken two or three times a day for 10 days (such as amoxicillin), particularly if both are available in generic forms. Another example is when a medicine needs to be taken as often or as long as other choices, but a single drug replaces one or more other treatments, or one dose is a combination of more than one drug (improving compliance).

c) *Intensity*: The intensity value proposition also occurs under three circumstances:

    (1) When a medicine allows reduction in the level of care. For example, if it allows a hospitalized patient to be treated in a "regular" bed instead of in an intensive care unit.

    (2) When a medicine allows care to be provided in a lower-cost, different site. For example, a once daily, injectable antibiotic can be administered to a patient in an outpatient setting rather than requiring the patient to be hospitalized.

    (3) When a better and/or less costly new medicine replaces an older one. The classic example in this category is the introduction of generic alternatives.

"Recent drug spending growth has largely been due to new brands [higher intensity], high prices for existing drugs, and fewer patent expiries [lower potential for generics, another intensity issue]."[32]

## EVOLVING STRUCTURE OF THE BIOPHARMACEUTICAL INDUSTRY

### *Bringing medicines to market*

The worldwide pharmaceutical market was worth nearly $1.3 trillion in 2019 and the top 10 companies accounted for about one-third of sales ($392.5 billion). Before looking at restructuring trends, it is necessary to understand the current functions that are needed to bring a drug to market. Figures 8.4 and 8.5 outline the new drug development process and highlights are explained next.

1. Basic research/discovery: Companies have traditionally carried out this function themselves "in-house" or by contracts with university partners. Recognizing the financial potential of such deals, universities have established technology transfer offices to handle such relationships. For example, in 2007, Northwestern sold the rights to about half of its Lyrica royalties for $700 million. Total royalties amounted to about $1.4 billion, including annual payments plus the value of the rights the university sold. Lyrica has recently been responsible for as much as 18% of the $10 billion Northwestern endowment.[33]

2. Clinical trials: "Clinical trials are conducted in a series of steps, called phases—each phase is designed to answer a separate research question.

    *Phase I*: Researchers first test a new drug or treatment in a small group of people for the first time to evaluate its overall safety, determine a safe dosage range, and identify side effects.

    *Phase II*: The drug or treatment is given to a larger group of people to see if it is effective and to further evaluate its safety.

    *Phase III*: The drug or treatment is given to large groups of people to confirm its effectiveness, monitor side effects, compare it to commonly used treatments, and collect information that will allow the drug or treatment to be used safely."[34]

3. Patent application: Depending on when the developer realizes the potential success of the product, it applies for patent protection; this protection is separate from the market exclusivity the FDA can grant in certain cases.

4. Regulatory application: The common types of drug applications to the FDA[35] are:

    a) Investigational New Drug (IND)

    Federal law requires that a drug be the subject of an approved marketing application before it is transported or distributed across state lines. Because a sponsor (the manufacturer or licensee or company) will probably need to ship the investigational drug to clinical investigators in many states, it must seek an exemption from that legal requirement. The IND is the means through which the sponsor technically obtains this exemption from the FDA.

    b) New Drug Application (NDA)

    When the sponsor of a new drug believes that enough evidence on the drug's safety and effectiveness has been obtained to meet the FDA's requirements for marketing approval, the sponsor submits an NDA to the

FDA. The application must contain specific technical data for review, including chemistry, pharmacology, medical, biopharmaceutics, and drug trial statistics. If the NDA is approved, the product may be marketed in the U.S. For internal tracking purposes, all NDAs are assigned an NDA number.

c) Abbreviated New Drug Application (ANDA)

An ANDA contains data that, when submitted to FDA's Center for Drug Evaluation and Research (CDER), Office of Generic Drugs, provides for the review and ultimate approval of a generic drug product. Generic drug applications are called "abbreviated" because they are generally not required to include preclinical (animal) and clinical (human) data to establish safety and efficacy. Instead, a generic applicant must scientifically demonstrate that its product is bioequivalent (i.e., performs in the same manner as the innovator drug).

d) Over-the-Counter Drugs (OTC)

OTC drug products are those drugs that are available to consumers without a prescription. There are more than 80 therapeutic categories of OTC drugs, ranging from acne drug products to weight control drug products. As with prescription drugs, CDER oversees OTC drugs to ensure that they are properly labeled and that their benefits outweigh their risks

e) Biologic License Application (BLA)

Biological products are approved for marketing under the provisions of the Public Health Service (PHS) Act. The Act requires a firm which manufactures a biologic for sale in interstate commerce to hold a license for the product. A biologics license application is a submission that contains specific information on the manufacturing processes, chemistry, pharmacology, clinical pharmacology, and the medical effects of the biologic product. If the information provided meets FDA requirements, the application is approved and a license is issued allowing the firm to market the product.

5. Manufacturing: This process ranges from sourcing of raw materials (including biologic substrates) to finished product production to packaging.

6. Marketing and sales: These functions range from internal company planning to managing a salesforce to price negotiations with public and private entities to ultimate product sales.

7. Post-market surveillance (Phase IV study): After the technology reaches the marketplace it is constantly monitored for adverse reactions ranging from mild side effects to death.

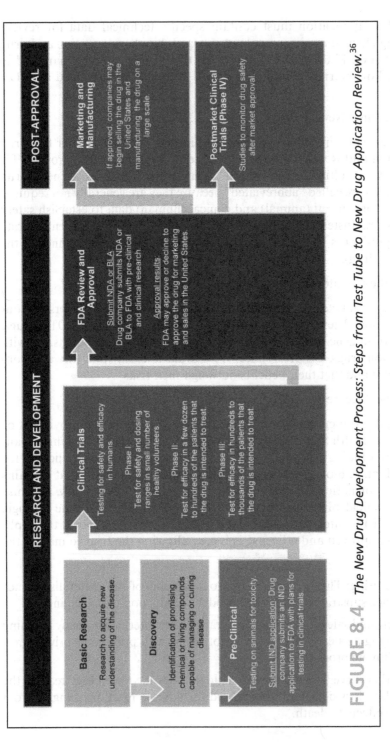

**FIGURE 8.4** *The New Drug Development Process: Steps from Test Tube to New Drug Application Review.*[36]

BLA = biologic license application; FDA = Food and Drug Administration;
IND = investigational new drug; NDA = new drug application

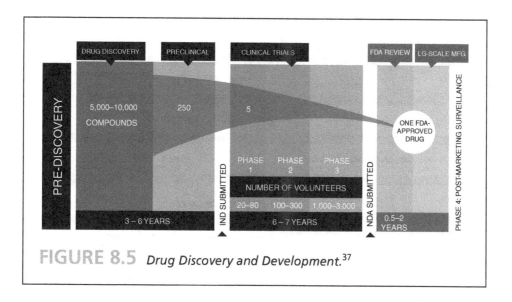

**FIGURE 8.5** *Drug Discovery and Development.*[37]

## Evolving industry structure

All of the functions listed in the previous subsection had traditionally been performed by the company itself in an integrated, single-entity, business model. However, the structure of the biopharma sector (as well as health care technology in general) has been changing in at least two major ways:

1. Merger, acquisition, and alliance: These activity trends have been taking place since the start of the century. See Figure 8.6 for many prominent examples. A principal, though not exclusive, reason for these combinations is the desire of companies to fill their pipelines with new products as the older ones go off patent. (Please see the section below on environmental forces.) The effectiveness of these strategies has been questioned since the late 2000s and the research results do not provide clear cut answers. Some of the problems that confound evaluation include:

   ■ The *nature of the companies* can differ. Examples include: large pharmaceutical company mergers, large pharmaceutical companies acquiring small ones, small biotech firms merging, and pharmaceutical companies buying biotech firms. Since the characteristics of each of the original firms are different, one would expect the results to vary.

   ■ Some businesses may go into a new arrangement from strength while others may do so because they are distressed.

   ■ The *specific reasons* for the combination also matter. For example, one company may have an unpromising pipeline and seeks another company with many potential products. Another company may have a promising research agenda but wants to diversify into a new class of products it

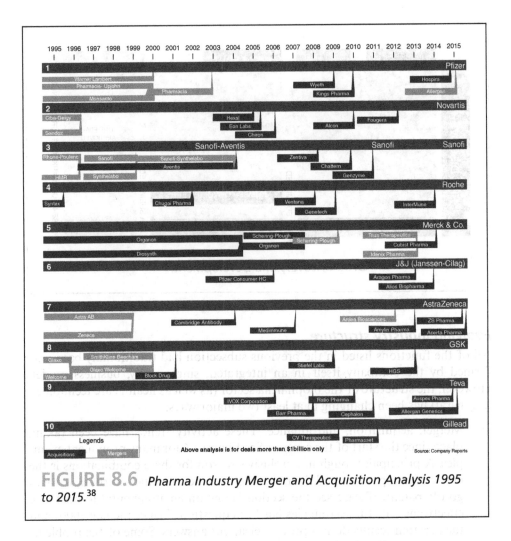

**FIGURE 8.6** *Pharma Industry Merger and Acquisition Analysis 1995 to 2015.*[38]

had not previously investigated. This latter reason has been a common one when large pharmaceutical companies wish to enter the biotech field.

■ The *operational nature* of the deals also varies. For example, there can be great differences among the mergers of large companies, the acquisition of one company by another, and an alliance based on mutual performance results. Further, among these models, cultural compatibilities can have varying degrees of importance.

■ The *measures of success* across studies varies. For example, is success measured by the number of new patents, number of drugs that reach a particular clinical trial stage, number of new drug applications, or product revenue? Also, when one or more of these metrics are used, what is the time period over which they are measured?

Given these caveats about the structure of the deals and outcomes measurements, according to Bain & Co., "in the late 1990s, pharma companies spent an average of $1.1 billion to develop and launch a new drug. A decade later, that investment has doubled to $2.2 billion. At the same time, R&D productivity, measured in the number of new molecular entities and biologic license applications per R&D dollar spent, declined by 21% a year."[39] In other words, despite growing company combinations, drugs are twice as expensive to develop and there are fewer of them.

Large company mergers have achieved short-term cost savings through economies of scale of operational activities; however, there is "little evidence to date that they've increased long-term R&D performance or outcomes. By contrast, the empirical research on *alliances* [emphasis added] between smaller biotech firms and larger pharmaceutical entities is more encouraging in nature."[40]

Further, "products developed in an alliance have a higher probability of success in the more complex late stage trials, particularly if the licensee is a large firm."[41] The reason for this latter finding may be that large scale trials and regulatory expertise at a *global level* are required to assure the critical factor of speed to market for these products.

2. Specialization by function is a second trend: As companies discovered the downsides of these mergers and the effectiveness of alliances, with the large pharmaceutical companies playing the role of coordinator, questions arose concerning: what functions should companies outsource and which should they keep in-house? A diversity of opinions and actual company actions highlight attempts to answer these questions. Using the categories of product development, we can address the industry's current status.[42]

- Basic research/discovery. The Bain & Co. study also explains why this task should be moved, to a large degree, outside the company: "Innovation is one area where scale doesn't work. Innovation can't be manufactured; it must be nurtured in a highly entrepreneurial environment. That argues for acquiring new compounds from a large global pool of smaller, independent, innovation-focused companies. In fact, the big pharma deals have better odds of success if the companies involved move quickly to reduce the scale of their internal research. They should shift 40% to 50% of their current innovation budgets to outside their newly merged companies."

  Indeed, because of the riskiness of these new product developments (particularly for biotech drugs), there has been a trend toward larger companies using smaller ones as sources of new products. (This risk is highlighted by the fact that in 2019, 11 biotech firms went bankrupt, and an additional 31 were at high risk for the same fate in 2020.[43]) The financial deals usually take the form of some combination of upfront payments, milestone payments, and royalties.

  Another trend in this area is for larger companies to spin off parts of R&D functions into smaller companies. For example, in 2010, GSK spun off a biotech research group Convergence Pharmaceuticals in which it took an 18% stake.[44] It is also important to note the evolving role of academia in basic research/discovery. Significant breakthroughs have always come from such sources, e.g., the discoveries of insulin at the University of Toronto and penicillin at St. Mary's Hospital in London.

However, until recently these finds were picked up by biopharma companies and commercialized, leaving the pioneers with only the prestige of their breakthroughs. Starting in the latter part of the twentieth century, the science became more complex and expensive, so universities established "offices of technology transfer" to negotiate financial deals for their products with commercial companies. As mentioned above, perhaps the most well-known example is Northwestern University's $700 million in royalties for Pfizer's drug Lyrica.

More recently, other academic models have developed. In one arrangement, academia hosts nascent biopharma companies, e.g., in 2019 NYU Langone Health became the home for 22 biotech and life science companies.[45] In another model, the academic entity sponsors its own biopharma startup. An example is the 2019 partnership between Duke University and Deerfield Management Company to created Four Points Innovation.[46] The new company will not only develop new products, but take it through the IND submission to the FDA. Both of these new organizational models pose challenges to traditional biopharma companies which must create newer cooperative (and costlier) arrangements.

- Clinical trials. As companies seek to predict research costs and avoid staffing-up for particular clinical trials, they are increasingly hiring outside firms to manage their clinical trials. The outside organizations they employ are called Contract Research Organizations (or CROs). Companies may also hire outside firms (called functional service providers, or FSPs) for *portions* of these trials. "The global CRO market value reached $39 billion in 2018 and is expected to reach $44 billion by 2021."[47] Some observers of this trend disagree with its logic as a business strategy. For example, Christiansen et al.[48] believe a "far better strategy would be to focus on the place in the value chain that is becoming decommoditized: the management of clinical trials, which are now an integral part of the drug research process and so a critical capability for pharmaceutical companies. Despite this, most drugmakers have been outsourcing their clinical trials to contract research organizations such as Covance and Quintiles, better positioning those companies in the value chain. Acquiring those organizations, or a disruptive drugmaker like Dr. Reddy's Laboratories, would help reinvent big pharma's collapsing business model." In addition to outsourcing the performance of trials, large companies are increasingly also taking on investment partners to pay for the trials to mitigate their riskiness. Examples include NovaQuest Capital Management, LLC and Avillion, LLC.[49]

■  Regulatory filing and compliance. Outsourcing regulatory affairs is particularly useful for small companies which do not have experience dealing with the FDA. On the other hand, this function is a core competency of larger firms. For both types of businesses, however, it is often helpful to hire an outside company to help with part of the process if they are filing outside the U.S.

External expertise with such tasks as language translation, application formatting, and identification of appropriate governmental agencies can be very helpful.[50]

■  Sales and Marketing. This function has been the traditional province of large, well-established companies. Smaller firms, however, can incur large fixed costs by staffing-up to promote just one product. Consequently, these firms often hire companies which can detail their products to potential purchasers or prescribers. Sometimes these outside firms are larger companies in the same business which have a business arrangement to co-promote a product.

■  Manufacturing. Given the global nature of the sources or components of health care products, it is difficult for companies to directly own and control the manufacturing process from start to finish. Consider, for example, a pill. The raw ingredients, often coming from India or China, are transformed into a therapeutic chemical entity, after which it is crafted into a form (tablet, capsule, etc.) that can be swallowed. The final product must then be bottled, labeled, and shipped. All of these processes may be done at different sites by different companies.

With these restructuring trends comes an increase in system complexity. Even after the product has come to market the relationships can be equally complex. See Figure 8.7 for relationships in the pharmaceutical industry. Coordination of activities has become much more important to decrease the likelihood that errors will occur, perhaps leading to more and more costly regulation.

A newer and important development in this category is provider organizations "manufacturing" their own products. In September 2018, CivicaRx[51] was formed by a consortium of hospital and systems (which now represent about 30% of all U.S. hospital beds) to address drug shortages. The nonprofit company contracted with Hikma Pharmaceuticals PLC, a multinational generic pharmaceutical company, in July 2019 to produce the medications. In October 2019 Vancomycin became its first product from this business to be administered to a patient.

By December, the company announced 14 other products would become available. The reason for listing these dates is to highlight the speed with which

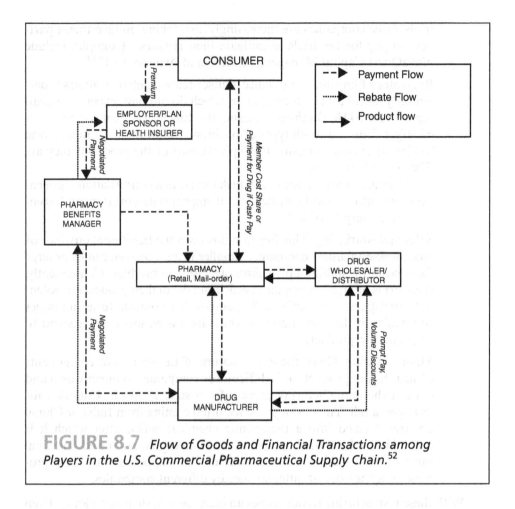

**FIGURE 8.7** *Flow of Goods and Financial Transactions among Players in the U.S. Commercial Pharmaceutical Supply Chain.*[52]

this challenge to traditional biopharma companies can develop. While many of these medications are in short supply because larger companies do not find them profitable, more lucrative off-patent products can also be manufactured in short order. Biopharma companies should keep this development on their marketing screens and, if they have excess capacity, perhaps offer to participate in manufacturing for these customers/new competitors.

## ENVIRONMENTAL CHALLENGES AND MARKETING STRATEGY RESPONSES

Many environmental challenges involve periodic disruptions, such as supply chain interruptions caused by natural disasters, and manufacturing problems that produce product safety issues. Examples include Hurricane Maria in September 2017

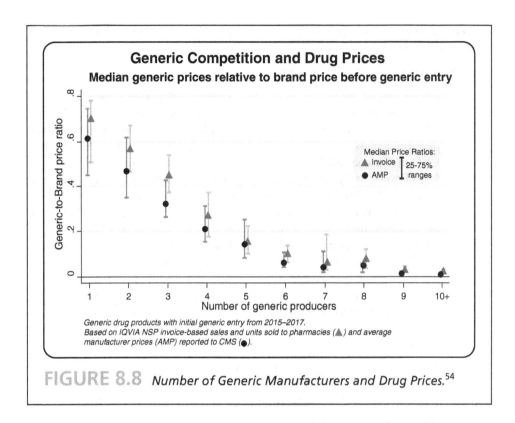

**FIGURE 8.8** *Number of Generic Manufacturers and Drug Prices.*[54]

which severely disrupted production in Puerto Rico (a significant source of mainland U.S. medical products), and the COVID-19 pandemic of 2019–2020. Consequences of both of those events are still being felt as of this writing. However, two overriding issues that have shaped the biopharma industry since the late 2000s and loom large in the future are the *need for new products* and *pressures on the prices* of those medications.

### New Product Development

The reason biopharma companies have accelerated their quests for new products is the many significant patent expirations that have recently occurred and will hit in the near future. When a drug loses patent protection, competition can cause dramatic reductions in sale price; for that reason, the event is often called a "patent cliff." In 2019, such well-known drugs as Rituxin, Lyrica, Herceptin, Avastin, and Advair were slated to go off patent. Between 2019–2024, more than $198 billion is at risk from patent expirations.[53] The effect on price of multiple competitors is highlighted in Figure 8.8. While one generic manufacturer causes price to decrease by 39%, when at least six firms are in the market prices decline by 95%.

The marketing strategies biopharma companies have taken include the following measures:

1. Deciding which drugs to develop:

   a) Prior to about 2000, companies had the philosophy that if they made new and interesting (whatever that term meant) products, they would sell themselves. Realization of meeting stakeholder value propositions in drug development is more recent. For example, in 2008, Andrew Witty, then CEO of GlaxoSmithKline invited a group of health care officials from the UK, France, Italy and Spain to London to examine the drugs the company was developing. "[It] was an opportunity for us to say, 'Look, here's what the development pipeline at (Glaxo) looks like, here's what these drugs are going to be ... which one of these do you think?' This is exactly where I would prioritize health care dollars," Witty was quoted as saying.

   The officials who were mostly looking at the drugs Glaxo was testing in small, intermediate human trials, gave blunt feedback on which drugs to prioritize and what sort of data Glaxo would need to show to make state health care systems willing to buy the drugs.[55] Unfortunately many companies have not used this insightful method to guide drug development.

   b) In a variation on the previous strategy of targeting selected drugs for development, some companies are narrowing their focus to certain disease categories. A recent example of this strategy is Sanofi's exit from cardiovascular and diabetes products.[56]

   c) Another prevalent strategy companies have used to decide which drugs to develop reflects a shift in their profit models: from high volume, low-cost products (such as antibiotics and antihypertensives) to much lower volumes, but very high-cost products (such as drugs of biologic origin). Many of these drugs are called "orphan drugs" because, prior to the Orphan Drug Act in 1983, their potential market for sales did not warrant the cost of clinical trials to prove safety and efficacy to allow them to obtain approval under an NDA. Since they were neither reviewed nor withdrawn, they were called "orphan" drugs; the diseases treated by these medications were thus called orphan diseases. Legislation gave a boost to this strategic shift when Congress passed the Orphan Drug Act to encourage development of potentially unprofitable drugs and respond to lobbying by organizations representing patients with rare conditions.[57] The law provided pharmaceutical companies with: (1) federal funding of grants and contracts to perform clinical trials of orphan products, (2) a tax credit of 50% of clinical testing costs, (3) an exclusive right to market the orphan drug for seven years from the date of marketing approval, (4) enhanced coordination with the FDA throughout the drug's development,

(5) priority FDA review, and (6) a waiver of drug application fees.[58] Initially, the Act was aimed at drugs for which there was "no reasonable expectation" that U.S. sales would support their development. The vagueness of that description and lack of resultant company interest caused passage of a 1984 Amendment changing the definition of the targeted products to those used for "rare diseases," defined as any disease or condition which: "(A) affects less than 200,000 persons in the United States, or (B) affects more than 200,000 in the United States and for which there is no reasonable expectation that the cost of developing and making available in the United States a drug for such disease or condition will be recovered from sales in the United States of such drug."[59]

Of note is that the Orphan Drug Act does not allow deviation from regulatory requirements applied to non-orphan drugs and does not extend product patent life (it only extends *marketing exclusivity*). A 1988 Amendment to the Act requires sponsors to apply for orphan drug designation *before* submitting a new drug application or a product license application to the FDA. The regulatory administration of this Act is carried out by the Office of Orphan Product Development.[60]

The success of this Act can be measured by the number of medications brought to market as the result of its enactment. Because of the high cost of development and lengthy approval process (about 90 months in 1982–1983, two-thirds of which was taken up with clinical trials[61]), pharmaceutical companies brought to market fewer than 10 drugs for rare conditions between 1973 and 1983.[62] Today, the Orphan Drug Product designation database[63] contains about 3,800 entries. Further, the FDA says its Orphan Grants Program has been used to bring more than 45 products to marketing approval.

The effect of this law has tremendous implications for increasing costs of medical care. According to the health insurance trade group AHIP:

- "From 1998 to 2017, the average per-patient annual cost for orphan drugs increased 26-fold, while the cost for specialty and traditional drugs merely doubled

- The average annual orphan drug cost rose from $7,136 in 1997 to $186,758 in 2017

- Orphan drugs are 25x more expensive than non-orphan drugs

- Today, 88% of orphan drugs cost more than $10,000 per year per patient

- In 2017, 7 out of 10 best-selling drugs had orphan indications."[64]

The regulatory reasons for this problem include the following loopholes in the Orphan Drug Act (of which pharma companies are acutely aware and exploit):

- Orphan status requires prevalence data from the U.S. tax benefits and market exclusivity does not consider foreign product sales, which, for example, in the case of some infectious diseases (such as tropical parasites), may be considerable.

- Market exclusivity is much broader protection than patent protection. The former grants a treatment monopoly to prevent entrance of competitors whose products have similar effects on the disease; the latter merely protects the chemical entity. The only way a new medication can challenge the market protection of the established orphan drug is if the company "provides a reasonable hypothesis that their product is 'clinically superior' to the approved product by means of greater effectiveness, greater safety, or that it provides a major contribution to patient care (MC-to-PC)."[65] The FDA emphasizes that a claim of clinical superiority will be "evaluated on a case-by-case basis for each drug product," that is, there is no prescription for making this determination when comparing it to the existing orphan drug.[66] However, *clinical superiority cannot be claimed based on lower cost, greater patient compliance, or increased quality of life.*

- The Act specifies that the only circumstance that allows the FDA to categorically grant permission to another company to offer another drug in this category is when the market exclusivity holder "cannot assure the availability of sufficient quantities of the drug to meet the needs of persons with the disease or condition for which the drug was designated."

- A drug can obtain orphan status for more than one indication if *each* condition affects fewer than 200,000 people. This loophole encourages companies to separate disease categories as much as possible, even if the drug treats a broad group. It is, difficult, therefore, to classify *overall* drug use by disease or category. As examples, medications used to treat one autoimmune disease may also be used to treat a different autoimmune condition. Further, it may also be used to treat a different class of disease, such as cancers.

- A pharmaceutical company can obtain orphan drug designation if one of the indications is a rare disease and other indications are for much more prevalent conditions. Another variant on this theme is that a company can obtain orphan status for a rare condition and physicians can prescribe the drug for "off label" (non-approved) indications. In either case, the pharmaceutical company charges orphan drug (that is, high) prices for all uses. As an example of these practices, Daniel et al. state: "rituximab, which was initially FDA approved for use in the treatment of follicular non-Hodgkin's lymphoma, is the number 1 selling medication approved as an orphan drug. It is currently used to treat a wide variety of conditions, ranks as the 12th all-time bestselling medication in the United States, and generated over $3.7 billion in US sales in 2014."[67] The overall significance of this issue was highlighted in a report by AHIP:[68] of 46 orphan drugs available between 2012 and 2014, 22 were used for non-orphan diseases; prices for orphan drugs used primarily for non-orphan diseases increased by 37%, while those used primarily for orphan indications rose by 12%; and almost half of all drugs approved by the FDA in 2015 were orphan drugs.

▪ Orphan status is granted based on disease prevalence *at the time of approval*. Regulations do not take into account growth of the affected population over the life of the market exclusivity. This problem was highlighted when AZT was approved as a drug for AIDS.

▪ Orphan drug status can be granted to a company that does not develop the drug and also for a drug which is not new. In other words, if new research shows an older, generic drug can be used to treat a rare condition in the U.S., a company other than the one who developed it can obtain orphan designation and market exclusivity. For example, by 1993, thalidomide received orphan drug status for treatment of leprosy and a complication of bone marrow transplants.[69] In 1998, Celgene received orphan drug designation for thalidomide for treatment of the blood disease multiple myeloma.[70]

Not all high-cost medications are orphan drugs. The previously-explained specialty drugs fall into this category.

2. Deciding who will develop new drugs: As already mentioned, biopharma companies can develop their own products, partner with other companies, acquire/merge with other companies, or license rights. Obviously, the cost and speed to market are major considerations in deciding which of these tactics are appropriate for each product.

3. Expediting new drug discovery: A variety of new techniques have been used to expedite new drug discovery, most recently the use of AI[71] to sort out likely useful molecules. Two newer methods stand out. First, rather than develop their own AI capabilities, biopharma companies are partnering with firms that have that expertise. For example, Pfizer, Novartis, and Johnson & Johnson are using IBM Watson for Drug Discovery.[72]

A second unprecedented innovation is cooperation among companies for drug development. A prime example is the consortium called MELLODDY (machine learning ledger orchestration for drug discovery). According to its website:[73]

"The MELLODDY project aims to establish a machine learning platform that would make it possible to learn from multiple sets of proprietary data while respecting their highly confidential nature, as data and asset owners will retain control of their information throughout the project.

Through this innovative, blockchain-based solution, the pharmaceutical companies in the project aim to demonstrate the feasibility of this approach with an unprecedented volume of competitive data in the form of over a billion drug-development-relevant data points, and hundreds of terabytes of image data that annotate the biological effects of more than 10 million small molecules. The platform would also take a federated machine learning approach, meaning that the learning effort is not centralized but spread over different, physically separated partners."

## Price pressures

Because medicines have become much more expensive, payers and other stakeholders have adopted a variety of strategies to control costs. (These methods apply to all expensive technologies, not just specialty drugs.) The biopharma marketer must understand which of the measures explained here are being used in order to develop a strategic plan to ensure product success.

1. Employing disease management: Payers have internal units or hire outside companies to attend to patients with rare, high-cost diseases or conditions which are very common (such as diabetes and heart failure). The hope is that this special attention will result in more appropriate use of high cost medications. These arrangements can pose opportunities or threats to biopharma companies depending on whose products the company uses.

2. Contracting with a specialty PBM: Payers either have subsidiaries or contract with independent companies that manage pharmacy benefits on their behalf. Certain firms specialize in tracking and managing specialty pharmaceuticals. Prominent examples include: BriovaRX, which is a subsidiary of OptumRX, owned by UnitedHealth Group; CVS Caremark Specialty Pharmacy, owned by CVS Health; and Accredo, a division of Express Scripts. Contracts usually include management fees as well as incentives to control costs. Providers (such as physicians) must order the drugs from one of these companies. Favorable contract terms are obviously important.

3. Requiring prior authorization: When a drug is expensive, and often when it is first launched, payers want the option to review its necessity by using pre-determined protocols. For example, a physician may need to call a special phone number (frequently staffed by a PBM) to get authorization to prescribe a medication. Obtaining this permission often does not prevent the drug's use, but does determine whether the payer will cover its expense. Assuring that prescribers have an easy time getting such authorization will enhance the likelihood of new product use.

4. Restricting off-label or experimental uses/narrowing indication: While an FDA-approved medication can be used for non-approved indications, payers will often check to make sure the patient's disease is one of the *approved* indications as a precondition for payment.[74] Experimental medications are often covered by the company running the clinical trial. An example of a narrowed indication is that an insurance company approved the use of bupropion for depression but not smoking cessation.

5. Implementing physician-developed guidelines: When a treatment is very new and appears to effectively treat a disease, national guidelines may not be available. Payers will, therefore, often convene local experts to decide on appropriate use. The process may be ad hoc or as part of an ongoing review by the payer's Pharmacy and Therapeutics (P&T) Committee which makes formulary decisions. The appropriateness decision may be that the newer (and presumably more expensive) drug should be used only after established and less costly treatments are tried first. (See point 15. for step therapy.)

6. Changing the benefit design: On average, specialty pharmaceuticals are paid 60% from pharmacy benefits and 40% medical benefits.[75] (Variations from these figures can occur by insurer, e.g., Medicare, Medicaid, private payer as well as by site of care, e.g., hospital, physician's office, home, etc.) For example, a patient may only be responsible for a physician's office co-payment while receiving a medication billed at tens of thousands of dollars. Some plans have moved the basis for payment to the pharmacy benefit at a level that requires the patient to pay a co-insurance—often thousands of dollars. Other strategies for changing the benefit design include increasing deductibles or co-payments for these medications. (Patient responsibility is, of course, subject to annual out-of-pocket limits.) This cost-control method is, however, flawed in the long run for payers and patients. Making patients responsible for any costs for goods or services only works if they can make choices about their care. Since these medications are often used for chronic and, frequently, life-threatening indications, there is no discretionary component. In fact, creating a financial barrier to their use may result in greater expenses for the payer if the patient does not take the medications.

   One way pharmaceutical companies are responding to these increased out-of-pocket expenses is by a method called "couponing." These companies raise their charges for medications but provide patients with coupons to cover their increased out-of-pocket expenses. Some insurance plans have responded by banning the use of the coupons or making their use less appealing for patients. For example, in 2018, PBM "Express Scripts and others introduced a new 'copay accumulator' approach for its corporate customers. The programs prevent copay card funds from counting toward a patient's required out-of-pocket spending before insurance kicks in on expensive specialty drugs, such as arthritis and HIV treatments."[76] CMS has taken retaliation a step further by suing offenders. For example, when Pfizer contributed to a charity that helped patients pay for the company's drugs, CMS won a $23.85 million judgment. As U.S. Attorney Andrew Lelling commented, "Pfizer knew that the third-party foundation was using Pfizer's money to cover the co-pays of patients taking Pfizer drugs, thus generating more revenue for Pfizer and masking the effect of Pfizer's price increases."[77]

7. Selective contracting with infusion centers: Since some providers charge more than others, insurance companies look to selective contracting to provide volume in return for lower prices for care. Biopharma companies must maintain a close relationship with these centers and make sure their products are priced appropriately for these customers.

8. Bundling with service payment: Instead of paying separately for the service component and medication, payers are contracting with providers to bundle the entire episode of care into one fee. For example, Medicare's End Stage Renal Dialysis program requires injectable medications (such as erythropoietin) be billed with the global episode of dialysis. Other such initiatives include courses of treatment for cancers. It should be noted that part of this bundling process assumes that payment is made for services that occur over a period of time, not just one encounter. Consider another example: treatment of high blood pressure. Instead of paying by episode, bundling would take into account such treatment components as additional medications required to achieve the target pressure, laboratory tests needed to monitor the medication (for example, to prevent side effects), and handling adverse reactions. In this setting, biopharma companies must realize their products are only one of many components of the ultimate payment.

9. Removing "buy and bill" incentives: Physicians buy many in-office administered medications (such as traditional chemotherapy and specialty pharmaceuticals) directly from the manufacturer. They then bill the insurance company at rates that are often significantly higher than acquisition cost. (The exception is Medicare Part B, which allows only a 6% markup over national average sales price.) Some insurers have instituted a process by which the physician orders the drugs and the company pays the PBM the acquisition cost. Obviously, this change has caused much resentment from physicians whose revenue largely depends on those markups, e.g., oncologists. This change also upsets the long-standing relationships the biopharma companies have with their physician customers.

10. Establishing pay-for-performance metrics: Insurance companies pay not only for the medications that work, but those that do not. To mitigate this problem, insurers have contracted with pharmaceutical companies to only pay for the treatment courses that achieve a predetermined goal. For example, Merck "agreed to peg what the insurer Cigna pays for the diabetes drugs Januvia and Janumet to how well Type 2 diabetes patients are able to control their blood sugar."[78] Similar deals have been applied to more expensive medications, like those that treat multiple sclerosis.[79]

11. Sequencing multiple therapeutically equivalent medications: Some treatment classes contain medications with similar efficacy and rates of side effects. However, the costs for each of these medications can vary significantly. For example, in 2018, the wholesaler acquisition cost (WAC) of a

30-day course of maintenance treatment for rheumatoid arthritis could range from about \$1,500 for infliximab (Renflexis, Merck) to \$14,100 for etanercept (Enbrel, Amgen).[80] Having physicians choose the lowest effective drug in a class, and then the next most expensive if the first fails, can achieve significant savings.

12. Incentivizing prescription of generic medications: Many terms have been applied to generic, biologic, specialty medications. Differences among these terms are important because their approval and usage indications can vary. With respect to the "reference product" (original branded medication) *biosimilars* are very similar in structure, do not have any clinically meaningful differences in safety and effectiveness, are allowed to have only minor differences in clinically inactive components, and cannot be automatically substituted. Biosimilars are sometimes called *follow-on biologics*. *Bioequivalent* or *interchangeable* medications are biosimilar but also meet other standards that allow a pharmacist to substitute them for the reference product without the order of the prescriber. *Biobetter* medications are based on the reference product but claim to offer improvements.

Savings from these medications will be determined by their development and production costs, which are substantially more than non-biologic medications. As a result, while generic non-biologics are typically discounted by about 80%, biosimilars and bioequivalents may only be discounted by 15–30%.[81] However, because the reference drugs are so expensive, even this smaller reduction can be significant. "Cumulative potential savings to health systems in the European Union (EU) and the U.S., as a result of the use of biosimilars, could exceed EUR50 billion in aggregate over the next five years and reach as much as EUR100 billion."[82] Some major specialty drugs losing patent protection include: Herceptin (trastuzumab), June 2019; Avastin (bevacizumab), July 2019; Aranesp (darbepoetin alfa), May 2024; and Enbrel (etanercept), November 2028.

The incentives occur at two levels: patient and prescriber. For the patient, out-of-pocket expenses, such as co-payments, are greater for branded than generic drugs. Patients will therefore often request generics when they receive prescriptions. Prescribers have two types of incentives. The first is saving time. Often patients request the generic when at the pharmacy, prompting the pharmacist to call the office and take precious practitioner time redoing the order. Second, some payers have bonus payment arrangements with physicians who meet certain generic prescribing targets.

In order to combat generic competition, biopharma companies have undertaken a number of strategies, including:

a) *When a generic drug company files an ANDA, it must notify the NDA sponsor or patent holder*. However, the NDA sponsor or patent holder usually has several patents on the same product, not all of which run concurrently; therefore, within 45 days of receipt of notice, the patent holders can file a patent infringement suit against the ANDA applicant. Unless the courts reach an earlier decision, the FDA may not give final approval to the ANDA for at least 30 months from the date of the notice. Companies have used this tactic to slow the ANDA approval, sometimes claiming the last patent on the drug has not expired (even if that particular patent is not material to generic production of the chemical entity).[83]

b) *Improved formulations of a drug are often planned in a company's product pipeline.* By introducing this improvement before the old drug's patent expiration (a process called *next-generation preempt*), the branded pharmaceutical company can make generic production of its initial drug less desirable. An example of this practice was Forest Laboratory's (now part of Actavis) drug Celexa (citalopram). Several years before this antidepressant lost patent protection, the company launched its L-isomer escitalopram (Lexapro), which was at least as effective as Celexa but had fewer side effects.

c) *When a company's drug goes off patent, it can obtain another patent on a modified form, which has its own patent life.* This strategy is called *product extension*. A classic example was the Marion Merrell Dow (now part of Sanofi) drug Cardizem (diltiazem), used for hypertension and heart rhythm problems. The drug was originally administered three or four times a day; when the patent life expired, the company introduced a twice-daily product (Cardizem SR). When this latter formulation was due to go off patent, Cardizem CD, a once-daily product, was brought to market.

d) *When a company's brand is very strong and its drug is about to go off patent, the firm may want to introduce its own generic product, called a branded generic.* For example, for many years, the McNeil Consumer Health Care Division of Johnson & Johnson marketed the Motrin brand of ibuprofen. When the drug became a generic, the company still marketed it under the Motrin brand and preserved some sales.

e) *If a branded drug company faces patent expiration, it can manufacture the medication in partnership with a generic drug company.* The advantage derives from cooperation in not challenging an ANDA filing. If the partnering generic drug company is the first applicant to file a substantially complete ANDA and the patent holder does not challenge it, the generic product will be eligible for a 180-day period of exclusivity beginning from the date it begins commercial marketing. Since only one generic drug company is marketing the product, this time period affords significant profitability potential for the branded company because it can continue its manufacturing and maintain some of its pricing power. The generic drug maker saves money in litigation and manufacturing costs while sharing in the pricing benefit of the period of exclusivity. This strategy is sometimes called producing an *authorized generic*. In a variation of this process, the patent holder may partner with a generic drug company once another company has its generic product approved. This process is called *flanking*. GSK employed this strategy in 2003 when Apotek launched a generic version of the antidepressant Paxil; GSK then partnered with generic drug company Par Pharmaceutical to supply it with generic Paxil in return for royalties on U.S. sales.

f) *If a generic drug maker achieves the 180-day period of exclusivity, the branded drug manufacturer can pay that firm to withhold its product introduction.* This process is called *pay for delay*. According to an FTC study, these anticompetitive deals cost consumers and taxpayers $3.5 billion in higher drug costs every year.[84] For many years the FTC has sued companies that engage in the practice, claiming illegal anticompetitive behavior. In a June 2013 Supreme Court ruling, the Court stated "that the deals could potentially be a violation of antitrust law" but refused the FTC's request to declare them to be presumed to be illegal.[85] Despite the lack of definitive guidance, the FTC noted that there were fewer pay-for-delay deals in fiscal year 2014 (21) compared to 2012 (40).[86]

In a potentially more far-reaching decision, in November 2016, the Supreme Court declined to hear an appeal by Glaxo of a ruling concerning a delay deal that did not involve an explicit cash payment.

Teva sought to make a generic version of Lamictal, a drug used to treat epilepsy and bipolar disorder, which prompted Glaxo to file a patent infringement lawsuit. The drug makers later reached a deal, but Glaxo did not make a cash payment to Teva. Instead, Glaxo agreed to allow Teva to sell generic chewable and tablet forms of Lamictal before its patent expired. Moreover, Glaxo also agreed not to sell its own so-called authorized generic version of Lamictal, which would have competed with a version sold by Teva. This was the central issue, because payers that filed their own lawsuit [in addition to the FTC's] against the drug makers charged the settlement was unfair. How so? They maintained the deal paved the way for higher prices than if Teva had proceeded to sell a lower-cost generic.[87]

Despite these rulings, the FTC is still pursuing individual actions. State-based action has also occurred. In 2019, California enacted a law prohibiting this practice.[88]

g) *When all other periods of exclusivity have lapsed on an approved and marketed product, if a branded drug maker can show it has studied the product's safety and efficacy for use in children, then it can receive an additional*

*6 months of exclusivity*. This extension is obtained through the FDA's Written Request (WR) process. This tactic originated in 1997 with the FDA Modernization Act (FDAMA).

h) *In order to avoid generic competition, a branded drug can go from prescription to OTC status*. The original drug maker can then keep its brand identity as a sales advantage, be a first mover in marketing its OTC version, and have a cost advantage because it is already manufacturing the drug. Examples of this approach include such companies as Astra Zeneca, which moved its branded gastrointestinal product Prilosec to OTC status.

13. Enabling pharmacists to substitute generics: Once interchangeable medications are available, allowing pharmacists to substitute them for the reference products can save payers and patients money. Enabling laws to allow this substitution are the province of individual states and will be subject to much lobbying by pharmaceutical companies and others whose profits are lowered by this practice. This practice is also good for the pharmacies because, despite their lower prices, profit margins are *greater for generics* than branded medications.

14. Using pharmacogenomics: With advances in understanding how genes determine the effectiveness of therapies, physicians can better predict who will benefit from certain treatments, particularly very expensive ones. For example, the HER2-neu receptor protein predicts the response to Herceptin in breast cancer patients. Both clinicians and payers now require genetic profiles where drug choices depend on their results. Biopharma companies have also used this technology to re-patent older drugs, *viz.* when a medication is found to successfully treat patients with a specific genetic profile, the product can be (re)patented for that narrow indication. In fact, this tactic is part of a larger trend, with one study finding that 78% of drugs getting new patents are already on the market.[89]

15. Requiring step therapy: For many conditions, successful treatment is often not achieved with a single dose of one medication. Instead, these diseases are treated with a series of medications in a step-wise fashion—escalating doses and/or use of more medications that may be more expensive and have more adverse effects. Payers often insist that practitioners follow guidelines for adjusting therapy before the most expensive medication is prescribed. For example, a patient with chronic asthma might be sequentially treated with an inhaled corticosteroid, long acting beta agonist, and leukotriene receptor antagonist before omalizumab (Xolair) is administered.[90] The marketing professional should understand where the company's products fit into this scheme.

16. Mandating specialist evaluation/use: For some specialty medications, payers will authorize use only by practitioners with certain expertise and experience.

Using the asthma example above, some insurers will only pay for omali-zumab if it is prescribed and administered by an allergist or pulmonologist. This tactic reduces the products' channels for use but also enhances the ability to target market physician customers.

17. Reducing waste: Ordering just the right dose for individual patients can save costs. For example, if a practitioner orders a multi-dose vial for more than one course of treatment, there is often extra medication left over. Payment for more than a patient needs is costly. However, this extra medication can be used in other patients at no additional cost to the specialist. Strictly speaking, this practice is illegal when treating Medicare patients; however, enforcement is often lax. Marketers must be aware of how their injectable products are being used in this fashion in order to plan better packaging and pricing strategies.

18. Pricing using reference products or indexes: To combat high prices, payers (especially government-sponsored insurance plans outside the U.S.) use a variety of reference and indexing techniques. This type of pricing is one method of cost control currently under consideration in the U.S. This tactic forces marketers to take a more global view of pricing strategies:

    - Lowest priced identical chemical entity—active ingredient formulation, such as generics (generic referencing); examples: U.S., Canada (some provinces), Sweden, Spain, Denmark

    - Lowest price in therapeutic class (therapeutic referencing); examples: Germany, the Netherlands, New Zealand, British Columbia

    - Representative drug in class as benchmark for payment; examples: most European countries

    - Market basket of prices from different countries; example: Canada (Patented Medicine Prices Review Board)

    - Maximum price lowest of list of comparison countries; example: Brazil

    - Total cost per time period comparisons; examples: weighted average monthly treatment cost (WAMTC) in therapeutic categories (Australia, e.g., for ACE inhibitors, statins, CCBs, PPIs, and SSRIs) and defined daily dose (DDD) cost of therapy, average cost within a category (Germany)

    - Additional opportunity for pharmacist ability/mandate to substitute—generic and/or therapeutic class; examples: notify patient of generic equivalent, patient decides (Finland, South Africa, and Slovakia) on a mandatory substitution of lowest cost generic alternative (Sweden)

    A variation on this method for lowering costs applies exclusively for the patient's benefit. Many U.S. insurance companies forbid pharmacists to tell patients if their drugs are cheaper when they pay out-of-pocket than if they use their insurance and pay a co-payment (or co-insurance). This prohibition is called a "gag clause." Legislators are currently looking into such arrangements and making the practice illegal.[91]

19. Importing medications from other, lower-cost, countries: In the U.S., retail purchasing from another country, e.g., Canada, is illegal. However, pending rule changes at the FDA will make this option available, geared particularly to states seeking to lower their Medicaid drug costs.[92] Biopharma companies can combat this practice by keeping foreign sales to historic levels, thereby cutting the potential for reimportation into the country.

20. Requiring price transparency: Patients do not often know how much their medications will cost until they pick them up at the pharmacy or receive them in the mail. Therefore, they cannot discuss alternate choices with their physicians or decide where to purchase their medications. This lack of transparency along with payer pushback against Direct to Consumer (DTC) advertising[93] has led to the call for more price transparency. In May 2019, CMS issued its final rule requiring drug price transparency:

*This final rule revises the Federal Health Insurance Programs for the Aged and Disabled by amending regulations for the Medicare Parts A, B, C and D programs, as well as the Medicaid program, to require direct-to- consumer (DTC) television advertisements of prescription drugs and biological products for which payment is available through or under Medicare or Medicaid to include the Wholesale Acquisition Cost (WAC or list price) of that drug or biological product. This rule is intended to improve the efficient administration of the Medicare and Medicaid programs by ensuring that beneficiaries are provided with relevant information about the costs of prescription drugs and biological products so they can make informed decisions that minimize their out-of-pocket (OOP) costs and expenditures borne by Medicare and Medicaid, both of which are significant problems.[94]*

In reaction to these regulations, Merck & Co Inc, Eli Lilly and Co., and Amgen Inc. sued the federal government. In deciding the case in favor of the plaintiffs, Judge Amit P. Mehta explained:

It is the agency's incursion into a brand-new regulatory environment, and the rationale for it, that make the rule so consequential. This case is not just about whether HHS can force drug companies to disclose their list prices in the name of lowering costs. Rather, the WAC Disclosure Rule represents a significant shift in HHS's ability to regulate the health care marketplace. Congress surely did not envision such an expansion of regulatory authority when it granted HHS the power to issue regulations necessary to carry out the 'efficient administration' of the Medicare and Medicaid programs.[95]

This decision and reasoning were upheld by the U.S. Court of Appeals for the District of Columbia Circuit in June, 2020. Despite the judicial decision, Congress can pass legislation requiring such pricing disclosure.

21. Restricting in-person detailing and marketing materials: Concerns about drug company representatives influencing physicians' decisions to prescribe costlier medications has led some hospitals and medical groups to severely restrict or prohibit product detailing visits. Many also forbid medication sampling.

      In a similar vein, many academic articles conclude that gifts to physicians (such as pens, mugs, and meals) enhance the likelihood of prescribing the gift-giver's product.[96] Acting on the threat of legislation banning all such activities, the trade group PhRMA issued a Code on Interactions With Health Care Professionals, which went into practice in January 2009. (It has most recently been updated in October 2019.[97]) The health care marketer should be totally familiar with this code before designing promotional campaigns.

      To add transparency to this voluntary code, as part of the ACA, CMS issued the rule titled: Medicare, Medicaid, Children's Health Insurance Programs; Transparency Reports and Reporting of Physician Ownership or Investment Interests.[98] Among other requirements, the rule requires companies to report the value of gifts and names of physicians receiving them. Included also are speaking fees. Lists by physicians of such amounts can be accessed on a CMS-sponsored website.[99]

      The Covid-19 pandemic has further accelerated the trend away from in-person visits. In January 2020 there were 40.7 million global in-person sales rep visits; by April 2020 the number dropped to 22.2 million.[100] This decline was accompanied by a marked increase in email communication and online meetings.

22. Providers deciding what products to use based on price (cost/benefit decisions): Traditionally, payers have been the source of cost-reduction measures. In recent years, however, providers and organizations have recognized their ethical responsibility to keep medications affordable. Two notable initiatives are the American Society of Clinical Oncology (ASCO) Value Framework[101] and Memorial Sloan Kettering's Drug Abacus.[102]

## BIOPHARMA ADVERTISING

In previous sections, the role of such factors as PBMs, formularies, and outpatient drug charges were discussed with respect to medication choices. Here, advertising to physicians and consumers is considered in its role to promote drug use.

### Advertising to Physicians

Advertising to physicians uses several different channels. For example, ads in journals and other educational publications (both print and electronic media) frequently promote the effectiveness of the drug and include full prescribing information, including side effects. In-person detailing by pharmaceutical representatives often includes the same promotional material used in ads, but also incorporates discussions of competitors' products.

Unlike many other sectors, biopharma advertising is highly regulated by the government and the industry itself. The governmental regulation comes from the FDA's Office of Prescription Drug Promotion (OPDP),[103] whose mission is:

> To protect the public health by ensuring that prescription drug information is truthful, balanced, and accurately communicated. This is accomplished through a comprehensive surveillance, enforcement, and education program, and by fostering better communication of labeling and promotional information to both healthcare professionals and consumers.

The OPDP defines two types of promotion: advertisements and promotional labeling, which are treated differently. *Advertisements* generally appear in:

- Print periodicals, such as journals, magazines, and newspapers
- Broadcast media, such as television and radio, as well as through telephone systems

*Promotional labeling* differs from advertising in the way it is distributed. Promotional labeling includes additional types of materials and ways to get them to the consumer, for example:

- Brochures and booklets
- Mailed materials, including letters to patients
- Videotapes
- Refrigerator magnets, cups, and other giveaways that show a drug's name

Promotional labeling about a drug is said to "accompany" that drug, even if the promotional labeling is not physically attached to a drug container. Promotional labeling must be accompanied by the drug's "prescribing information."[104] The industry's policing of promotional activities started in earnest on July 1, 2002, when the PhRMA issued its Code on Interactions with Health Care Professionals.[105] Prior to issuance of this code, the public (including lawmakers) were confronted with stories of companies that provided exotic trips, gifts, and lucrative "consulting" contracts to physicians in order to garner their prescriptions.

The Code specifies that promotional materials "provided to health care professionals by or on behalf of a company should: (a) be accurate and not misleading; (b) make claims about a product only when properly substantiated; (c) reflect the balance between risks and benefits; and (d) be consistent with all other Food and Drug Administration (FDA) requirements governing such communications." The specific areas governed by the code are listed below:

a) Informational Presentations by Pharmaceutical Company Representatives and Accompanying Meals

b) Prohibition on Entertainment and Recreation

c) Pharmaceutical Company Support For Continuing Medical Education

d) Pharmaceutical Company Support for Third-Party Educational or Professional Meetings

e) Consultants

f) Speaker Programs and Speaker Training Meetings

g) Health Care Professionals Who Are Members of Committees That Set Formularies or Develop Clinical Practice Guidelines

h) Scholarships and Educational Funds

i) Prohibition of Non-Educational and Practice-Related Items

j) Educational Items

k) Prescriber Data

l) Independence and Decision Making

m) Training and Conduct of Company Representatives

Since the effect of this Code on encouraging prescribing was still not clear, in 2010 the ACA included a provision called "The Sunshine Act," which requires that manufacturers of drugs and devices report to CMS payments and "transfers of value" to physicians, teaching hospitals, and other entities (such as group purchasing organizations) which participate in federal programs (Medicare, Medicaid, and CHIP). These considerations can be for activities such as research, consulting, travel, and gifts.

Starting September 30, 2014, the data from this reporting was published online at a CMS website called Open Payments.[106] The initiative was extended in 2018 with passage of the SUPPORT for Patients and Communities Act,[107] which was passed in response to the opioid addiction crisis. Specifically, this legislation extended the definition of "covered recipients" to include physician assistants, nurse practitioners, clinical nurse specialists, certified registered nurse anesthetists, and certified nurse midwives.

It also mandated that the "Medicare Payment Advisory Commission must report on Medicare payment for opioid and non-opioid pain management treatments, *current incentives for prescribing opioid and non-opioid treatments* [emphasis added], and how opioid use is currently tracked and monitored."

Despite these legal, ethical, and transparency requirements, biopharma's promotional activities continue to successfully influence physician prescribing. For example, using the Open Payments database and Medicare Part D claims from 2013 to 2015, research found physician payments led to a nearly 4% increase in prescribing.[108] The spending was higher overall for drugs in classes that had five or fewer promoted drugs. Further, there was "no evidence that paid physicians transitioned their patients to generics more slowly than physicians who don't get payments. However, paid physicians are more likely to put patients on a new formulation of a drug." As far as impact on patients, the researchers concluded that "we do not find clear evidence that such payments are harmful to patients, only that they do not seem to be obviously helpful."

Physicians were always free to ask a company for more information about FDA-*approved* indications for its products; however, requests for *non-approved* (off-label) use were prohibited. The opposing opinions on this prohibition cited the First Amendment's freedom of speech guarantees versus the government's regulatory authority. Two actions opened up the flow of information for biopharmaceuticals. First, on January 13, 2009, the FDA issued a new guidance that permitted manufacturers to distribute academic journal reprints that discussed off-label uses. Second, in 2011, the Supreme Court decision in *Sorrell v. IMS Health* upheld the Second Circuit's decision that "speech in aid of pharmaceutical marketing ... is a form of content-based expression protected by the Free Speech Clause of the First Amendment."[109] Some limitations still exist on this form of promotion.[110]

### Advertising to Patients

This category is most frequently called Direct to Consumer Advertising, or DTCA. The opposing forces that have governed this channel are information and the public's "right to know" versus the role of government to assure ads are not deceptive. Regulations that apply to DTCA are not only determined by the *medium* used (as described above for OPDP review) but also the *content* of the message. These messages can fall into three basic categories:

1.  *General information about a medical condition*: These ads mention a medical condition and state that a treatment is available. Products are not named and (as with almost all DTCA) patients are instructed to "ask your doctor." For example, one of the earliest ads for Rogaine highlighted a treatment for baldness but did not mention the drug. Many other countries have legalized such promotions.

2.  *Reminders about products*: These ads mention the product name and may include pricing or dosage (like one-pill-a-day advantage). The first television DTCA was of this type and aired on May 19, 1983; it was for Boots' drug Rufen.[111] The ad merely mentions the drug's name and said it was a generic form of ibuprofen that costs less than the branded version.

This type of ad can also hint at the product's benefit but not explicitly state it. For example, a televised commercial appeared in the early 2000s showing middle aged men happily getting out of bed in the morning; the well-known erectile dysfunction drug Viagra was then mentioned without reference to what it does.

3. *Product claim/product education ad*: This form of DTCA is the most common and tells the public what the drug does. However, such an expansion of information requires disclosure of side effects and risks. When DTCA became legal in the U.S. in 1985, the requirements for those caveats were extensive. When the FDA Modernization Act of 1997 relaxed them, this category of ads greatly expanded. While New Zealand is the only country other than the U.S. to legalize this form of DTCA, the internet and cable television allow U.S. promotions to have a wider reach. For example, some U.S. television channels are readily accessible to the majority of Canadian residents.

DTCA is also governed by a code of ethics by the industry itself.[112] For example, actors cannot play doctors on ads and those who say they use the product must actually do so.

The proposed regulatory requirement of DTCA listing prices of medications was discussed above.

DTCA spending is now more than $6 billion per year, with the average American seeing nine drug ads on TV every day.[113] Spending on television ads alone exceeded $200 million in January 2020,[114] with AbbVie's Humira topping the list for the past several years.[115] The effectiveness of DTCA is indicated by results of the following market research and academic studies. In 2018 The Decision Resource Group published a study of *consumer behavior* regarding searches for drug information and *actions following DTCA exposure*.[116] The major findings were:

- Nearly two in three U.S. adults say they recall seeing advertising in the past 12 months.

- Among the 65% of U.S. patients who recall seeing or hearing DTCA in the past 12 months, nearly two-thirds remembered seeing TV ads and half (49%) remembered seeing ads online. Among the 65% of patients who recalled seeing or hearing TV ads about prescription drugs in the past 12 months, 22% had requested a specific drug. Among the 49% of patients who recalled seeing or hearing online ads, 42% had requested a specific prescription drug.

- The data suggest that online ads are as effective as TV ads at prompting online searchers to ask their doctor about a specific prescription drug.

- Among the 61% of patients who had researched prescription drugs online in the past 12 months, 34% had requested a specific prescription drug at least once. Among patients who had requested an Rx, 25% were prompted to do so by a TV ad and 25% by ads seen online.

- TV or online ads may be particularly effective at reaching some condition groups. Among online searchers requesting a prescription, patients with multiple sclerosis, hypertension, and Alzheimer's disease were particularly likely to cite TV ads as the impetus for their request, while patients with hepatitis C, type 1 diabetes, and severe asthma were more likely to cite online ads. Rheumatoid arthritis patients who conducted online research were much more responsive to both TV and online ads than were patients generally.

- Brand recall for TV ads tracked closely with spending—AbbVie's immunosuppressant Humira, the most-advertised brand on TV in 2017, was the brand that most patients recalled seeing.

- The data indicate that while patients are more likely to visit general health websites like WebMD or Everyday Health, those visiting pharma websites are more likely to request a specific drug.

- Patients visiting pharma websites early in the treatment journey are more likely to request a specific medication. For example, 52% of patients using pharma websites to prep for a doctor visit had requested a specific drug, while 33% of those using general health websites for the same purpose had requested a prescription.

The implications of these findings were summarized by Rory Stanton, head of patient research at DRG Digital:

We've seen in our studies that advertising is really good at sparking that initial awareness. But websites are even more effective at getting patients to "ask their doctor," pharma websites most of all. So the task for pharma brands is to utilize that advertising to drive patients to their digital properties while also investing in other touchpoints, like paid search and sponsored content on general health websites, to meet them in many places as they go about gathering information to make a treatment decision … We're advising clients to invest in paid and organic search strategies to drive patients to their websites in the pre-doctor's visit stage and at the point of care.

He also noted that nearly 1 in 10 patients recalled viewing Rx ads on a digital device at the point of care.

The *economic benefit* of DTCA to biopharma companies and effects on patients was highlighted in 2015 by the National Bureau of Economic Research study.[117] The findings are:

- The authors estimate that a 10% increase in advertising exposure increased the number of prescriptions purchased by about 5%.

- About 70% of this increase is due to new prescriptions while the other 30% is due to increased drug adherence among existing patients. Therefore, the 10% increase in advertising only increases adherence by about 1–2%. (This finding is important because increased education, leading to increased adherence, is one of the arguments companies make for the benefit of DTCA.)

- Those patients initiating treatment because of DTCA are *less* adherent than average.

As *media choice*[118] for DTCA has become more complex, further research provides some guidance. Liu et al.[119] found that:

"[a]s measured by new patient visits with physicians, DTCA has a greater impact on patients with more severe versus milder conditions. Severely affected patients may anticipate more adverse effects from inaction and are therefore more likely to seek medical information and visit their physicians to discuss their health conditions ... print DTCA is more effective in driving patients with more severe versus milder afflictions to visit physicians. Because reading a message in print is cognitively more demanding, print media are more suitable for influencing patients that are actively seeking medical information.

On the other hand, television DTCA is more effective for patients with milder versus more severe afflictions. Television ads require less processing and hence are better suited for patients with low involvement who are more likely to be influenced by verbal and visual messages. Our findings on the role of television versus print DTCA can potentially be extended to understanding the role of Internet-based DTCA in influencing patients' behaviors because both print and non-video-Internet–based advertising requires consumers' active participation.

Also, many companies have increased their online advertising (including on social media), because they find advantages over other media in cost as well as the ability to target customers and measure responses."[120]

*Content framing* is also important in delivering the message. For example, Aiken et al.[121] presented 215 adult participants with a self-reported diagnosis of diabetes with a series of choices: "Each choice pair represented a prescription diabetic nerve pain drug with a different efficacy level and one of the two had a market claim of '#1 Prescribed'. Participants indicated which drug they would prefer if they had to choose one. Results showed an advantage of '#1 Prescribed.' A drug without this claim needed at least 1.23% greater efficacy to be chosen over a drug with this claim."

Finally, De Frank et al.[122] conducted a systematic review of DTC research which raised cautionary notes about research studies. They found that studies:

- "Seldom included a meaningful comparison group (e.g., patients who were not exposed to or influenced by DTCA). Therefore, it is difficult to know if the frequency with which patients reported outcomes would have been higher or lower among those not exposed to DTCA."

- "Often asked patients to recall past behaviors, which is prone to recall bias."

■ "Rarely included those with lower educational backgrounds or those who speak English as a second language"

■ Frequently "assume a somewhat simplistic model of behavior change, where exposure to DTCA is thought to influence thought, which in turn leads to behavior. Communication Theory suggests that a more complex interaction of factors is at play. For example, exposure to DTCA may have a stronger influence for some population segments (e.g., those who actively seek drug information for a diagnosed condition) than others, or after repeated exposures through multiple channels, or in the presence of other social or institutional factors."

More controlled research studies that include diverse populations need to be conducted to assess the true worth of DTCA.

## CHAPTER SUMMARY

While biopharmaceuticals compromise only about 10% of U.S. health care costs, the industry has become a major target for cost-containment initiatives. Using the information here and in other chapters, future developments are clear.

Demographic trends clearly point to aging global populations and an increase in products to treat or prevent chronic conditions, such as Parkinson's and Alzheimer's diseases. At the same time, older medications need to be replaced with safer or more effective products, e.g., antibiotics.

The political and legal sectors will continue to focus on lowering prices. The debate will still revolve around the merits of the free market versus government regulation. Lobbying by significant stakeholders will have an important role in the balance of these two approaches. Further, regulatory activities will continue to try to balance quick introduction of new products to help current patients against unforeseen side effects.

This latter balance will become more difficult as newer technologies, such as genetic manipulation, become possible. Biopharma interface with medical products and diagnostics will further blur lines that define what is a drug.

Finally, socio-cultural forces will demand better value in these products. In addition to price, value propositions include patients' inputs into what *they* think important features of biopharma products should be.[123] As providers take on more financial risk for delivering their services, they want to know that the medications they use will be cost effective. In order to address these diverse stakeholder value demands, biopharma marketing professionals must be prepared to craft product strategies that can provide financial guarantees the medications will be affordable and effective.

## DISCUSSION QUESTIONS

1.   Your company is about to launch a specialty pharmaceutical. Who are your stakeholders? What are their value propositions? Outline a plan to overcome the measures that payers will implement to mitigate the high cost of this product.

2.   Your company is launching a new drug treatment for a specific type of cancer (you can choose the disease category). What target markets would you identify and what media would you use to reach those targets? How would you involve non-government organizations (NGOs) to support your efforts?

3.   Read some of the references for this chapter and do some additional research to recommend what measures can be taken to streamline the FDA approval process for traditional medications. As a VP of marketing/legislative action for a biopharma alliance, who are your key allies in this process? Who would be against these measures?

4.   Since the biopharma market is international in scope, pick a country where you think your new product would have a good marketing opportunity and outline the drug approval process and marketing channels for that country.

## CASE: MARKETING ETHICS AND THE OPIOID EPIDEMIC

Aggressive promotion of opioids by pharmaceutical companies[124] coincided with changing practice recommendations in pain management.[125] These changes can be dated to James N. Campbell's presidential address to the American Pain Society in 1995:

> *Today, nurses and physicians routinely assess the vital signs of pulse, blood pressure, core temperature, and respirations in evaluating patients. We should consider pain the fifth vital sign... We need to train doctors and nurses to treat pain as a vital sign. Quality care means that pain is measured. Quality of care means that pain is treated.*[126]

Also, in 1995, the FDA reviewed the New Drug Application (NDA) for Purdue Pharma's OxyContin,[127] a long-acting version of the opioid oxycodone, for use in chronic, low back and cancer-related pains. The new version was approved for twice a day dosing, instead of four times a day, but was not more effective.[128] After its launch in 1996, Purdue aggressively promoted OxyContin using such marketing measures as:

■   Training more than 5,000 physicians, pharmacists, and nurses to participate in a national speaker bureau to promote the drug as a safe and effective pain treatment. These all-expense paid meetings were held at resorts and the company paid participants for any subsequent talks they delivered about the product. This type of program is well-known to influence prescribing habits of attendees. Some of the physicians were already the highest opioid prescribers in the country.

- Increasing its internal sales force from 318 sales representatives to 671, and its call list from approximately 39,000 to approximately 82,000 physicians.

- Providing generous sales bonuses that *averaged* $71,500 by 2001. (Total sales bonuses that year totaled $40 million.)

- Offering starter coupons that provided patients with a free, limited-time prescription for a 7- to 30-day supply of the drug. By 2001, when the program was ended, approximately 34,000 coupons had been redeemed nationally.

- Rolling out a promotional gift campaign with the slogan "Get in the Swing With OxyContin." Items that sales reps gave to prescribers included fishing hats, stuffed plush toys, and music compact discs.[129]

- Sponsoring a program called Partners Against Pain (PAP), which the company described as an international alliance "that serves patients, caregivers, and health care professionals to help alleviate unnecessary suffering by advancing standards of pain care through education and advocacy."[130]

Throughout these efforts, Purdue's marketing materials omitted key information on efficacy. In various clinical studies, published as early as 1997, OxyContin did not consistently relieve pain for the entire 12-hour dosing interval, causing many patients to take short acting oxycodone for relief. Other patients had a delayed response, so a 12-hour dosing schedule could cause drug accumulation and overdosing. Instead of describing the wide range of patient responses and the importance of individual dose titration, to maintain its marketing "advantage," Purdue told physicians that if their patients weren't experiencing 12 hours of pain relief, they should increase the q12 dose as a response to pain breakthrough. This recommendation resulted in a much higher q12 dose escalation in some patients who instead should have received lower, more frequent dosing.[131] Further, Purdue's own MS Contin had been abused in the late 1980s in a fashion similar to how OxyContin was later to be used. Further, Purdue's own testing in 1995 had demonstrated that "68% of the oxycodone could be extracted from an OxyContin tablet when crushed."[132] Despite the above problems, the twice-daily "advantage" was not challenged. Instead, in 1997, the company encountered a different problem: Medco (a pharmaceutical benefit management company, or PBM, now part of Express Scripts) started to voice concerns about the growing costs of OxyContin's use in non-cancer pain. Further, some physicians said they were worried that prescribing the drug would become more difficult as utilization controls were implemented. To combat that worry, Purdue considered two options. The first option was to convince the PBMs and payers that the drug was a cost-effective treatment to relieve pain. However, after high-level discussions, the company decided on a campaign to promote OxyContin's safety vis-à-vis other opioids. Their message was that the longer-acting form of oxycodone was less abusable. But the unchallenged credibility of that message did not last long.

When OxyContin entered the market in 1996, the FDA approved its original label, which stated that iatrogenic [physician-caused by prescribing] addiction was "very rare" if opioids were legitimately used in the management of pain. But at least by 1999, even Purdue was aware of the abuse potential. In November of that year a sales representative emailed Dr. J. David Haddox, a Purdue executive, about the growing concern among physicians about news reports of the diversion and abuse of OxyContin, including people extracting the oxycodone in the tablet for "mainlining" illegally. "While many sales people have sold controlled-release opioids as having less abuse potential, the current situation has put us in an awkward situation," the sales rep wrote. "I feel like we have a credibility issue with our product. Many physicians now think, OxyContin is obviously the street drug all the drug addicts are seeking."[133]

Despite the above problems, the marketing plan was working and sales increased from $48 million at launch to $1.1 billion by 2000. But the success was not solely due to Purdue's marketing efforts. The medical community had strengthened its commitment to pain treatment.

For example, in October 2000, the Veterans Administration published *Pain as the 5th Vital Sign Toolkit* in order to "offer guidelines for the completion of comprehensive pain assessments."[134] Further, the Joint Commission, which accredits hospitals and other health care organizations, launched its new pain assessment and management standards on January 1, 2001. To help promote the drug, in 2000 Purdue sent each sales rep 50 copies of the 1999 American Pain Society treatment guidelines to give to physicians.

Given this treatment mandate, Purdue found it easy to expand promotion of OxyContin to primary care physicians for non-cancer-related pain. (By 2003, almost half of all physicians prescribing OxyContin were primary care physicians.) This expansion contributed to a nearly 10-fold increase in OxyContin prescriptions for this type of pain, from about 670,000 in 1997 to about 6.2 million in 2002, whereas prescriptions for cancer-related pain increased about fourfold during that same period. Combined 2001 and 2002 sales grew to nearly $3 billion.

By 2001, knowledge of OxyContin's abuse potential began to grow further, and in July the FDA required a label change to state that data were not available for establishing the true incidence of addiction in chronic-pain patients. In August, The Kentucky OxyContin Task Force issued its recommendations to curb illegal use; the report noted that "representatives from Purdue Pharma have joined the task force and have committed time and money for education on diversion aspects."[135]

The first serious challenge to Purdue came in 2004, when generic versions started to become available.[136] In response to loss of patent protection, Purdue changed its calculation for sales bonuses—they would be based not only on the prescriptions for OxyContin but also on the size of the overall market.[137] The "rising tide lifts all boats" strategy was calculated to give reps the ability to convert prescriptions to their product.

The second major challenge came as result of the company's ongoing misrepresentation of OxyContin's addiction potential. "On May 10, 2007, Purdue Frederick Company Inc, an affiliate of Purdue Pharma, along with three company executives, pled guilty to criminal charges of misbranding OxyContin by claiming that it was less addictive and less subject to abuse and diversion than other opioids" and was ordered to pay $634 million in fines.[138] The settlement included a non-prosecution agreement that there would "be no further criminal prosecution or forfeiture action by the United States for any violations of law, occurring before May 10, 2007." Any subsequent action against the company would, therefore, have to be based on its actions after that date.

Six months after the settlement, the Sackler family (Purdue's owners) incorporated Rhodes Pharma. According to an FDA database, "Rhodes Pharmaceuticals makes a wide range of opioid products containing highly addictive opiates such as morphine, oxycodone and hydromorphone. Although registered as a separate entity from Purdue, employees say that little distinction is made internally between the two companies."[139] Despite Purdue's working closely with the state of Kentucky, the growing concern over illegal use of OxyContin (and unethical promotion of the drug) prompted a lawsuit against the company in 2007 by former Attorney General Greg Stumbo.[140]

Still, in the following two years, the drug maker regrouped, hiring more than 100 new sales reps to boost revenues from OxyContin, and by 2010 the medicine was pulling in more than $3bn a year. One Purdue executive said: "They did not listen to their critics and insisted they had just a few isolated problems. After the settlement, they didn't change the way the sales force was managed and incentivized, everything stayed the same."[141] In the next few years, prescribers continued to order opioids inappropriately.[142]

One impetus for the improper prescribing was brought to light in 2020: "Practice Fusion [a unit of Allscripts Healthcare Solutions, Inc.] began soliciting payments from Pharma Co. X in late 2013 in exchange for creating a physician alert designed to boost opioid prescriptions by suggesting doctors focus on assessing and treating a patient's pain symptoms with opioid medication as a preferred option."[143] Pharma Co. X is alleged to be Purdue Pharma. The computerized alert was triggered 230 million times from July 2016 to spring 2019. By 2015, more than 33,000 Americans had died as a result of an opioid overdose and about 2 million people had substance use disorders related to prescription opioid pain relievers.

As a result of these deaths and disorders, in November 2016 CMS announced that it was "finalizing the removal of the pain management dimension of the Hospital Consumer Assessment of Healthcare Providers and Systems (HCAHPS) survey for purposes of the Hospital Value-Based Purchasing Program to eliminate any financial pressure clinicians may feel to overprescribe medications."[144]

In August 2017, CMS announced that effective January 1, 2018, it would replace the previous HCAHPS pain questions with three new questions that comprise a new composite measure called "Communication About Pain."[145] On October 27, 2017, President Trump called the opioid epidemic a "national shame" and a public health emergency. In the private sector, the Joint Commission issued new and revised pain assessment and management standards effective January 1, 2018.[146]

Given the growing public attention to opioid deaths and addiction, and revision in clinical recommendations, more states, as well as counties and municipalities, started to sue opioid manufacturers on grounds of misleading marketing of safety and effectiveness. Further, suits were initiated against the major drug wholesalers (McKesson Corp., Cardinal Health, Inc., and AmerisourceBergen Corp.) and pharmacy chains, such as Walgreens and CVS.

In September 2019, Purdue filed for Chapter 11 bankruptcy and many plaintiffs are also going after the Sackler family's personal wealth. Liability of all defendants is estimated in the tens of billions of dollars, but as of early 2020 most settlements have not been reached, e.g., in mid-February, more than 20 states rejected an $18 billion opioid offer from wholesalers.[147] In a further twist, pharmacy chains are now suing physicians in order to share the financial burden of plaintiffs' claims.[148]

The crisis is not only one of monetary and reputational penalties, but it has impeded new product introductions. In January 2020, a joint FDA advisory committee rejected three new opioid drugs in a week because of concerns of poor controls over abuse potential.[149]

## CASE QUESTIONS

1.  What were the critical times Purdue made marketing strategy choices? What were other strategic options the company had at those times?

2.  Given the information you would have had as a company executive at each of those times, what strategic marketing decisions would you have made? Make sure your answer includes addressing product characteristics and promotional activities.

3.  Think about the prevailing medical climate that mandated aggressive pain control. In that light, explain what company actions were ethical and which were unethical.

# CHAPTER

# SOCIAL CAUSE MARKETING IN HEALTH CARE

The term *social marketing* was first introduced in 1971.[1] The authors, Philip Kotler and Gerald Zaltman, defined social marketing as:

> *The design, implementation, and control of programs calculated to influence the acceptability of social ideas and involving considerations of product planning, pricing, communication, distribution, and marketing research.*

Note that social marketing aims to use marketing tools to influence the acceptability of social ideas. The tools include the 4Ps of product, price, place, and promotion. Within promotion, the tools will include advertising, sales force, public relations, and other influence-bearing tools. Advertising itself will be a blend of traditional advertising (e.g., TV, radio, newspapers, magazines, and billboards) and social media (e.g., Facebook, Twitter, YouTube). However, we must be careful to distinguish between *social marketing* and *social media marketing*, the latter describing using social media to promote a cause. Social marketing is much broader than social media marketing. Perhaps we should call social marketing *social cause marketing* or more simply *cause marketing*.

Let's consider a typical social cause. For generations Americans enjoyed smoking cigarettes. First the men took up the habit, then the women, and then teenagers as the tobacco industry strained to increase the number of smokers.

As information grew about the adverse health effects of smoking—it raises the blood pressure and increases the chances for a heart attack or stroke, damages the lungs causing emphysema and breathing problems, and causes a range of cancers—some smokers managed to stop smoking, but most continued because tobacco was an addiction and smokers continued to hear the tobacco industry challenge the evidence. The industry would point to many smokers in their 90s who smoked all their life and still were healthy.

For those who opposed smoking, there were two major courses of action. One was to prohibit the manufacture and purchasing of cigarettes. Criminalization, however, would probably be a failure as was the U.S. experience with banning the manufacture and sale of alcohol. Prohibition of alcohol was such a colossal failure that there were few advocates of banning tobacco.

The alternative was to use stronger means of persuasion and move to a *full marketing approach*. A full marketing approach involves using all 4Ps. These are the main tools used by companies to sell their products. These tools can be used by social organizations to "unsell" products. In the anti-tobacco case, one can advocate changing the product (e.g., requiring the product to be made with a bitter taste), raising the price of cigarettes to make smoking a more expensive habit, reducing the number of places where cigarettes could be purchased or smoked, and increasing the number and forcefulness of negative messages about smoking coming from doctors, concerned family and friends, and even highlighting the harmfulness of smoking right on the cigarette package with health warnings.

A full marketing approach actually starts earlier by distinguishing among different groups of smokers—teenage girls, pregnant mothers, males over 60, and others—and tailoring a different marketing plan for each group. This process is called *market segmentation, targeting, and positioning* (STP) and it recognizes that different motives and beliefs operate in different groups of smokers. By researching the main drivers of smoking in each group, the social marketer can carry out the 4P steps more effectively in dissuading smoking.

Smoking did go down drastically in the U.S. From a situation where nearly everyone smoked at work and at home, today fewer people smoke, and those few have to leave the building or even their home to have a quick smoke. Although we can't attribute all the reduction to social marketing efforts—other factors such as companies banning smoking in the factory or office, or not hiring smokers because of the higher health costs—social marketing nevertheless played a strong role. The Truth Campaign was the largest national youth smoking prevention campaign, and even the Tobacco Quit Line Campaign in Washington State had documented success.[2]

Today there are over 2,000 professional social marketers applying their skills around the world to help individuals, groups, and whole populations to adopt healthy behavior. Social marketers have gone from just wanting to change the acceptability of a social idea to actually succeed in *changing behavior*. We like this latest definition of social marketing:[3]

*Social marketing is a process that applies marketing principles and techniques to create, communicate, and deliver value in order to influence target audience behaviors that benefit society as well as the target audience.*

We can be more specific by distinguishing four types of behavior that can be the target of social marketing initiatives. Social marketers typically try to influence their target audience regarding four types of behavioral change:

- *Accept* a new behavior (e.g., composting food waste)
- *Reject* a potential undesirable behavior (e.g., starting smoking)
- *Modify* a current behavior (e.g., increasing physical activity from three to five days of the week),
- *Abandon* an old undesirable one (e.g., holding and talking on a cell phone while driving).[4]

## THE MAIN PUBLIC HEALTH ISSUES ATTRACTING SOCIAL MARKETING EFFORTS

Social marketers address a wide range of health problems where there is a strong public consensus that solutions must be found. In most cases, the solutions would benefit individuals, groups, and the society at large. Social marketing health care challenges are the result of events (accidents), the environment (Covid-19 pandemic), community problems (persuading non-compliant consumers to wear masks to reduce infection), and forces that reduce financial well-being (unemployment). These four forces affect the health status of the population, as do the following clinical health issues:

- Issues in maternity—Educating pregnant mothers not to smoke, reducing infant mortality through improving safe water
- Issues in disease prevention or reduction—Motivating behavior to reduce malaria, HIV/AIDs, river blindness, Guinea worm disease, and breast cancer
- Issues in healthy living—Exercising regularly, eating healthy food, getting adequate sleep, oral health, managing blood pressure, childhood immunization, avoiding tobacco, opioid abuse, obesity, and eating disorders.

## THREE EXAMPLES OF SOCIAL MARKETING IN HEALTH CARE

The best way to illustrate social marketing theory and practice is to describe several examples in different categories that illustrate successful social marketing outcomes. The following three examples will be described:

1. Preventing sickness: Providing safe water treatment devices (example 1)
2. Increasing healthy living: Sweden and Singapore health promotion (example 2)
3. Reducing the spread of a transmissible disease: HIV/AIDS (example 3)

## EXAMPLE 1 IMPROVING THE AVAILABILITY OF SAFE WATER

One of the looming health problems is whether there will be enough water available to human communities and whether the water will be safe. People in water-rich countries take daily showers and water their lawns while much of the world lacks water for drinking, cleaning, and bathing. Water is very scarce in parts of China, India, and the Middle East. Water is scarce in certain U.S. states and has to be allocated. California has periodically launched a "Use Less Water Campaign" to conserve on the limited supply of water which has to be used in agriculture but also has to flow into homes for washing, drinking, and watering needs. California entreats its citizens to shower less, water their lawns less, flush their toilets less, and adopt a variety of devices that will limit their water use.

The challenge of obtaining safe water faces at least half the world's population. Unsafe water and sanitation leads to diarrhea, Guinea worm, hookworm, and other diseases. About 5 million people die each year from poor drinking water, poor sanitation, or a dirty home environment.[5]

How can health social marketers make water safer in rural communities especially for poorer people? Consider the effort of PATH, an international nonprofit organization, that launched a Safe Water Project in 2006 in Andhra Predesh, India, with the support of the Bill and Melinda Gates Foundation.[6] PATH took on the task of promoting home devices for treating water using HWTS products (household water treatment and safe storage). PATH researchers placed five different durable products—a ceramic water pot, a stainless steel filter, two multistage filters, and one portable hollow fiber filter—in different low-income households to study their acceptability and use. PATH conducted a number of interviews and trials. They arrived at a number of findings on the impact of Product, Price, Place, and Promotion on low-income consumers' interest and choices of water treatment alternatives.

Regarding Product, PATH researched the product features and attributes that improved the user's experience of each product. PATH concluded that the best water treatment devices would use transparent containers or water level indicators so that the household would know how much safe water remained available. In addition, the product should be easy to clean and maintain. The shape of the product (cylindrical or angular) and its material (plastic or wood) made a difference.

Regarding Price, the five products were all aspirational products for poor people who could only hope to eventually buy a water treatment device. The decision was made to price these devices between $US11 and $US21.

Regarding Place, the products could be made available in formal and informal retail settings. Very low-income consumers were slightly intimidated by shops although shops added the element of confidence and aspiration. Low-income consumers were more likely to buy a water treatment device from informal mobile vendors who could help install the product, explain its use, and be available for replacement parts.

Regarding Promotion, the findings favored mass media to introduce low-income households to the alternative products. The advertising, however, would only create awareness but not drive purchase. Purchase was more likely to take place when low-income household members would see the filter in the house of a friend or relative and hear about its good performance.

This example shows how social marketers use marketing tools to research and sell a product or change behavior. Social marketing was able to improve the quality of water available to low-income consumers through effective Product, Price, Place, and Promotion strategies and tactics.

# EXAMPLE 2 SWEDEN AND SINGAPORE'S HEALTH PROMOTION INITIATIVES

Most countries do not develop a national policy to improve the health of their people. They simply establish hospitals, clinics, and hire medical personnel. Medical personnel and facilities are largely focused on curing the sick rather than on preventing sickness from occurring in the first place.

One of the earlier preventive health programs was undertaken in Sweden in the 1970s. As a welfare-oriented nation, Sweden launched a program that aimed to raise a nation of non-smokers. The program included anti-smoking education in the schools and maternity clinics, progressive restrictions on cigarette advertising, price increases through higher taxation, prohibiting smoking in public places, and special efforts to help people who wanted to stop smoking. Later efforts were launched to discourage alcohol consumption and addictive drugs, and to encourage Swedish people to eat healthier foods and undertake regular exercise.

What efforts did Sweden undertake to reduce the high level of alcohol consumption? Sweden couldn't do much to change the Product except to prevent the illegal manufacture of alcoholic products. Sweden made heavy use of Price by placing heavy taxes on the purchase of alcohol. Sweden also made heavy use of Place by restricting the sale of alcoholic products to state-owned and operated liquor stores, and through putting limits on the amount that a person could purchase. Finally, Sweden developed heavy Promotion campaigns to describe the harm done by heavy drinking. The authorities put in place strict punishments for driving while drunk that led Swedish people to appoint a designated driver who would drive them home.

This was a grand experiment to raise a nation of healthy people who would avoid the common vices of smoking, drinking, and drugs. But not everyone cooperated. Those who wanted to drink more would get their friends to buy alcohol for them, or they would travel to Denmark where they could buy and bring home much more liquor. In spite of this resistance, Sweden did succeed in lowering the rate of alcohol consumption and drunkenness.

Singapore provides another example of effective social marketing. Singapore introduced a program to encourage more healthful eating through the Singapore Health Promotion Board (HPB).[7] The target was Singaporeans who eat at least one meal outside their homes six or more times a week. The aim was to motivate these diners to ask for healthier food to be provided by vendors on the street and in food courts. Figure 9.1 shows the out-of-home signage placed in locations where food vendors were present.

The HPB persuaded food vendors to offer at least one appropriate healthier choice to its customers. The program was later extended to restaurants. HPB nutritionists offered a series of sessions and workshops to restaurant chefs and managers on national nutrition

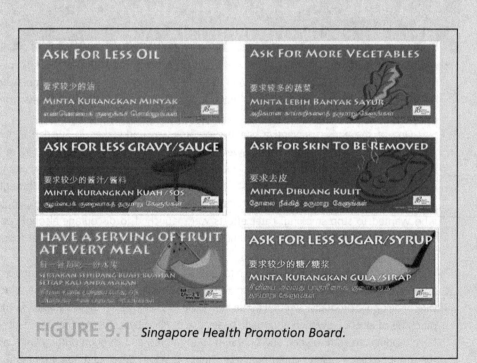

**FIGURE 9.1** *Singapore Health Promotion Board.*

and dietary guidelines to get them to add some healthy items to their menus. Once a critical mass of 150 restaurants had signed on for the Healthier Restaurant Programme, HPB embarked on a marketing communication campaign to draw diners to these restaurants.

An advertising campaign raised the profile of the cooperating restaurants, and it attracted additional restaurants to sign up for the program. The marketing communication program for the Healthier Restaurants Programme used a television and print advertisement campaign that was supported by promotional collateral including posters and tent-cards at all participating restaurants. Newspapers and magazines generated publicity by publishing feature articles on these restaurants.

An on-site promotion offered diners the chance to dine free if they ordered at least one healthier choice dish and entered their name for a lucky drawing. HPB worked with food critics from various radio stations to promote restaurants offering healthier choices. Participating radio stations also created contests and incentives for listeners to dine at these restaurants.

What was the outcome? The HPB Research and Evaluation Department conducted a survey and found that two out of five respondents (42.6%) asked for healthier modifications when buying food on the street or in food courts. Of table orders in restaurants, 45% ate a healthier dish.

Clearly the key to altering behavior is to create consumer motivation and help food vendors and restaurants to provide healthy choices. An aggressive marketing communication campaign helped to attract participating restaurants. The "Ask for Healthier Food" and "Healthier Restaurants" programs helped drive consumer traffic.

## EXAMPLE 3 HIV/AIDS

The third example examines the application of social marketing to fight the spread of a transmissible disease, in this case HIV/AIDS (hereafter AIDS). An effective social marketing strategy to control the AIDS pandemic is similar to a social marketing strategy to control the Covid-19 pandemic.

At the outbreak of the global AIDS pandemic some countries went into denial, not unlike a number of countries during the Covid-19 pandemic. The South African President Mbeki denied that there was a problem and delayed a positive response from taking place for several years, resulting in the unnecessary deaths of many South Africans.

A more common response to fight AIDS was for a country to launch an information campaign about the disease and to propose ways to avoid it. In 1988, the Surgeon General of the United States, C. Everett Koop, mailed an eight-page brochure to every U.S. household. The brochure posed and answered questions such as:

- How do you get AIDS?
- What is all the talk about condoms?

- What does someone with AIDS look like?
- Should you get an AIDS test?

The idea that just distributing information about the disease would reduce the problem was an example of naïve "social marketing." What is the right way to mount a social marketing campaign against an emerging epidemic? In the case of AIDS, the first step is to gather information about what groups are most susceptible to contracting AIDS. The effort is to understand these groups and then launch a campaign to reach them and commit them to safer behavior.

The most susceptible groups are LGBTQ + people, intravenous drug users, sex workers, sexually active teens and young adults, drivers, and soldiers, among others. Demographically, ethnicity played a role in AIDS infection rates in New York City with 46% White, 31% Black, and 23% Latinx.[8] A single social marketing campaign could never be effective in reaching diverse groups about the dangers of AIDS and motivating them to plan to protect themselves. Social marketers must research each susceptible group separately to understand that specific group's knowledge, attitudes, beliefs, and behavior. Based on the findings, social marketers would prepare a separate long-term strategy for being effective with each susceptible group.

How does AIDs spread through a population? One person who has contracted AIDS may or may not know that they have the disease. If this person has unprotected sex with another person, there is a good chance that the other person will contract AIDS. This sexual event may take place between two strangers, or a dating couple, or a married couple. The other way AIDS is spread is when a drug addict borrows the needle of another drug addict who is infected with AIDS.

Given the knowledge of how AIDS is spread, there are three major approaches applied by social marketers to contain the spread of AIDS:

1. Educate and motivate persons to use condoms in any sexual encounter.
2. Motivate every sexually active person to seek a test as to whether they are infected so that they don't spread the disease and get early treatment.
3. Involve various organizations and institutions to take steps to promote AIDS awareness and facilitate protective behaviour.

Let's examine how each of these solutions can be applied.

## ADVOCATE THE USE OF CONDOMS

Condoms are available for both men and women and are highly effective when used to protect the other partner. But their use is not widespread for a number of reasons. First, they involve a cost that is high for low-income people. One solution is for the state to provide free condoms to the most susceptible groups. Second, many sexual encounters involve a strong passionate moment without the time to pause for using a condom and often the condom is not available at that moment. Third, men say that they do not enjoy sex as much when wearing a condom and that it compromises their spontaneity and macho self-image. Fourth, women feel diffident about insisting that the male wear a condom as if it would lower the male's view of the woman's desirability.

Each of these objections to using condoms suggests the kind of social marketing approach that would be required. First, bring down the cost of condoms even to the extent of distributing them free. Second, make condoms available as broadly as possible including getting women to have condoms available even if their male partners are without them. Third, convince males to feel more responsible to the partner and more protected personally by using a condom. Fourth, educate women to be stronger in insisting on protection in a sexual encounter.

Those who are likely to practice more protected sex would be high on four conditions:

- They would be high on *perceived susceptibility*. Those who know that their behavior is risky are more likely to use condoms.

- They would be high on *perceived severity*. They are aware of how deadly AIDS can be to their life.

- They would be high on *perceived response efficacy*. They believe that condoms offer great protection against contracting the disease.

- They would be high on *perceived self-efficacy*. They believe that they have the ability to always use a condom before engaging in a sexual activity.

Let's examine the steps taken by the city of New York to promote the use of condoms. New York City had a very high rate of cases of AIDS that was three times the U.S. average rate as the leading cause of death for residents ages 35 to 54. Mayor Michael Bloomberg decided that NYC should confront this problem with an intense social marketing campaign that would become a national and global model. The NYC Commission on AIDS aimed to "make condoms much more widely available." During Valentine's Day 2007, community volunteers distributed more than 150,000 NYC Condoms across the five boroughs. As the campaign continued, it engaged various NYC establishments—health clubs, coffee houses, bars, hair salons, nail salons, hair braiding shops, wine and liquor stores, laundromats, minimarts, bath houses, spas, tattoo shops, theaters, bars, taverns, saloons, ethnic centers, even churches—to become partners. They set up the number 311 for information and the health department stood ready to deliver free NYC-branded condoms in bulk. Note that this campaign addressed all 4Ps: Product (NYC Condoms), Price (free), Place (all these establishments), and Promotion (posters, radio ads, t-shirts, TV ads and promotion, and so on).

## GETTING PEOPLE TO TAKE AN AIDS TEST

The second challenge in the fight against AIDS was to motivate persons who were sexually active with more than one partner to take an AIDS test. Many resisted doing this. When asking what keeps them from getting tested, there were two big factors. One was fear: the fear of knowing, of dying, or being rejected. The second was the inconvenience and long waiting period before they got the results. They would not know for a week or two whether they had AIDS and this would create considerable anxiety, another Covid-19 similarity.

To counter the resistance to testing, health social marketers would promote the strong benefits of persons knowing their condition. If they were not infected, this would be good news and they could be more careful. If they were infected, they could get early treatment before it was too late. Medical treatment was improving rapidly. They would also have the benefit, if they were infected, of not infecting their partners.

In addition, diagnostic advances were reducing the time to receive test results. The *Chicago Tribune* on January 2, 2004 ran the headline: "Rapid HIV Tests Offered Where Those at Risk Gather: Seattle Health Officials Get Aggressive in AIDS Battle by Heading into Gay Clubs, Taking a Drop of Blood and Providing Answers in 20 Minutes." Now there was no waiting for results. And this led health officials to take a more proactive stand by visiting bathhouses and gay sex clubs to encourage these more highly susceptible persons to be tested.[9]

One dramatic instance of trying to highlight the importance of testing for AIDS occurred when Barak Obama visited Kenya and took a public HIV test and spoke about his trip on World AIDS Day:

> So, we need to show people that just as there is no shame in going to the doctor for a blood test or a CAT scan or a mammogram, there is no shame in going for a HIV test. Because while there was once a time when a positive result gave little hope, today the earlier you know, the faster you can get help. My wife Michelle and I were able to take the test on our trip ... by getting a simple 15-minute test, we may have encouraged as many as half-a-million Kenyans to get tested as well.[10]

Another problem to be faced is with intravenous drug addicts who often use the same needle or share a needle that could spread infection. To combat this problem, many cities distributed free needles to reduce the risk of needle exchanges.

### Involving Community Organizations

Social marketers distinguish between three levels of social marketing: *downstream social marketing* which aims to change the behaviour of individuals; *midstream social marketing* which aims to use peer influence on the target market; and *upstream social marketing* which aims to get major institutions to influence and facilitate target market behavior.

Here the role of upstream social marketing is illustrated in trying to influence the target market. Social marketers need to develop marketing plans to incentivize major community organizations to use their influence on the target market. Consider the potential influence of the following organizations:

- The public school system can prepare curricula that will address the problem of the spreading epidemic of AIDS and how male and female students should avoid unprotected sexual behavior and other actions that might spread the disease.

- Physician groups can get their member physicians to advise their patients about unprotected sex and encourage highly susceptible patients to take an HIV/AIDS test.

- Pharmacies need to make condoms easily available and also facilitate HIV/AIDS testing.

- The media should be engaged in reporting trends and personal stories and even insert AIDS into storylines (i.e., "edutainment") that might dramatize the AIDS problem.

- Community leaders and clergy should be engaged to address the issue and explain how this deadly disease spreads from unprotected sex and other causes.

- Operators of bathhouses and gay sex clubs need to be approached to help their clientele understand how to protect themselves and to test themselves periodically.

- Operators of hair salons and barber shops can be especially effective in high-lighting the AIDS issue to their clients.

- Local governments need to increase funding for research, condom availability, and free testing facilities.

## DEVELOPING A SOCIAL MARKETING CAMPAIGN: STEP BY STEP

Having told the three stories, we now need to describe the typical steps in developing a social marketing campaign. In *Social Marketing: Influencing Behaviors for Good*, Kotler and Lee[11] divided the development of a typical social marketing campaign into 10 steps and illustrated each step in great detail. Here, we will describe these steps and present them concisely.

***Step 1:*** *Define the problem, purpose, and focus*

Any social marketing health campaign needs a clear statement of the specific public health *problem*, which might be a severe epidemic (AIDS or Covid-19), an evolving issue (increases in opioid use), or a justifiable need (public education on the prevention of HPV). Adequate background information is needed at this step. It is critical to identify the program's sponsor(s) and to summarize the factors that led to developing such a program.

Once the public health problem is defined, a *purpose statement* is needed to make it clear what impact and benefits the social marketing campaign, when successful, would generate.

A *focus* is needed to narrow down the scope of the social marketing campaign to make the best use of the available resources, maximize the campaign impact, and ensure the campaign feasibility. The campaign focus is selected from a number of options that have some potential to help achieve the campaign purpose.

**Step 2:** *Conduct a situation analysis*

Typically, a SWOT analysis (strengths, weaknesses, opportunities, and threats) is conducted to provide a quick audit of *organizational* strengths and weaknesses and *environmental* opportunities and threats. Strengths to maximize and weaknesses to minimize include internal factors such as levels of funding, management support, current partners, delivery system capabilities, and the sponsor's reputation. Opportunities to take advantage of and threats to prepare for include major trends and events outside your influence—those often associated with demographic, psychographic, geographic, economic, cultural, political, legal, and technological forces. At this step, you will also conduct a literature review and environmental scan of current and prior campaigns, especially those with similar efforts, and summarize their major activities conducted, major effects achieved, and major lessons learned.

**Step 3:** *Select target audiences*

A *target audience* is quite like the bull's eye. It is selected through *segmentation*, a process to divide a broad audience (population) into homogeneous sub-audiences (groups), called *audience segments*. An audience segment is identified and aggregated by the shared characteristics and needs of the people in a broad audience, including similar demographics, psychographics, geographic locations, behaviors, social networks, community assets, and stage of change.

It is ideal that a social marketing campaign focuses on one primary target audience, but secondary audiences are often identified, based on the marketing problem, purpose, and focus of the campaign defined earlier. An estimated size and informative description of the target audience(s) is needed at this step. An ideal description of the target audience will make you believe that if a member of the audience walked into the room, you would "recognize" her or him.

**Step 4:** *Set marketing objectives and goals*

A social marketing campaign needs clear marketing goals. Specifying desired behaviors and changes in knowledge, attitudes, and beliefs, *marketing goals* always include a *behavior goal*—something the target audience is desired to do as a result of the campaign. Marketing goals also often include a *knowledge goal* which makes clear the information or facts that the target audience needs to know, and a *belief goal*, which relates to the things the target market needs to believe in order to "change its mind."

A social marketing campaign also needs to establish quantifiable measures, called *marketing objectives*, that correspond to the marketing goals. Marketing objectives, responding to behavior objectives, knowledge objectives, and belief objectives respectively, should be ideally SMART—specific, measurable, achievable, relevant, and time-bound in terms of knowledge, attitudes, and behavior changes.[12] What is determined here will have strong implications for budgets, guide marketing mix strategies, and direct evaluation measures in the later planning process in a social marketing campaign.

### Step 5: Identify factors influencing behavior adoption

The social marketer needs to understand what the target audience is doing or prefers to do, and what is affecting its behaviors and preferences. Specifically, barriers, benefits, competitors, and the influencers need to be identified at this step.

*Barriers* refer to reasons, real or perceived, why the target audience may not want to adopt the behavior, or think that it cannot be adopted. *Benefits* are the "gains" the target audience could see through adopting the targeted behavior. *Competitors* refer to any related behaviors that the target audience is currently engaged in, or prefers, rather than the ones being promoted. *Influencers* include any "important others" who could have some influence on the target audience, such as family members, social networks, the entertainment industry, and religious leaders.

### Step 6: Craft a positioning statement

A *positioning statement* describes what the target audience is wanted to feel and think about the targeted behavior and its related benefits. A positioning statement, together with brand identity, is inspired by the description of the target audience and its barriers, competitors, and influencers. It differentiates the targeted behavior from alternative or preferred ones. Effective positioning will guide the development of the marketing mix strategies in the next step, helping ensure that the offer will land on and occupy a distinctive place in the minds of the target audience.

### Step 7: Develop marketing mix strategies: The 4Ps

The traditional marketing toolbox includes the 4Ps of product, price, place, and promotion. Social marketers use these tools to create, communicate, and deliver values for their targeted behaviors.

The 4Ps should be developed and presented with the product strategy at the beginning and the promotion strategy at the end. Promotion is at the end because it ensures that the target markets become aware of the targeted product, its price, and its accessibility, which need to be developed prior to the promotion strategy. Great attention is called for the "mix" of the 4Ps, which should be highly integrated and reinforcing.

*1. Product strategy:* It is essential to have a clear description of the product in a social marketing campaign, at core, actual, and augmented levels. A *core product* comprises the benefits that the target audience will experience or expect in exchange for performing the targeted behavior (e.g., a healthier life and the reduc-tion in the risk of becoming obese or overweight). An *actual product* is the desired behavior, often embodied by its major features and described in specific terms (such as healthy foods or beverages available at vending machines). An *augmented product* refers to any additional tangible objects and/or services that will be included in the offer and promoted to the target market. An augmented product helps perform the targeted behavior or increase its appeal (e.g., information on healthy products available at vending machines).

*2. Price strategy*:    A price strategy sums up the costs that the target audience will "pay" for adopting the desired behavior that leads to the promised benefits. These costs could be monetary such as those for tangible goods and services. Most of the time, however, social marketers sell behaviors that require something else in exchange: time, effort, energy, psychological costs, or physical discomfort. A sen-sible price strategy is aimed at minimizing these costs in relation to the benefits.

*3. Place strategy*:    Place is largely where and when the target audience will be encouraged to perform the desired behavior and to obtain tangible products or services associated with the campaign. Place can be regarded as the delivery sys-tem or a distribution channel for a social marketing campaign. Place strategies aim to ensure that the offer will be as convenient and pleasant as possible for the customer to engage in the targeted behavior.

*4. Promotion strategy*:    Information on product benefits and features, fair price, and easy accessibility needs effective and efficient communication to bring to the target audience and inspire action. Promotion strategy is needed to maximize the success of the communication. The development of the communication is a pro-cess beginning with the determination of key messages, continues with the selec-tion of messengers and communication formats and channels, moves on to the creation of communication elements, and ends up with the implementation of those communications.

The key *messages* need to be aligned with marketing goals, because they deliver what the target audience is to know, believe, and do. Information on bar-riers, benefits, competitors, and influencers will help shape message choices. *Messengers* are those who deliver the messages. Credibility, expertise, and likeabil-ity are some key considerations for selecting messengers.

Messages are delivered through various *communication channels*, such as advertising (including public service advertising, simply called PSA), public rela-tions, social media, events, sponsorships, and personal selling and word of mouth. Media channels can be online, offline, or both. Popular online media vehicles used to communicate social marketing messages are email, websites, blogs, podcasts, Twitter, Instagram, or Facebook groups. Traditional media include print, radio, and television, as well as direct mail, billboards, transit (e.g., buses, taxes, and subways), and kiosks. The most effective medium choice for a social marketing message is the one the target market prefers.

Social marketers need to have a good idea of the media budget and media options before choosing the communication elements. *Creative elements* translate the content of intended, desired messages into specific communication elements, which include copy, graphic images, and typeface as well as interactive features and audio and video for online media.

### *Step 8: Outline a plan for monitoring and evaluation*

A plan for monitoring and evaluating a social marketing campaign is needed before final budget and implementation plans are made. It needs to refer back to the goals established for the campaign. *Monitoring* is a measurement conducted sometime after the launch of a new campaign, but before its completion. Monitoring is executed to determine if mid-course corrections are needed to ensure that marketing goals of the program will be reached. An *evaluation* refers to a measurement and a final report on what happened through the campaign. It needs to address questions like: Were the marketing goals reached? What components of the campaign can be linked with outcomes? Was the program on time and within budget? What worked well and what did not? What should be done differently next time?

Measures fall into three categories—*output* measures for program activities; *outcome* measures for target audience responses and changes in knowledge, beliefs, and behavior; and *impact* measures for contributions to the plan purposes (e.g., many more people are willing to buy healthy foods and beverages due to a social marketing campaign).

In the development of a monitoring and evaluation plan, five basic questions need to be answered:

- Why will this measurement be conducted? For whom?
- What inputs, processes, outcomes, and impacts will be measured?
- What methods (such as an individual in-depth interview, focus group, survey, or online tracking) will be used for these measurements?
- When will these measurements be conducted?
- What is the cost of these measurements?

### *Step 9: Establish budgets and find funding sources*

The budgets for a social marketing campaign reflect the costs for implementing it, which include those associated with marketing mix strategies (the 4Ps), and additional costs anticipated for monitoring and evaluation. In ideal objective-and-task budgeting, these anticipated costs become a preliminary budget based on what is needed to achieve the established marketing goals.

When the preliminary budget exceeds available funds, however, options for additional funding and the potential for adjusting campaign phases (such as spreading out costs over a longer period of time), revising strategies, or reducing behavior change goals may need to be considered. Additional funding sources

# NOTES

## PREFACE

1. "U.S. Health Care from a Global Perspective, 2019: Higher Spending, Worse Outcomes?" Roosa Tikkanen and Melinda K. Abrams, The Commonwealth Fund, January 30, 2020, www.commonwealthfund.org/publications/issue-briefs/2020/jan/us-health-care-global-perspective-2019, accessed 4/23/20.
2. "Seven in 10 Maintain Negative View of U.S. Healthcare System," Gallup Poll Social Series, January 14, 2019, https://news.gallup.com/poll/245873/seven-maintain-negative-view-healthcare-system.aspx, accessed 4/23/20.

## CHAPTER 1

1. Zyman, S., *The End of Marketing As We Know It*, New York, HarperBusiness, 1999.
2. Sheth, J. N. and Sisodia, R. S., *4Ps of Marketing*, Chicago, IL, American Marketing Association, 2008.

## CHAPTER 2

1. Tim Calkins, *Breakthrough Marketing Plans*, New York, Palgrave Macmillan, 2008, pp. 48–70.
2. Tally E. Lassiter, MD, Edward D. Ricks, Haiying Fan, and Thomas Slaughter, "Shoulder Shop: The Shoulder Care Specialists," Summer 2007.
3. *Best, Market Based Management & Hot Topics & EBIZ PKG*, 2nd ed., Copyright 2001. Electronically reproduced by permission of Pearson Education, Inc., Upper Saddle River, NJ (KSS first edition, p. 232).
4. Kotler, *Kotler on Marketing*, New York, Free Press, 1999.
5. Kotler and Keller, *A Framework for Marketing Management*, 3rd ed., New York, Pearson/Prentice Hall, 2006, p. 30.
6. Kotler and Keller, *A Framework for Marketing Management*, 3rd ed., New York, Pearson/Prentice Hall, 2006, p. 66.
7. Macchiette, B. and Abhijit, R., "Sensitive Groups and Social Issues," *Journal of Consumer Marketing*, 11 (4), 1994, pp. 55–64.
8. "Ex-Drug Company CEO Martin Shkreli to Speak at Harvard," Associated Press, February 12, 2017, http://abcnews.go.com/US/wireStory/drug-company-ceo-martin-shkreli-speak-harvard-45444233, accessed 2/13/17.
9. Ries, A. and Trout, J., *Positioning: The Battle for Your Mind*, New York, Warner Books, 1982.
10. Clancy, Kevin J., "Whatever Happened to Positioning," Copernicus Marketing Consulting & Research, 2001.

11. Kotler, P. and Keller, K. L., *Marketing Management*, 12th ed., Upper Saddle River, NJ, Pearson Prentice-Hall, 2006, pp. 275–276.

12. Adapted from a table in Kotler, P., *A Framework for Marketing Management*, 2nd ed., Upper Saddle River, NJ, Prentice-Hall, 2003, p. 217.

13. Kotler, P. and Keller, K. L., *Marketing Management*, 12th ed., Upper Saddle River, NJ, Pearson Prentice-Hall, 2006, pp. 371–372.

14. This discussion is adapted from Theodore Levitt, "Marketing Success through Differentiation of Anything," *Harvard Business Review*, January–February, 1980, pp. 83–91. The first level, core benefit, has been added to Levitt's discussion.

15. Harper W. Boyd Jr. and Sidney Levy, "New Dimensions in Consumer Analysis," *Harvard Business Review*, November–December, 1963, pp. 129–140.

16. Dagmara Scalise, "The Patient Experience," *Hospitals and Health Networks*, December 2003, 41–47.

17. The Birthplace at Caromont Regional Medical Center, www.caromonthealth.org/Services/Womens-Health/The-Birthplace.aspx, accessed 4/15/20.

18. Shantanu Dutta, Mark J. Zbaracki, and Mark Bergen, "Pricing Process as a Capability: A Resource Based Perspective," *Strategic Management Journal*, 24 (7), 2003, pp. 615–630.

19. "Seven Factors Driving Up Your Health Care Costs," *Kaiser Health News*, October 24, 2012, www.pbs.org/newshour/rundown/seven-factors-driving-your-health-care-costs/, accessed 2/20/17.

20. "The Lesson of EpiPens: Why Drug Prices Spike, Again and Again," *New York Times*, September 2, 2016, www.nytimes.com/2016/09/04/opinion/sunday/the-lesson-of-epipens-why-drug-prices-spike-again-and-again.html?_r=0, accessed 2/13/17.

21. "Mylan Tries Again to Quell Pricing Outrage by Offering Generic EpiPen," *New York Times*, August 29, 2016, www.nytimes.com/2016/08/30/business/mylan-generic-epipen.html, accessed 2/25/17.

22. Anne T. Coughlan, Erin Anderson, Louis W. Stern, and Adel I. El-Ansary, *Marketing Channels*, 7th ed., Upper Saddle River, NJ, Prentice Hall, 2007.

23. "Medicare Home Visit Program Associated with Fewer Hospital and Nursing Home Admissions, Increased Office Visits," *Health Affairs*, 34 (12), 2015, pp. 2138–2146.

24. IndUShealth Pricing, www.indushealth.com/pricing/, accessed 3/23/17.

25. John R. Rossiter and Larry Percy, *Advertising and Promotion Management*, 2nd edition, New York, McGraw-Hill, 1997.

26. Stephanie Thompson, "Minimal Hype Nets Max Buzz at Kiehl's," *Advertising Age*, April 5, 2004, pp. 4, 33.

27. "What's a Pound of Prevention Really Worth?" D. Leonhardt, *New York Times*, January 24, 2007, pp. C1, C4.

## CHAPTER 3

1. www.informationweek.com/strategic-cio/can-argonaut-project-make-exchanging-health-data-easier/a/d-id/1318774, accessed 4/6/15.

2. Andreasen, Alan, "'Backward' Market Research," *Harvard Business Review*, May 1985.

3. Catherine Arnold, "Global Perspective: Synovate Exec Discusses Future of International Research," *Marketing News*, May 15, 2004, p. 43; Michael Erard, "For Technology, No Small World after All," *New York Times*, May 6, 2004; Deborah L. Vence, "Global Consistency: Leave It to the Experts," *Marketing News*, April 28, 2003, p. 37.

4. Kevin J. Clancy and Peter Krieg, *Counterintuitive Marketing: How Great Results Come from Uncommon Sense*. New York, The Free Press, 2000.

5. U.S. and World Population Clock, U.S. Census Bureau, www.census.gov/popclock, accessed 12/13/19.

6. "Statistical Brief #481: The Concentration and Persistence in the Level of Health Expenditures over Time—Estimates for the U.S. Population, 2012–2013," Agency for Healthcare Research and Quality, September 2015, https://meps.ahrq.gov/data_files/publications/st481/stat481.pdf, accessed 12/13/19.

7. "Total Professionally Active Physicians," Kaiser Family Foundation, Special data request for information on active state licensed physicians from Redi-Data, Inc, March 2019, http://kff.org/other/state-indicator/total-active-physicians/?currentTimeframe=0&sortModel=%7B%22colId%22:%22Location%22,%22sort%22:%22asc%22%7D, accessed 12/13/19.

8. National Health Expenditures 2018 Highlights, CMS,www.cms.gov/files/document/highlights.pdf; www.cms.gov/Research-Statistics-Data-and-Systems/Statistics-Trends-and-Reports/NationalHealthExpendData/NationalHealthAccountsHistorical, accessed 1/1/20.

9. "Employer Costs for Employee Compensation," Bureau of Labor Statistics, 3/17/17, www.bls.gov/news.release/ecec.nr0.htm, accessed 9/11/17.

10. Centers of Excellence | For Patients | JAMA | The JAMA Network, September 4, 2013, jamanetwork.com/journals/jama/fullarticle/1734706, accessed 4/21/17.

11. "Emerging Trends in Health Care Survey," Towers Watson, January 2015, www.towerswatson.com/en-US/Insights/IC-Types/Survey-Research-Results/2015/04/infographic-top-four-employer-health-care-trends, accessed 4/21/17.

12. "Uninsured Rate Rose in 2018, Says Census Bureau Report," Katie Keith, Health Affairs, September 11, 2019, www.healthaffairs.org/do/10.1377/hblog20190911.805983/full, accessed 11/21/19.

13. "American Medical Association's Study of Nation's 25 Largest Health Insurers Indicates that Biggest Companies Hold Dominant Market Share in Most Regional Markets," *Dark Daily*, www.darkdaily.com/american-medical-associations-study-of-nations-25-largest-health-insurers-indicates-that-biggest-companies-hold-dominant-market-share-in-most-regional-markets-109#ixzz4ffgOeVg1, accessed 4/29/17.

14. Allan D. Shocker, "Determining the Structure of Product-Markets: Practices, Issues, and Suggestions," in *Handbook of Marketing*, Barton A. Weitz and Robin Wensley (eds.), Sage Publications, 2002, pp. 106–125. See also Bruce H. Clark and David B. Montgomery, "Managerial Identification of Competitors," *Journal of Marketing*, 63 (July), 1999, pp. 67–83.

15. Jeffrey F. Rayport and Bernard J. Jaworski, *e-Commerce*, New York, McGraw-Hill, 2001, p. 53.

16. Gerald Celente, *Trend Tracking*, New York, Warner Books, 1991.

17. www.modernhealthcare.com/article/20141008/NEWS/310089966, accessed 3/9/15.

18. United Nations and the U.S. Census Bureau, www.worldometers.info/world-population/, accessed 4/18/17.

19. 2015 Revision of World Population Prospects, United Nations, July 29, 2015. www.un.org/en/development/desa/population/events/other/10/index.shtml, accessed 4/18/17.

20. "Fact Sheet: Aging in the United States," Population Reference Bureau, January 2016, www.prb.org/Publications/Media-Guides/2016/aging-unitedstates-fact-sheet.aspx, accessed 4/18/17.

21. Population Distribution by Race/Ethnicity, Kaiser Family Foundation, 2018, www.kff.org/other/state-indicator/distribution-by-raceethnicity/?currentTimeframe=0&sortModel=%7B%22colId%22:%22Location%22,%22sort%22:%22asc%22%7D, accessed 1/1/20.

22. "Key Findings About U.S. Immigrants," Pew Research Institute, June 17, 2019, www.pewresearch.org/fact-tank/2019/06/17/key-findings-about-u-s-immigrants/, accessed 1/1/20.

23. www.uhclatino.com/content/lat-muhclati/uhc-latino/es/planbien.html, accessed 4/19/17.

24. "What Growing Life Expectancy Gaps Mean for the Promise of Social Security," Barry P. Bosworth, Gary Burtless, and Kan Zhang, Brookings Institute, February 12, 2016, www.brookings.edu/research/what-growing-life-expectancy-gaps-mean-for-the-promise-of-social-security/#recent/, accessed 4/29/17.

25. "National Health Expenditure Data, CMS, December 5, 2019," www.cms.gov/Research-Statistics-Data-and-Systems/Statistics-Trends-and-Reports/NationalHealthExpendData/NHE-Fact-Sheet, 12/13/19.

26. National Health Expenditure Data 2018 Fact Sheet, CMS, www.cms.gov/files/document/nations-health-dollar-where-it-came-where-it-went.pdf, accessed 1/1/20.

27. "$10,345 Per Person: U.S. Health Care Spending Reaches New Peak," *PBS News Hour*, July 13, 2016, www.pbs.org/newshour/rundown/new-peak-us-health-care-spending-10345-per-person, accessed 12/13/16.

28. *Quality Matters: Profile: Heartland Regional Medical Center ACO*, The Commonwealth Fund, June/July 2014.

29. "Credit Cards and Finance Lines for Medical Care," Consumer Reports, April 2012, www.consumerreports.org/cro/2012/04/overdose-of-debt/index.htm#, accessed 5/1/17.

30. Altarum Institute Survey of Consumer Health Care Opinions—Spring 2014.

31. http://kaiserhealthnews.org/news/retail-health-care-spurs-innovation-in-south-florida, accessed 3/12/15.

32. www.usnews.com/news/articles/2015/02/06/mmr-vaccine-is-less-effective-for-mumps-than-measles-rubella, accessed 3/12/15.

33. http://dupress.com/articles/2012-survey-of-u-s-health-care-consumers-five-year-look-back/, accessed 3/12/15.

34. http://dictionary.reference.com/help/faq/language/d24.html, accessed 3/17/15.

35. www.cdc.gov/vhf/ebola/outbreaks/2014-west-africa/case-counts.html, accessed 3/17/15.

36. www.webmd.com/cold-and-flu/what-are-epidemics-pandemics-outbreaks, accessed 3/16/15.

37. www.flu.gov/images/clip_image002_com.jpg, accessed 3/16/15.

38. Global COVID-19 Pandemic Notice, CDC, wwwnc.cdc.gov/travel/notices/warning/coronavirus-global, accessed 4/16/20.

39. http://en.wikipedia.org/wiki/Hospital-acquired_infection, accessed 3/17/15.

40. http://molecular.roche.com/assays/Pages/cobasMRSASATest.aspx, accessed 3/17/15.

41. Christensen, C. M., *The Innovator's Prescription*, New York, McGraw-Hill, 2009, pp. 3–6, 227.

42. "Biologists Propose to Sequence the DNA of All Life on Earth," *Science*, February 24, 2017, www.sciencemag.org/news/2017/02/biologists-propose-sequence-dna-all-life-earth, accessed 5/4/17.

43. South Carolina Department of Health and Human Services, presentation at South Carolina's 17th Annual Rural Health Conference, reported in "Top Health Industry Issues of 2015," PwC, pp. 5, 12–14.

44. "The Truth About the Uninsured Rate in America," *CNN Money*, March 14, 2017, http://money.cnn.com/2017/03/13/news/economy/uninsured-rate-obamacare, accessed 5/8/17.

45. "U.S. Uninsured Rate Rises to Four-Year High," *Gallup*, January 23, 2019, https://news.gallup.com/poll/246134/uninsured-rate-rises-four-year-high.aspx, accessed 1/1/20.

46. "Key Facts about the Uninsured Population," Kaiser Family Foundation, September 29, 2016. http://kff.org/uninsured/fact-sheet/key-facts-about-the-uninsured-population/, accessed 5/8/17.

47. www.advisory.com/daily-briefing/2014/05/01/cms-proposes-million-in-medicare-cuts-requires-hospitals-to-post-their-chargemasters, accessed 4/1/15.

48. "Top Health Industry Issues of 2015," PwC, 12/14, p. 7.

49. "House Bill Seeks to Add Mandatory Drug Recall Authority to FDA's Arsenal," Regulatory Affairs Professional Society, February 1, 2017, www.raps.org/Regulatory-Focus/News/2017/02/16/26852/House-Bill-Seeks-to-Add-Mandatory-Drug-Recall-Authority-to-FDA%E2%80%99s-Arsenal/, accessed 5/7/17.

50. "History of NAHAC," Joanna Smith, LCSW, MPH, CHA, http://nahac.memberlodge.com/history, accessed 5/7/17.

# CHAPTER 4

1. George Belch and Michael Belch, *Advertising and Communication Management*, 6th ed., 2003, Homewood, IL, Irwin.

2. "Mortality in the United States, 2014," NCHS Data Brief No. 229, National Center for Health Statistics, Center for Disease Control, December 2015, www.cdc.gov/nchs/products/databriefs/db267.htm, accessed 6/12/17.

3. OECD (2020) *Life Expectancy at Birth (Indicator)*, doi: 10.1787/27e0fc9d-en, accessed 2/14/20.

4. OECD (2019) *Health at a Glance 2019: OECD Indicators*, Paris, OECD Publishing, https://doi.org/10.1787/4dd50c09-en, accessed 2/14/20.

5. "Trends in Out-of-Hospital Births in the United States, 1990–2012," National Center for Health Statistics, Center for Disease Control, www.cdc.gov/nchs/data/databriefs/db144.htm#x2013;2012</a>, accessed 9/8/16.

6. "Morbidity vs. Mortality," Diffen, www.diffen.com/difference/Morbidity_vs_Mortality, accessed 5/17/17.

7. "Prevalence of Obesity Among Adults and Youth: United States, 2015–2016," NCHS Data Brief No. 288, October 2017, www.cdc.gov/nchs/data/databriefs/db288.pdf, accessed 2/11/20.

8. "Comorbidity and the Use of Primary Care and Specialist Care in the Elderly," Annals of Family Medicine, American Academy of Family Physicians, www.ncbi.nlm.nih.gov/pmc/articles/PMC1466877/#!po=7.14286, accessed 1/13/20.

9. "Characteristics of Office-Based Physician Visits, 2016," NCHS Data Brief, No. 331, January 2019, CDC, www.cdc.gov/nchs/data/databriefs/db331-h.pdf, accessed 1/13/20.

10. "Mortality in the United States, 2018," NCHS Data Brief No. 355, National Center for Health Statistics, Center for Disease Control, January 2020, www.cdc.gov/nchs/products/databriefs/db355.htm, accessed 2/6/20.

11. "Key Statistics for Lung Cancer," American Cancer Society, www.cancer.org/cancer/non-small-cell-lung-cancer/about/key-statistics.html, accessed 5/15/17.

12. "Key Injury and Violence Data," CDC, September 19, 2016, www.cdc.gov/injury/wisqars/overview/key_data.html, accessed 5/16/17.

13. "Diabetes Type 1 and 2," MedicineNet.com, www.medicinenet.com/diabetes_mellitus/article.htm, accessed 5/17/17.

14. "Kidney Disease Statistics for the United States," National Institute of Diabetes and Digestive and Kidney Diseases, December 6, 2016, www.niddk.nih.gov/health-information/health-statistics/kidney-disease, accessed 5/17/17.

15. "Suicide Statistics," American Foundation for Suicide Prevention, 2015, https://afsp.org/about-suicide/suicide-statistics/, accessed 5/17/17.

16. "Medical Errors Now 3rd Leading Cause of Death in U.S., Study Suggests," *CBS News*, May 4, 2016, www.cbsnews.com/news/medical-errors-now-3rd-leading-cause-of-death-in-u-s-study-suggests/, accessed 5/17/17.

17. "NHE Fact Sheet," CMS, December 5, 2019, www.cms.gov/research-statistics-data-and-systems/statistics-trends-and-reports/nationalhealthexpenddata/nhe-fact-sheet, accessed 2/20/20.

18. "OECD Data, Health Spending, 2018," https://data.oecd.org/healthres/health-spending.htm, accessed 2/1/20.

19. "IOM Report Focuses on $750 Billion in Inefficient Health Care Spending," KHN, September 6, 2012, http://khn.org/news/iom-report-focuses-on-750-billion-in-inefficient-health-care-spending; "Best Care at Lower Cost: The Path to Continuously Learning Health Care in America," 2013, accessed 5/22/17.

20. www.modernhealthcare.com/article/20141008/NEWS/310089966, accessed 3/9/15.

21. "We Spend $750 Billion on Unnecessary Health Care—Two Charts Explain Why," *The Washington Post*, September 7, 2012, www.washingtonpost.com/news/wonk/wp/2012/09/07/we-spend-750-billion-on-unnecessary-health-care-two-charts-explain-why/?utm_term=.cf942610c432, accessed 5/22/17.

22. "We Can Do Better—Improving the Health of the American People," Steven A. Schroeder, M.D., *New England Journal of Medicine*, September 20, 2007, www.nejm.org/doi/full/10.1056/NEJMsa073350#t=article, accessed 5/24/17.

23. "Connected Health and the Rise of the Patient-Consumer," William H. Frist, *Health Affairs*, 33 (2), 2014, pp. 191–193.

24. Fuchs, Victor, *Who Shall Live?*, New York, Basic Books, 1974, pp. 54–55.

25. "Multicultural Healthcare Marketing," *EthnoConnect*, Dublin, CA, www.ethnoconnect.com/articles/5-multicultural-healthcare-marketing, accessed 5/25/17.

26. Richard P. Coleman, "The Continuing Significance of Social Class to Marketing," *Journal of Consumer Research* 10, 1983, pp. 265–280; Richard P. Coleman and Lee P. Rainwater, *Social Standing in America: New Dimension of Class*, New York, Basic Books, 1978.

27. "Social Class as Culture," Association for Psychological Science, August 8, 2011, www.psychologicalscience.org/news/releases/social-class-as-culture.html, accessed 2/19/20.

28. Glen Llopsis, "The Cultural Demographic Shift is Changing the Business of Healthcare," *Forbes*, July 13, 2015, http://onforb.es/1Mptazg, accessed 10/5/16.

29. "Do Friends, Family Affect Your Health?" Insight, Dana-Farber Cancer Institute, May 19, 2014, http://blog.dana-farber.org/insight/2012/05/do-friends-family-affect-your-health/, accessed 5/25/17.

30. *Social Determinants of Health 101 for Health Care: Five Plus Five*, National Academy of Health, https://nam.edu/social-determinants-of-health-101-for-health-care-five-plus-five/, accessed 2/21/20.

31. *Social Determinants of Health, Healthy People 2020*, www.healthypeople.gov/2020/topics-objectives/topic/social-determinants-of-health, accessed 2/18/20.

32. *Top Health Industry Issues of 2019: The New Health Economy Comes of Age*, PwC Health Research Institute, p. 24, www.pwc.com/us/en/industries/health-services/pdf/pwc-us-healthcare-top-health-industry-issues-2019.pdf, accessed 2/18/20.

33. Leon G. Schiffman and Leslie Lazar Kanuk, *Consumer Behavior*, 10th ed., Upper Saddle River, NJ, Prentice Hall, 2010.

34. Kay M. Palan and Robert E. Wilkes, "Adolescent-Parent Interaction in Family Decision Making," *Journal of Consumer Research* 24, 1997, pp. 159–169; Sharon E. Beatty and Salil Talpade, "Adolescent Influence in Family Decision Making: A Replication with Extension," *Journal of Consumer Research* 21, 1994, pp. 332–341.

35. "Cardiac Rehabilitation and Survival in Older Coronary Patients," *Journal of the American College of Cardiology*, 54 (1), 2009, pp. 25–33.

36. "Cardiac Rehabilitation Using the Family-Centered Empowerment Model versus Home-Based Cardiac Rehabilitation in Patients with Myocardial Infarction: A Randomized Controlled Trial," *Open*

*Heart* 3, 2016, doi:10.1136/openhrt-2015-000349, www.researchgate.net/publication/299602642_Cardiac_Rehabilitation_using_the_Family-Centered_Empowerment_Model_Verses_Home-Based_Cardiac_Rehab_in_Patients_with_Myocardial_Infarction_A_Randomized_Controlled_Trial, accessed 10/5/16.

37. Center for Financing, Access, and Cost Trends, AHRQ, Household Component of the Medical Expenditure Panel Survey, 2012, http://meps.ahrq.gov/mepsweb/data_files/publications/st448/stat448.shtml, accessed 4/5/16.

38. "America's Families and Living Arrangements: 2012," U.S. Census Bureau, www.census.gov/prod/2013pubs/p20-570.pdf, accessed 10/11/16.

39. "Growing Number of People Living Solo Can Pose Challenges," Pew Charitable Trust, September 11, 2014, www.pewtrusts.org/en/research-and-analysis/blogs/stateline/2014/09/11/growing-number-of-people-living-solo-can-pose-challenges, accessed 10/11/16.

40. "Americans Again Cite Cost and Access as Top Health Issues," *Gallup*, November 18, 2015, www.gallup.com/poll/186722/americans-again-cite-cost-access-top-health-issues.aspx?g_source=CATEGORY_HEALTHCARE&g_medium=topic&g_campaign=tiles, accessed 3/23/16.

41. "3 Types of Nonprofit Healthcare Organization Brand Personalities," Pinpoint for Health, September 4, 2014, http://pinpoint-for-health.com/3-types-of-npho-brand-personalities/, accessed 5/29/17.

42. M. Joseph Sirgy, "Self Concept in Consumer Behavior: A Critical Review," *Journal of Consumer Research* 9, 1982, pp. 287–300.

43. Navarro, Frederick, *The PATH Model: Understanding the Health Care Consumer*, Fontana, CA, The PATH Institute, 2004.

44. Navarro, Frederick, *The PATH Model: Understanding the Health Care Consumer*, Fontana, CA, The PATH Institute, 2004.

45. Navarro, Frederick, *Medical Expenditures Effects from Increasing Behavioral Conformity to Patterns of Health-Related Behavior*. Self-published, 2015, www.researchgate.net/publication/283017392_Medical_Expenditure_Effects_from_Increasing_Behavioral_Conformity_to_Patterns_of_Health-Related_Behavior, accessed 7/6/16; Navarro, Frederick, *Patterns of Health-Related Behavior as Predictors of Medical Expenditures*, Walden University, 2014. UMI: 3631562, http://dissexpress.umi.com/dxweb/results.html?QryTxt=&By=Frederick+Navarro&Title=Patterns+of+Health-Related+Behavior+as+Predictors+of+Medical+Expenditures&pubnum=, accessed 7/6/16; Navarro, Frederick, *Pattern of Health*, New York, Quantum House, 2014.

46. "Health Belief Model," University of Twente, www.utwente.nl/en/bms/communication-theories/sorted-by-cluster/Health%20Communication/Health_Belief_Model/, accessed 5/31/17.

47. "Theory at a Glance, A Guide For Health Promotion Practice," 2nd ed., U.S. Department of Health and Human Services, National Institutes of Health, Spring 2005, pp. 13–14.

48. "Theory at a Glance, A Guide For Health Promotion Practice," 2nd ed., U.S. Department of Health and Human Services, National Institutes of Health, Spring 2005, p. 14.

49. John R, Anderson, *The Architecture of Cognition*, Cambridge, MA, Harvard University Press, 1983; Robert S. Wyer, Jr. and Thomas K. Srull, "Person Memory and Judgement," *Psychological Review*, 96 (1), 1989, pp. 58–83.

50. "Brand Concept Maps: Measuring What Your Brand Means to Consumers," Carlson School of Management, University of Minnesota, 5/19/06.

51. For additional discussion, see John G. Lynch Jr. and Thomas K. Srull, "Memory and Attentional Factors in Consumer Choice: Concepts and Research Methods," *Journal of Consumer Research*, 9, 1982, pp. 18–36; and Joseph W. Alba, J. Wesley Hutchinson, and John G. Lynch, Jr., "Memory and

Decision Making," in *Handbook of Consumer Theory and Research*, Harold H. Kassarjian and Thomas S. Robertson (eds.), Englewood Cliffs, NJ, Prentice Hall, Inc., 1992, pp. 1–49.

52. Shapiro, B., Rangan, V. K., and Sviokla, J., "Staple Yourself to an Order," *Harvard Business Review*, July-August, 1992, pp. 113–122. See also Heilman, C. M., Bowman, D., and Wright, G. P., "The Evolution of Brand Preferences and Choice Behaviors of Consumers New to a Market," *Journal of Marketing Research*, May, 2000, pp. 139–155.

53. Howard, J. A., and Sheth, J. N., *The Theory of Buyer Behavior*, New York, Wiley, 1969; Engel, J. F., Blackwell, R. D., and Miniard, P. W., *Consumer Behavior*, 8th ed., Fort Worth, TX, Dreyden, 1994; Luce, M. F., Bettman, J. R., and Payne, J. W., *Emotional Decisions: Tradeoff Difficulty and Coping in Consumer Choice*, Chicago: University of Chicago Press, 2001.

54. Putsis, W. P. Jr., and Srinivasan, N., "Buying or Just Browsing? The Duration of Purchase Deliberation," *Journal of Marketing Research*, August, 1994, pp. 393–402.

55. Chem L. Narayana and Rom J. Markin, "Consumer Behavior and Product Performance: An Alternative Conceptualization," *Journal of Marketing*, October, 1975, pp. 1–6. See also Wayne S. DeSarbo and Kamel Jedidi, "The Spatial Representation of Heterogeneous Consideration Sets," *Marketing Science* 14 (3), pt. 2, 1995, pp. 326–342; Lee G. Cooper and Akihiro Inoue, "Building Market Structures from Consumer Preferences," *Journal of Marketing Research* 33 (3), 1996, pp. 293–306.

56. See Paul E. Green and Yoram Wind, *Multiattribute Decisions in Marketing: A Measurement Approach*, Hinsdale, IL, Dryden, 1973, ch. 2; Leigh McAlister, "Choosing Multiple Items from a Product Class," *Journal of Consumer Research*, December, 1979, pp. 213–224; Richard J. Lutz, "The Role of Attitude Theory in Marketing," in *Perspectives in Consumer Behavior*, Harold H. Kassarjian and Thomas S. Robertson (eds.), Englewood Cliffs, NJ, Prentice-Hall, Inc., 1991, pp. 317–339.

57. Solomon, M. R., *Consumer Behavior: Buying, Having, and Being*, Upper Saddle River, NJ, Prentice Hall, 2001.

58. Jagdish N. Sheth, "An Investigation of Relationships among Evaluative Beliefs, Affect, Behavioral Intention, and Behavior," in *Consumer Behavior: Theory and Application*, John U. Farley, John A. Howard, and L. Winston Ring (eds.), Boston, MA, Allyn & Bacon, 1974, pp. 89–114.

59. Fishbein, M., "Attitudes and Prediction of Behavior," in *Readings in Attitude Theory and Measurement*, M. Fishbein (ed.), Hoboken, NJ, Wiley, 1967.

60. Raymond A. Bauer, "Consumer Behavior as Risk Taking," in *Risk Taking and Information Handling in Consumer Behavior*, Donald F. Cox (ed.), Boston, MA, Division of Research, Harvard Business School, 1967; James W. Taylor, "The Role of Risk in Consumer Behavior," *Journal of Marketing*, April, 1974, pp. 54–60.

61. Priscilla A. La Barbera and David Mazursky, "A Longitudinal Assessment of Consumer Satisfaction/Dissatisfaction: The Dynamic Aspect of the Cognitive Process," *Journal of Marketing Research*, November, 1983, pp. 393–404.

62. www.cdc.gov/chronicdisease/overview/index.htm, accessed 3/24/16.

63. "Chronic Diseases: The Leading Causes of Death and Disability in the United States," Centers for Disease Control and Prevention, www.cdc.gov/chronicdisease/overview/, accessed 4/2/16.

64. "Chronic Care: Making the Case for Ongoing Care," Robert Wood Johnson Foundation, February 2010, www.rwjf.org/pr/product.jsp?id=50968. *Note: Chronic Care: Making the Case for Ongoing Care—all of the information is available for use and reproduction without charge; permission from the authors to use the charts is not necessary.*

65. Ward, B. W., Schiller, J. S., and Goodman, R. A., "Multiple Chronic Conditions Among US Adults: A 2012 Update," Prev Chronic Dis. 2014, doi: http://dx.doi.org/10.5888/pcd11.130389.

66. www.cdc.gov/chronicdisease, accessed 4/2/16.

67. "Chronic Care: Making the Case for Ongoing Care," Robert Wood Johnson Foundation, February 2010, www.rwjf.org/pr/product.jsp?id=50968. *Note: Chronic Care: Making the Case for Ongoing Care—all of the information is available for use and reproduction without charge; permission from the authors to use the charts is not necessary.*

68. McGinnis, J. M. and Foege, W. H., "Actual Causes of Death in the United States," *Journal of the American Medical Association*, 270 (18), 1993, pp. 2207–2212.

69. "The Four Domains of Chronic Disease Prevention," National Center for Chronic Disease Prevention and Health Promotion, CDC, 2015, www.cdc.gov/chronicdisease/pdf/four-domains-factsheet-2015.pdf, accessed 5/16/16.

70. "Healthcare Costs Top Financial Problem for U.S. Families," Jeffrey F. Jones, Gallup, Inc, May 30, 2019, https://news.gallup.com/poll/257906/healthcare-costs-top-financial-problem-families.aspx, accessed 2/21/20.

71. 2018 Milliman Medical Index, May 2018, p. 3, www.milliman.com/-/media/Milliman/importedfiles/uploadedFiles/insight/Periodicals/mmi/2018-milliman-medical-index.ashx, accessed 2/21/20; and 2019 Milliman Medical Index, July 2019, p. 4, www.milliman.com/insight/2019-Milliman-Medical-Index, accessed 20/21/20.

72. Employer Health Benefits 2019 Annual Survey, Kaiser Family Foundation, 2019, p. 8, www.kff.org/health-costs/report/2019-employer-health-benefits-survey/, accessed 2/24/20.

73. Ibid.

74. "49% Don't Understand Health Plan Costs," *HealthLeaders Media News*, September 2016, www.healthleadersmedia.com/finance/49-dont-understand-health-plan-costs, accessed 10/15/16.

75. "Consumer Intelligence Series: The Wearable Life 2.0," PwC, May 2016, www.pwc.com/us/en/industry/entertainment-media/publications/consumer-intelligence-series/wearables.html, accessed 6/26/17.

76. "Engaged Employees Less Likely to Have Health Problems," Gallup-Healthways Well-Being Index, December 18, 2015, www.well-beingindex.com/engaged-employees-less-likely-to-have-health-problems, accessed 5/16/16.

77. "Gallup Editors Rank Important Survey Findings," Gallup-Healthways Well-Being Index Study, *Quirks Marketing Research Review*, February 2016, pp. 18–19.

78. Kaiser/HRET Survey of Employer-Sponsored Health Benefits, 1999–2015; KPMG Survey of Employer-Sponsored Health Benefits, 1993, 1996; The Health Insurance Association of America (HIAA), 1988, p. 197.

79. "Workplace Wellness Programs Can Generate Savings," *Health Affairs*, 29 (2), 2010, pp. 304–311.

80. "One Doctor's Entrepreneurial Quest to Reinvent Medicine," Bryant McBride, Worth, January 8, 2019, www.worth.com/contributor/one-doctors-entrepreneurial-quest-to-reinvent-medicine/, accessed 2/25/20.

81. "The Doctor Is In. Co-Pay? $40,000," *New York Times*, Nelson D. Schwartz, June 12, 2017, www.nytimes.com/2017/06/03/business/economy/high-end-medical-care.html?_r=0, accessed 6/22/17.

82. "Family Physicians, Psychiatrists—Top List of Most in Demand Doctors," Merritt Hawkins, June 6, 2017, www.merritthawkins.com/uploadedFiles/MerrittHawkins/Pdf/2017_Physician_Incentive_Review_Merritt_Hawkins.pdf, accessed 6/19/17.

83. "Drug Deaths in America are Rising Faster Than Ever," Josh Katz, *New York Times*, June 5, 2017, www.nytimes.com/interactive/2017/06/05/upshot/opioid-epidemic-drug-overdose-deaths-are-rising-faster-than-ever.html, accessed 6/19/17.

84. "Sports and Exercise," Bureau of Labor Statistics, May 2008, www.bls.gov/spotlight/2008/sports/, accessed 6/19/17.

85. "Early Release of Selected Estimates Based on Data From the 2018 National Health Interview Survey," Centers for Disease Control and Prevention, May 30, 2019, www.cdc.gov/nchs/nhis/releases/released201905. htm#7a, accessed 2/2720.

86. "Support or Competition? How Online Social Networks Increase Physical Activity—A Randomized Controlled Trial," *Preventive Medicine Report*, 4, 2016, pp. 453–458, www.sciencedirect.com/science/ article/pii/S2211335516300936?via%3Dihub, accessed 2/27/20.

87. "Want To Exercise More? Get Yourself Some Competition," Annenberg School for Communication, University of Pennsylvania, Ocotber 27, 16, www.asc.upenn.edu/news-events/news/competition-vs-support, accessed 3/2/20.

88. The study was funded by the National Cancer Institute's Center of Excellence in Cancer Communication Research grant to the Annenberg School for Communication.

89. "Study Identifies No. 1 Source of Motivation to Exercise More," *Psychology Today*, Christopher Bergland, October 30, 2016, www.psychologytoday.com/us/blog/the-athletes-way/201610/study-identifies-no-1-source-motivation-exercise-more, accessed 3/2/20.

## CHAPTER 5

1. "The Patient Experience and Health Outcomes," Matthew P. Manary, William Boulding, Richard Staelin, Seth W. Glickman, *New England Journal of Medicine*, December 26, 2012, at NEJM.org.

2. FSMB Census of Licensed Physicians in the United States, 2018, Federation of State Medical Boards, 2019, p. 12, www.fsmb.org/siteassets/advocacy/publications/2018census.pdf, accessed 1/4/20.

3. "Total of Professionally Active Physicians," Kaiser Family Foundation, March 2019, www.kff.org/ other/state-indicator/total-active-physicians/?currentTimeframe=0&sortModel=%7B%22colId%22:% 22Location%22,%22sort%22:%22asc%22%7D, accessed 1/4/20.

4. 2019 State Physician Workforce Data Report, Association of American Medical Colleges, Washington, DC, https://store.aamc.org/downloadable/download/sample/sample_id/305/, accessed 1/4/20.

5. "American Community Survey (ACS)," U.S. Census Bureau, https://datausa.io/profile/soc/291060/ #demographics, accessed 6/26/17.

6. "The Complexities of Physician Supply and Demand: Projections from 2013 to 2025," Association of American Medical Colleges, March 2015. The shortage range for physicians overall is smaller than the sum of the ranges for primary and non-primary care, reflecting that future demand for health care services will be provided by physicians, but in some instances, it is uncertain whether that care will be provided by a primary care physician or by a specialist.

7. "American Community Survey (ACS)," U.S. Census Bureau, https://datausa.io/profile/soc/291060/ #demographics, accessed 1/4/20.

8. Licensed Physicians in the United States and the District of Columbia by Gender and Age, FSMB Census of Licensed Physicians in the United States, 2018, Federation of State Medical Boards, 2019, p. 17. www.fsmb.org/siteassets/advocacy/publications/2018census.pdf, accessed 1/3/20.

9. Health Resources and Services Administration Bureau of Health Profession, "The Physician Workforce: Projections and Research into Current Issues Affecting Supply and Demand," U.S. Department of Health and Human Services, 2008.

10. Medscape Physician Compensation Report 2019, www.medscape.com/slideshow/2019-compensation-overview-6011286#4, accessed 1/4/20.

11. "Graduation Rates and Attrition Factors for U.S. Medical School Students," Analysis in Brief, Association of American Medical Colleges, 14, 5, 2014.

12. "Understand Physician Culture to Facilitate Change," Shari Welch, MD, Healthcare Executive, May/June 2010, www.thequalitymatters.com/media/Quality_Matters%2DUnderstanding_Physician_Culture.pdf, accessed 6/29/17.

13. Abraham Verghese, MD, Wikipedia, https://en.wikipedia.org/wiki/Abraham_Verghese, accessed 7/3/17.

14. Groopman, Jerome, *How Doctors Think*, Boston, Houghton Mifflin Co., 2007, p. 34.

15. Ibid.

16. "Letting Go," Atul Gawande, MD, *The New Yorker*, 8/2/10, p. 2.

17. "Letting Go," Atul Gawande, MD, *The New Yorker*, 8/2/10, p. 3.

18. "Letting Go," Atul Gawande, MD, *The New Yorker*, 8/2/10, p. 5.

19. "The Status of Baby Boomers' Health in the United States—The Healthiest Generation?" *JAMA Internal Medicine*, 173 (5), 2013, pp. 385–386.

20. 2018 Survey of America's Physicians, The Physicians Foundation and Merritt Hawkins, September 16, 2018, https://physiciansfoundation.org/research-insights/the-physicians-foundation-2018-physician-survey/, accessed 1/5/20.

21. Ibid.

22. 2016 Survey of America's Physicians, The Physicians Foundation and Merritt Hawkins, September 16, 2016, p. 20, www.physiciansfoundation.org, accessed 7/13/17.

23. 2019 Review of Physician and Advance Practitioner Recruiting Incentives, Merritt Hawkins, 2019, p. 51, www.merritthawkins.com/uploadedFiles/MerrittHawkins_2019_Incentive_Review.pdf, accessed 7/20/20.

24. "What is the MACRA Quality Payment Program?" HealthIT.gov, October 22, 2019, www.healthit.gov/topic/meaningful-use-and-macra/macra, accessed 7/20/20.

25. "Physician Compare Initiative," CMS.gov, 6/22/20, www.cms.gov/Medicare/Quality-Initiatives-Patient-Assessment-Instruments/physician-compare-initiative, accessed 7/20/20.

26. "Physician Attributes Commonly Used by Consumers to Choose Doctors Mostly Unrelated to Physician Quality, September 13, 2010, www.commonwealthfund.org/publications/press-releases/2010/sep/physician-attributes-commonly-used-by-consumers-to-choose-doctors, accessed 9/16/16.

27. 2016 Survey of America's Physicians, The Physicians Foundation and Merritt Hawkins, September 16, 2016, pp. 23–25, www.physiciansfoundation.org, accessed 7/13/17.

28. *Effects of Health Care Payment Models on Physician Practice in the United States*, Santa Monica, CA, RAND Corporation, 2015, www.rand.org/content/dam/rand/pubs/research_reports/RR800/%85/RAND_RR869.pdf, accessed 8/11/17; and *Factors Affecting Physician Professional Satisfaction and Their Implications for Patient Care, Health Systems, and Health Policy, 2013*, Santa Monica, CA, RAND Corporation, 2013, www.rand.org/content/dam/rand/pubs/research_reports/RR400/%85/RAND_RR439.pdf, accessed 8/11/17.

29. National Association of ACOs, Welcome, www.naacos.com/, accessed 7/20/20.

30. "Organizing Care: In Depth," RAND Corporation, June 1, 2015, www.rand.org/health/key-topics/organizing-care/in-depth.html, accessed 9/10/15.

31. *Effects of Health Care Payment Models on Physician Practice in the United States*, Santa Monica, CA, RAND Corporation, 2015, www.rand.org/content/dam/rand/pubs/research_reports/RR800/%85/RAND_RR869.pdf, accessed 8/11/17.

32. *Effects of Health Care Payment Models on Physician Practice in the United States*, Santa Monica, CA, RAND Corporation, 2015, www.rand.org/content/dam/rand/pubs/research_reports/RR800/%85/RAND_RR869.pdf, accessed 8/11/17.

33. Groopman, Jerome, *How Doctors Think*, Boston, Houghton Mifflin Co., 2007, p. 36.

34. "The Damaging Culture of Medicine and Physician Suicide," by Gabriel Perna, May 1, 2017, www.physicianspractice.com/worklife-balance/damaging-culture-medicine-and-physician-

suicide?GUID=0C6E097D-4055-495F-BA51-3F2643916A53&rememberme=1&ts=02052017, accessed 6/29/17.

35. Medscape National Physician Burnout & Suicide Report 2020, slide 2, www.medscape.com/slideshow/2020-lifestyle-burnout-6012460#2, accessed 7/20/20.

36. Lovelock, Christopher, *Services Marketing: People, Technology, Strategy*, 4th ed., Upper Saddle River, NJ, Prentice Hall, 2001, p. 494.

37. Heskett, James, et al. "Putting the Service-Profit Chain to Work," Harvard Business Review, 2000.

38. The Institute for Healthcare Improvement had proposed the "Triple Aim" to increase health care value in 2007. This innovative model gave providers new financial incentives for (1) improving clinical outcomes, (2) reducing the per capita cost of health care, and (3)managing the health of a defined patient population. www.ihi.org/communities/blogs/_layouts/ihi/community/blog/itemview.aspx?List=81ca4a47-4ccd-4e9e-89d9-14d88ec59e8d&ID=63, accessed 9/1/15.

39. "The Complexities of Physician Supply and Demand: Projections from 2013 to 2025," Prepared for:Association of American Medical Colleges by IHS Inc., March 2015, www.kff.org/wp-content/uploads/sites/3/2015/03/ihsreportdownload.pdf, accessed 9/1/15.

40. www.medscape.com/features/slideshow/compensation/2012/public, accessed 7/24/17.

41. "Millennials Want a Work-Life Balance—Their Bosses Just Don't Get Why," *Washington Post*, May 5, 2015, www.washingtonpost.com/local/millennials-want-a-work-life-balance-their-bosses-just-dont-get-why/2015/05/05/1859369e-f376-11e4-84a6-6d7c67c50db0_story.html?utm_term=.e43f70457ecf, accessed 7/24/17.

42. "Roadmap to the Development of the Vascular Center at Oklahoma Heart Institute," Farhan J. Khawaja, MD, 2013.

43. *The Lancet*, July 2013, www.medpagetoday.com/Cardiology/PeripheralArteryDisease/40803, accessed 6/23/15.

44. Laura Landro, "When Achy Legs are a Warning," *Wall Street Journal*, November 30, 2010.

45. Laura Landro, "When Achy Legs are a Warning," *Wall Street Journal*, November 30, 2010.

46. www.uspreventiveservicestaskforce.org/Page/Document/RecommendationStatementFinal/peripheral-arterial-disease-pad-and-cvd-in-adults-risk-assessment-with-ankle-brachial-index, accessed 6/23/15.

47. Berry, L. L., & Seltman, K. D., "Building a Strong Services Brand: Lessons from Mayo Clinic." *Business Horizons*, 50 (3), 2007, pp. 199–209.

48. Deloitte and Touche. "Vision in Manufacturing Study," Deloitte Consulting and Kenan-Flagler Business School, March 6, 1998; Nielsen, A. C., "New Product Introduction—Successful Innovation/Failure: Fragile Boundary," BASES and Ernst & Young Global Client Consulting, June 24, 1999.

49. Ansoff Matrix, Wikipedia, https://en.wikipedia.org/wiki/Ansoff_Matrix, accessed 11/9/17. Ansoff, I., "Strategies for Diversification," *Harvard Business Review*, 35 (5), 1957, pp. 113–124.

50. Kotler, P. and Keller, K. L., *Marketing Management*, 14th ed. Prentice-Hall, Upper Saddle River, NJ, 2012, chapter 20, p. 573.

51. "How At-Home Urgent Care Pays Off for Atrius Health," HealthLeaders Media, December 15, 2016, www.healthleadersmedia.com/physician-leaders/how-home-urgent-care-pays-atrius-health#, accessed 10/18/17.

52. "How Atrius Health is Making the Shift from Volume to Value," *Harvard Business Review*, December 13, 2016, https://hbr.org/2016/12/how-atrius-health-is-making-the-shift-from-volume-to-value, accessed 10/18/17.

53. "Virginia Doctor Tries Truck-Stop Medicine to Keep Family Practice Alive," *The Washington Post*, January 19, 2015, accessed 12/6/17; "From Delta Force to Country Doctor: 'He is a Hero'," *USA Today*, December 27, 2014, www.usatoday.com/videos/news/nation/2014/12/24/20771265/, accessed 12/6/17; White's Travel Center, company website, www.whitestravelcenter.com/raphine-medical-associates, accessed 12/6/17.

# CHAPTER 6

1. "The Role of Diagnosis Related Groups (DRGs) in Healthcare System Convergence," National Center for Biotechnology Information, www.ncbi.nlm.nih.gov/pmc/articles/PMC2773580/, accessed 7/21/20.

2. Stevens, Robert J., "Going to Market," *Marketing Health Services*, Summer 2005, p. 6.

3. AMC study sponsors included: Barnes-Jewish Hospital, Duke Health System, Emory Healthcare, Northwestern Memorial Hospital, Tufts—New England Medical Center, and Vanderbilt University Medical Center. The following AMCs participated in the study but did not sponsor it: Brigham and Women's Hospital, Johns Hopkins Medicine, University of California—San Francisco, University of California—Los Angeles, Yale—New Haven Hospital.

4. "Registration Requirements for Hospitals," AHA, 2008, www.aha.org/system/files/2018-02/REGISTRATION_FY_08.pdf, accessed 5/26/18.

5. "Fast Facts on U.S. Hospitals, 2020," AHA, 2018, www.aha.org/statistics/fast-facts-us-hospitals, accessed 3/12/20.

6. "Fast Facts on U.S. Hospitals, 2018," AHA Hospital Statistics, AHA Resource Center, February 2018, www.aha.org, accessed 2/26/18.

7. "Table 89 Hospitals, Beds, and Occupancy Rates Selected Years 1975–2014," *Health, United States*, 2016, p. 309.

8. "How Many Hospitals are in the US?" *Definitive Healthcare*, https://blog.definitivehc.com/how-many-hospitals-are-in-the-us, accessed 3/12/20.

9. "Urban and Rural Hospitals: How Do They Differ?" *Medicare & Medicaid Research Review*, 8 (2), 1986, pp. 77–85, www.ncbi.nlm.nih.gov/pmc/articles/PMC4191541, accessed 3/13/20.

10. "Fast Facts on U.S. Hospitals, 2020," AHA, www.aha.org/statistics/fast-facts-us-hospitals, accessed 3/12/20.

11. "How Many Hospitals Are in the US?" *Definitive Healthcare*, https://blog.definitivehc.com/how-many-hospitals-are-in-the-us, accessed 3/12/20.

12. National Center for Health Statistics (US). Health, United States, 2018 [Internet]. Hyattsville (MD): National Center for Health Statistics (US); 2019. Table 41, "Community Hospital Beds and Average Annual Percent Change, By state: United States, Selected Years 1980–2016," www.ncbi.nlm.nih.gov/books/NBK551099/table/ch3.tab41/, accessed 3/13/20. Most recent data available.

13. Table 89, "Hospitals, Beds, and Occupancy Rates, by Type of Ownership and Size of Hospital, U.S. Selected Years, 1975–2015," Health, United States, 2017, www.cdc.gov/nchs/data/hus/2017/089.pdf, accessed 3/13/20.

14. "AHA Data Show Hospitals' Outpatient Revenue Nearing Inpatient," *Modern Healthcare*, January 3, 2019, www.modernhealthcare.com/article/20190103/TRANSFORMATION02/190109960/aha-data-show-hospitals-outpatient-revenue-nearing-inpatient, accessed 3/16/20.

15. Table 89, "Hospitals, Beds, and Occupancy Rates, by Type of Ownership and Size of Hospital, U.S. Selected Years, 1975–2015," Health, United States, 2017, www.cdc.gov/nchs/data/hus/2017/089.pdf, accessed 3/13/20.

16. "Hospital Admissions per 1,000 Population by Ownership Type, KFF, 1999 and 2018," www.kff.org/other/state-indicator/admissions-by-ownership/?currentTimeframe=0&sortModel=%7B%22colId%22:%22Location%22,%22sort%22:%22asc%22%7D, accessed 3/15/20; and "Hospital Inpatient Days per 1,000 Population, KFF, 1999 and 2018," www.kff.org/other/state-indicator/inpatient-days-by-ownership/?currentTimeframe=19&sortModel=%7B%22colId%22:%22Location%22,%22sort%22:%22asc%22%7D, accessed 3/15/20.

17. "Hospital Outpatient Visits per 1,000 Population, KFF, 1999 and 2018," www.kff.org/other/state-indicator/outpatient-visits-by-ownership/?currentTimeframe=0&sortModel=%7B%22colId%22:%22Location%22,%22sort%22:%22asc%22%7D, accessed 3/15/20.

18. "AHA Data Show Hospitals' Outpatient Revenue Nearing Inpatient," *Modern Healthcare*, January 3, 2019, www.modernhealthcare.com/article/20190103/TRANSFORMATION02/190109960/aha-data-show-hospitals-outpatient-revenue-nearing-inpatient, accessed 3/16/20.

19. *AHA Trendwatch Chartbook 2018*, Chart 4.3, p. 38, and "AHA Data Show Hospitals' Outpatient Revenue Nearing Inpatient," *Modern Healthcare*, January 3, 2019, American Hospital Association's 2019 Hospital Statistics.

20. Ibid.

21. "Health System Growth Strategy for the Value-Based Market," Research Brief, The Advisory Board Company, p. 2, 2/27/14.

22. *Trendwatch Chartbook 2018*, American Hospital Association, Table 4.1, p. A-30. The estimates discussed in this section include hospital margins over the 1999–2016 period. The aggregate margin of hospitals in a particular year is equal to the sum of total revenues of all hospitals minus the sum of total costs of all hospitals, expressed as a percentage of total revenues. It is equivalent to the weighted average margin, with each hospital weighted by its total revenues.

23. "Hospital Operating Margins Decline 21% in 2019, Tracking Firm Finds," HFMA, December 30, 2019, www.hfma.org/topics/news/2019/12/hospital-operating-margins-decline-21-in-2019-tracking-firm-fi.html, accessed 3/18/20. Also, *Kaufman Hall Perspective*, Kaufman Hall, December 30, 2019, https://flashreportmember.kaufmanhall.com/kha-perspective-december-2019, accessed 3/18/20.

24. *Trendwatch Chartbook 2018*, American Hospital Association, Table 4.1, p. A-30.

25. "Health System Growth Strategy for the Value-Based Market," Advisory Board Company, p. 6, 2/27/14.

26. "What 146 C-suite executives told us about their top concerns—and how they've changed this year," Advisory Board Company, July 11, 2018, www.advisory.com/research/health-care-advisory-board/blogs/at-the-helm/2018/07/hcab-topic-poll, accessed 7/19/18.

27. Chapter 3, "Hospital Inpatient and Outpatient Services," Report to the Congress: Medicare Payment Policy, March 2018, p. 67, www.medpac.gov/docs/default-source/reports/mar18_medpac_ch3_sec.pdf?sfvrsn=0, accessed 6/6/18. For example, although hospitals are instructed to report all contributions and government transfers, some of those revenues may go unreported.

28. "Number of Bond Rating Upgrades and Downgrades Not-for-Profit Health Care, 1995–2015," Chart 4.9 (latest data available). American Hospital Association, *Trendwatch Chartbook 2016*.

29. "Have Hospitals Done Enough to Reduce Costs?" At the Margins, Advisory Board Company, 5/16/18.

30. "Health System Growth Strategy for the Value-Based Market," Research Brief, The Advisory Board Company, 2/27/14.

31. Lovelock, Christopher, *Services Marketing: People, Technology, Strategy*, 4th ed., New York, Pearson/Prentice Hall, pp. 494–496.

32. "Health System Growth Strategy for the Value-Based Market, Research Brief," The Advisory Board Company, 2014, p. 19.

33. The Consumer Loyalty Framework, Advisory Board Company, 2016, p. 6, www.advisory.com/-/media/Advisory-com/Research/MPLC/Research-Study/2016/Loyalty-study/34071_MIC_Consumer%20Loyalty_study.pdf, accessed 8/1/18

34. "Consumers' Use of HCAHPS Ratings and Word-of-Mouth in Hospital Choice," Health Services Trust, 45, 6, Part I (December 2010).

35. "Survey of HCAHPS Results by State, October 2012 to September 2013," www.hcahpsonline.org/files/Report_July_2014_States.pdf, accessed 10/19/16; HCAHPS Fact Sheet, June 2015, Centers for Medicare & Medicaid Services (CMS), Baltimore, MD, www.hcahpsonline.org/Facts.aspx., accessed 10/16/16.

36. "Competing on Consumer Experience," Advisory Board Company, 2015, p. 10. Calculation includes only Medicare patients and hospital-based services. Calculated as average of facilities with at least $10m annual inpatient revenue (n=3518), Source: Advisory Board Medicare Total Share Performance Assessment; Health Care Advisory Board Interviews and Analysis.

37. "Competing on Consumer Experience," Advisory Board Company, 2015, p. 20

38. "2018 State of Consumerism in Healthcare: Activity in Search of Strategy," Kaufman Hall & Associates, 2018, p. 10.

39. "2018 State of Consumerism in Healthcare: Activity in Search of Strategy," Kaufman Hall & Associates, 2018, p. 11.

40. "Competing on Consumer Experience," Advisory Board Company, 2015, p. 59.

41. "Competing on Consumer Experience," Advisory Board Company, 2015, p. 60.

42. "2018 State of Consumerism in Healthcare: Activity in Search of Strategy," Kaufman Hall & Associates, 2018, p. 10.

43. "Hospitals Must Now Post Prices. But it May Take a Brain Surgeon to Decipher Them," Robert Pear, *New York Times*, January 13, 2019, www.nytimes.com/2019/01/13/us/politics/hospital-prices-online.html, accessed 3/23/20.

44. "A Look Inside the Hospital Transparency Final Rule," Health Affairs Blog, Billy Wynne, Josh LaRosa and Taylor Cowey, November 18, 2019, www.healthaffairs.org/do/10.1377/hblog20191118.74200/full/, accessed 3/24/20.

45. "Trump Administration Proposes Transparency Rule For Health Insurers," Health Affairs Blog, Katie Keith, November 17, 2019, www.healthaffairs.org/do/10.1377/hblog20191117.364191/full/, accessed 3/24/20.

46. Source: Mehrota A, et al., "Visits to Retail Clinics Grew Fourfold from 2007 to 2009, Although Their Share of Overall Outpatient Visits Remains Low," Health Affairs, August 2012; MarketData Enterprises, "Retail Health Clinics & Urgent Care Centers Poised for Strong Growth—Market Worth $10 Billion," www.prweb.com, accessed 8/28/18.

47. "2018 State of Consumerism in Healthcare: Activity in Search of Strategy," Kaufman Hall & Associates, 2018, p. 5.

48. "2018 State of Consumerism in Healthcare: Activity in Search of Strategy," Kaufman Hall & Associates, 2018, p. 12.

49. "App Developed at UVA Improving HIV Care, Study Finds," *UVA Today*, June 12, 2018, https://news.virginia.edu/content/app-developed-uva-improving-hiv-care-study-finds, accessed 8/28/18.

50. "Consolidation and Health Systems in 2018: New Data From The AHRQ Compendium," Health Affairs Blog, 11/25/19, www.healthaffairs.org/do/10.1377/hblog20191122.345861/full/, accessed 3/17/20. Based on Compendium of U.S. Health Systems, 2018. Last reviewed December 2019. Agency for Healthcare Research and Quality, Rockville, MD, www.ahrq.gov/chsp/data-resources/compendium-2018.html, accessed 3/17/20.

51. "New Physicians Barraged by Job Offers," John Commins, *HealthLeaders*, May 14, 2019, www.healthleadersmedia.com/new-physicians-barraged-job-offers, accessed 3/18/20.

52. "2016 Survey of America's Physicians," The Physicians Foundation and Merritt Hawkins, 9/16, p.21,www.physiciansfoundation.org, accessed 7/13/17.

53. "2017 in Review—The Year M&A Shook the Healthcare Landscape," Kaufman Hall, www.kaufmanhall. com/sites/default/files/2017-in-Review_The-Year-that-Shook-Healthcare.pdf, accessed 7/9/18. Also, "2019 M&A in Review: In Pursuit of the New Bases of Competition," Kaufman Hall, 2020, p. 5, www. kaufmanhall.com/sites/default/files/documents/2020-01/2019_mergers_and_acquisitions_report_ kaufmanhall.pdf, accessed 3/18/20.

54. "Facing a financial squeeze, hospitals nationwide are cutting jobs," STAT, April 30, 2017, www. statnews.com/2017/04/30/hospitals-layoffs-national/, accessed 7/9/18.

55. "Financial Fallout from Covid-19: 10 Hospitals Laying off Workers," Becker's Hospital CFO Report, 6/11/20, www.beckershospitalreview.com/finance/financial-fallout-from-covid-19-10-hospitals-laying-off-workers.html, accessed 7/21/20.

56. "Hospital Culture and Clinical Performance: Where Next?" Russell Mannion and Judith Smith, BMJ Quality & Safety, 27, 2017, pp. 179–181, https://qualitysafety.bmj.com/content/qhc/27/3/179.full.pdf, accessed 8/17/20.

57. Robison, Jennifer, "Leading the Way to Better Patient Care," *Gallup Business Journal*, November 20, 2012, http://businessjournal.gallup.com/content/158,840/leading-better-patient-care.aspx, accessed 2/25/13.

58. "Leading the Way to Better Patient Care: How Cleveland Clinic Took Caregiving to a Higher Level with a Focus on Engaging Employees," *Gallup Business Journal*, November 20, 2012, https://news. gallup.com/businessjournal/158,840/leading-better-patient-care.aspx, accessed 8/20/18.

59. Nisen, Max, "Cleveland Clinic CEO Shares His Incredible Vision for the Future of Healthcare," *Business Insider*, December 5, 2012, www.businessinsider.com/business-innovation-in-healthcare-2012-12#ixzz39YOzxsTc, accessed 8/4/14.

60. "How We Engage," Cleveland Clinic, http://portals.clevelandclinic.org/ungc2017/Caregivers/Caregiver-Engagement/How-We-Engage#317,811,711-mytwocents- accessed 8/20/18.

61. "The Third-Leading Cause of Death in the U.S. Most Doctors Don't Want You to Know About," Ray Sipherd, special to CNBC.com, Published 9:31 am ET February 22, 2018, updated 9:39 am ET, February 28, 2018, www.cnbc.com/2018/02/22/medical-errors-third-leading-cause-of-death-in-america.html, accessed 8/20/18.

62. Gibson, C. and Nelson, K., "Obtaining Adolescents' Views about Inpatient Facilities Using Conjoint Analysis," *Paediatric Nursing*, 21 (2), 2009, pp. 34–37.

63. "Fable Hospital 2.0: The Business Case for Building Better Health Care Facilities," Hastings Center Report, 41 (1), 2011, pp. 13–23.

64. "Hospital of the Future's' Top 20 Features," Cheryl Clark, *HealthLeaders Media*, August 23, 2012, www. healthleadersmedia.com/print/QUA-283,716/Hospital-of-the-Futures-Top-20-Features, accessed 10/10/14.

65. "In Redesigned Room, Hospital Patients May Feel Better Already," Michael Kimmelman, *New York Times*, August 21, 2014.

66. "Report Finds Atlanta Has Some of World's Worst Traffic," The Atlanta Journal-Constitution, February 6, 2018, www.myajc.com/news/local-govt–politics/report-finds-atlanta-has-some-world-worst-traffic/PhkusU6Vq3buzATfC1hbPM/, accessed 8/21/18.

67. "WellStar Health System Presentation to East Cobb Civic Association," March 30, 2011, p. 15.

68. "2018 Employer Health Benefits Survey," Kaiser Family Foundation, October 3, 2018, www.kff.org/ report-section/2018-employer-health-benefits-survey-section-10-plan-funding/, accessed 3/29/20.

69. *Population HealthManagementA Roadmap for Provider-Based Automation in a New Era of Healthcare*, Institute for Health Technology Transformation, 2012. www.exerciseismedicine.org/assets/page_documents/PHM%20Roadmap%20HL.pdf, accessed 12/4/14.

70. "Using Risk Scores, Stratification for Population Health Management," Health IT Analytics, December 16, 2016, https://healthitanalytics.com/features/using-risk-scores-stratification-for-population-health-management, accessed 3/31/20.

71. "Population Health Service Organizations: Managed Care Gets a New 4-Wheel Drive Vehicle to Navigate the Value-based Terrain," Managed Care, November 24, 2018, www.managedcaremag.com/archives/2018/12/population-health-service-organizations-managed-care-gets-new-4-wheel-drive-vehicle, accessed 3/31/20.

72. "5-Part Strategy to Create a Population Health Services Organization," HealthLeaders Media, 10/31/19, www.healthleadersmedia.com/clinical-care/5-part-strategy-create-population-health-services-organization, accessed 3/30/20.

73. "Drivers of Consumer Choice: Implications from the 2007 Consumer Conjoint Survey," Advisory Board Company, 2007, p. 16.

74. "American Association of Physician Liaison's Program Survey, 2009," Marketing and Planning Leadership Council interviews and analysis.

75. "Advancing Physician Outreach Programs," Advisory Board Company, 2010, pp. 32–33.

76. Ibid, p. 40.

77. "The Consumer is the New Payer in Healthcare," NRC, 2017, pp. 6–7, https://nrchealth.com/wp-content/uploads/2017/05/The-New-Payer-White-Paper_V8.pdf, accessed 8/9/18.

78. "How Patients Actually Choose Providers," Healthgrades, February 24, 2017, https://hs.healthgrades.com/resources/february-2017/how-patients-actually-choose-providers, accessed 8/9/18.

79. "The Effects of Hospital Safety Scores, Total Price, Out-of-Pocket Cost, and Household Income on Consumers' Self-reported Choice of Hospitals," *Journal of Patient Safety*, 13 (4), 2017, pp. 192–198.

80. Kotler, P., *Marketing Management*, 11th ed., Upper Saddle River, NJ: Prentice Hall,2003, p. 567.

81. "2019–20 Best Hospitals Honor Roll and Medical Specialties Rankings," U.S. News & World Reports, July 29, 2019, https://health.usnews.com/health-care/best-hospitals/articles/best-hospitals-honor-roll-and-overview, accessed 4/1/20.

82. "Assessing Online Scheduling as an Emerging Trend in Physician Appointments," Healthgrades, January 12, 2018, https://partners.healthgrades.com/blog/assessing-online-scheduling-as-an-emerging-trend-in-physician-appointments, accessed 4/1/20.

83. Experian Health, www.experian.com/healthcare/products/payment-tools/online-patient-appointment-scheduling, accessed 4/2/20.

84. "Kaiser Permanente Building Infrastructure to 'Connect the Dots' for Social Determinants," FierceHealthcare, 5/8/19, www.fiercehealthcare.com/hospitals-health-systems/kaiser-permanente-launches-social-health-network, accessed 4/2/20.

85. Richard Owen and Laura L. Brooks, *Answering the Ultimate Question*, Jossey Bass, San Francisco, CA, 2009, p. 5.

86. Ibid., pp. 61–62.

87. Ibid., pp. 62–63.

88. Ibid., pp. 61–62.

89. *Would You Recommend This Hospital to a Friend?* Julie Coffman and Phyllis Yale, Bain & Company, 2007, p. 5.

90. *Would You Recommend This Hospital to a Friend?* Julie Coffman and Phyllis Yale, Bain & Company, 2007, p. 6.
91. Richard Owen and Laura L. Brooks, *Answering the Ultimate Question*, Jossey Bass, San Francisco, CA, 2009, pp. 111–114.
92. *Would You Recommend This Hospital to a Friend?* Julie Coffman and Phyllis Yale, Bain & Company, 2007, p. 4.
93. Ibid.,
94. "Linking the Customer Experience to Value," McKinsey & Company, March 2016.
95. By Anna Gorman April 13, 2017, this KHN story also ran in *Politico*. It can be republished for free (details).
96. "In Remote Idaho, a Tiny Facility Lights the Way for Stressed Rural Hospitals," Anna Gorman, April 13, 2017, Henry J. Kaiser Family Foundation, The Kaiser Family Foundation, Menlo Park, California, is a nonprofit, private operating foundation focusing on the major health care issues facing the nation and is not associated with Kaiser Permanente or Kaiser Industries, https://khn.org/news/in-remote-idaho-an-injection-of-hope-for-stressed-rural-hospitals, accessed 4/9/20.
97. By Anna Gorman April 13, 2017, this KHN story also ran in Politico. It can be republished for free (details).
98. "How to Turn a Critical Access Hospital Around," Amy Feldman, athenahealth, September 16, 2016, www.athenahealth.com/knowledge-hub/practice-management/lost-rivers-idaho-how-to-turn-a-critical-access-hospital-around, accessed 4/9/20.
99. "The Real Reason Loyalty Lacks in Healthcare," *Becker's Hospital Review*, May 2, 2018, www.beckershospitalreview.com/care-coordination/the-real-reason-loyalty-lacks-in-healthcare.html, accessed 4/13/20.
100. "Patient Leakage: A New Survey Highlights High Costs, Limited Control," Sage Consulting, October 2018, https://fibroblast.com/wp-content/uploads/2018/10/Patient-Leakage-A-new-survey-highlights-high-costs-limited-control-October-2018-1.pdf, accessed 4/13/20.
101. "Insights into Local Advertising—Healthcare Vertical," BIA Advisory Services, September 27, 2017, http://blog.biakelsey.com/index.php/2017/09/27/healthcare-advertising-spend-to-reach-10-85-billion-in-2017/, accessed 4/13/20.
102. "Hospitals Spend Big Bucks on Advertising—Here's a Look at the Cost of 8 Ad Campaigns," FierceHealthcare, 8/7/18, www.fiercehealthcare.com/hospitals-health-systems/hospitals-spending-big-bucks-advertising-a-look-cost-8-ad-campaigns, accessed 4/13/20.

## CHAPTER 7

1. "What is a Health Technology?" World Health Organization, www.who.int/health-technology-assessment/about/healthtechnology/en/, accessed 2/18/19.
2. https://ehrintelligence.com/news/most-hospitals-use-ehr-data-to-support-quality-improvement-efforts. https://dashboard.healthit.gov/quickstats/pages/physician-ehr-adoption-trends.php, accessed 10/21/19.
3. *A History of Medical Device Regulation & Oversight in the United States*, U.S. Food & Drug Administration, www.fda.gov/MedicalDevices/DeviceRegulationandGuidance/Overview/ucm618375.htm, accessed 2/26/19.
4. "Medical Devices Definition," World Health Organization, www.who.int/medical_devices/definitions/en/, accessed 2/18/19.

5. "The Medical Technology Industry Dossier," Statistica, p. 7. EvaluateMedTech—World Preview 2017, Outlook to 2022, p. 14, September 17.

6. *The U.S. Medical Device Industry: A Market Report*, Wallonia.be, Export Investment, January 2018, pp. 4–5.

7. "Medical Technology Spotlight—The Medical Technology Industry in the United States," Select USA, U.S. Department of Commerce, www.selectusa.gov/medical-technology-industry-united-states, accessed 2/11/19.

8. "Top 10 Most Successful Medical Device Companies," Global Healthcare, Shannon Lewis, February 11, 2018, www.healthcareglobal.com/top10/top-10-most-successful-medical-device-companies, accessed 2/16/19.

9. "Six Digit NAICS Codes and Titles," NAICS Association, www.naics.com/, accessed 2/21/19.

10. "Medical Technology Spotlight—The Medical Technology Industry in the United States," Select USA, U.S. Department of Commerce, www.selectusa.gov/medical-technology-industry-united-states, accessed 2/11/19.

11. "Six Digit NAICS Codes and Titles," NAICS Association, www.naics.com/, accessed 2/21/19.

12. "What's the Difference Between the FDA Medical Device Classes?" BMP Medical, February 2018, www.bmpmedical.com/blog/whats-difference-fda-medical-device-classes-2/, accessed 2/19/19.

13. "Understanding the Differences Between Class I, II and III Medical Devices," *Conelec*, https://conelec.net/understanding-differences-class-ii-iii-medical-devices/, accessed 2/20/19.

14. *Medical Technology Industry Dossier 2018*, Statistica, p. 26.

15. Health IT.gov, The Office of the National Coordinator for Health Information Technology www.healthit.gov/topic/health-it-basics/glossary, accessed 2/28/19.

16. *2016 Top Markets Report Health IT*, International Trade Administration, Department of Commerce, July 2016, p. 3, www.trade.gov/topmarkets/pdf/Health_IT_Top_Markets_Report.pdf, accessed 2/25/19.

17. *Digital Health—Global Market Outlook (2017–2026)*, Statistics Market Research Consulting, March 2018, www.strategymrc.com/report/digital-health-market, accessed 3/6/19.

18. *Revenue of Top 50 Health IT Companies in the U.S. 2018*, Statistica, August 9, 2019, www.statista.com/statistics/453472/leading-health-information-technology-companies-in-the-us-by-revenue/, accessed 10/24/19.

19. "Rock Health Funding Database," Rock Health, https://rockhealth.com/reports/2018-year-end-funding-report-is-digital-health-in-a-bubble/, accessed 3/11/19.

20. Ibid.

21. "Future of Electronic Medical Records: Experts Predict EMR Trends in 2019," Select Hub, https://selecthub.com/medical-software/emr/electronic-medical-records-future-emr-trends/, accessed 3/12/19.

22. "What Can Health Systems Do to Encourage Physicians to Embrace Virtual Care?" *Deloitte 2018 Survey of US Physicians*, July 18, 2018, www2.deloitte.com/insights/us/en/industry/health-care/virtual-health-care-health-consumer-and-physician-surveys.html, accessed 3/2/19.

23. "Is There a Difference Between Telemedicine and Telehealth?" mHealth Intelligence, June 3, 2016 https://mhealthintelligence.com/features/is-there-a-difference-between-telemedicine-and-telehealth, accessed 3/22/19.

24. *The Big-Data Revolution in US Health Care: Accelerating Value and Innovation*, McKinsey & Co., April 2013, www.mckinsey.com/industries/healthcare-systems-and-services/our-insights/the-big-data-revolution-in-us-health-care, accessed 3/21/19.

25. *Big Data in Health Care*, Advisory Board Company, 2017, p. 1.

26. "Healthcare IT Industry Landscape: Market Segments, Driver, and Trend Analysis," Healthcare Market Research and Consulting Services, iHealthAnalyst, February 13, 2017, www.ihealthcareanalyst. com/healthcare-industry-landscape-market-segments-drivers-trends-analysis/, accessed 2/27/19.

27. "What is Healthcare Revenue Cycle Management?" RevCycle Intelligence, June 16, 2016, https:// revcycleintelligence.com/features/what-is-healthcare-revenue-cycle-management, accessed 3/21/19.

28. Dev Culver, Executive Director, HealthInfoNet, 4/5/17.

29. *Promoting an Overdue Digital Transformation in Healthcare*, McKinsey & Co., June 2019, www. mckinsey.com/industries/healthcare-systems-and-services/our-insights/promoting-an-overdue-digital-transformation-in-healthcare?cid=other-eml-alt-mip-mck&hlkid=0232a39185994ed3 bea04dd115baacec&hctky=3,076,479&hdpid=a4dbf5bb-040c-4057-961a-ee591ea1ffb0, accessed 10/29/19.

30. "Two Months After Pilot, Apple Launches Personal Health Record Program to Boost Patient Engagement," MedCity News, March 29, 2018, https://medcitynews.com/2018/03/two-months-pilot-apple-launches-personal-health-record-program-boost-patient-engagement/, accessed 3/25/19.

31. "Human API and CMS Collaborate to Help Medicare Patients Share Claims Data in New Chapter for Blue Button," MedCity News, March 8, 2018, https://medcitynews.com/2018/03/medicare-patients-claims-data-and-blue-button-api/, accessed 3/25/19.

32. "2018 Telehealth Industry Trends," Advisory Board Company, slide 21.

33. "National Wearables Survey Shows Convergence of Wearables and Health Devices," Briodagh, IoT Evolution, November 29, 2018, www.iotevolutionworld.com/smart-home/articles/440,486-national-wearables-survey-shows-convergence-wearables-health-devices.htm, accessed 3/25/19.

34. *Telehealth Primer: Wearables*, Advisory Board Company, May 16, p. 16.

35. Ibid., pp. 16, 39.

36. *Digital Health Consumer Adoption Report 2019*, Stanford Medicine Center for Digital Health and Rock Health, October 2019, p. 6.

37. *Telehealth Primer: Wearables*, Advisory Board Company, May 2016, p. 4, www.wareable.com/wearable-tech/245-million-wearable-devices-sold-2019-1606, accessed 4/18/19.

38. *Beyond Wellness For the Healthy: Digital Health Consumer Adoption 2018*, Rock Health, 2019. https:// rockhealth.com/reports/beyond-wellness-for-the-healthy-digital-health-consumer-adoption-2018/, accessed 4/12/19.

39. Ibid.

40. "Patients Will Use Health Wearable to Reduce Trips to the Doctor: Survey," FierceHealthcare, June 25, 2019, www.fiercehealthcare.com/tech/patients-will-use-health-wearables-to-reduce-trips-to-doctor-survey, accessed 10/30/19.

41. InTouch, 2018 U.S. Telemedicine Industry Benchmark Survey, https://reachhealth.com/resources/ telemedicine-industry-survey/, accessed 10/30/192018.

42. "How is the Industry Trending in the US? Telehealth Services Industry in the US," IBIS World, www. ibisworld.com/industry-trends/specialized-market-research-reports/life-sciences/healthcare-services/ telehealth-services.html, accessed 4/19/20.

43. Medicare Provider/Supplier Purchase Summary Files, 2010–2017, Telehealth Industry Trends, Advisory Board Company, April 2019, slide 6.

44. *J.D. Powers Telehealth Satisfaction Study*, July 2019, www.jdpower.com/sites/default/files/2019185_ telehealth_usage_and_awareness.pdf, accessed 11/5/19.

45. "Telehealth Industry Trends," Advisory Board Company, April 2019, slide 18.

46. "Beyond Wellness For the Healthy: Digital Health Consumer Adoption 2017," Rock Health, 2018, https://rockhealth.com/reports/beyond-wellness-for-the-healthy-digital-health-consumer-adoption-2017/, accessed 4/12/19.

47. "Telehealth Industry Trends," Advisory Board Company, April 2019, slide 20.

48. "Telehealth Consumers Just Don't Know About You! Lessons for Health Systems," HealthLeaders, October 18, 2019, www.healthleadersmedia.com/innovation/telehealth-consumers-just-dont-know-about-you-lessons-health-systems, accessed 11/9/19.

49. *Digital Health Consumer Adoption Report 2019*, Rock Health/Stanford Medicine Center for Digital Health, p. 20.

50. "Mercer Capital's 5 Trends to Watch in the Medical Device Industry in 2018," *Mercer Capital*, p. 9, http://mercercapital.com/insights/newsletters/value-focus-industry-publications/medical-device-industry-newsletter/, accessed 4/12/19.

51. *Technology Vendor Worksheet, Digital Strategy Planning Guide*, Advisory Board Company, 2015.

52. Ibid.

53. "A Framework for Comprehensive Assessment of Medical Technologies—Defining Value in the New Health Care Ecosystem," AdvaMed, May 2017, p. 5, www.advamed.org/sites/default/files/resource/advamed-framework-comprehensive-assessment-medical-technologies-june2019.pdf, accessed 8/20/20.

54. "4 Digital Health Trends Set to Transform the Medical Device Market in 2019," Bigfoot Biomedical, Janaury 18, 2019, www.bigfootbiomedical.com/blog/4-digital-health-trends-set-to-transform-the-medical-device-market-in-2019, accessed 4/1/19.

55. "Winning with a Customer Focus in Medtech," Bain Consulting, 10/4/17, www.bain.com/insights/winning-with-a-customer-focus-in-medtech-forbes, accessed 11/11/19.

56. "Demonstrating Value," *EY Pulse of the Industry*, 2018, p. 12.

57. "Why Leading Medtech Companies are Putting Customers Ahead of Products," Bain Consulting, September 7, 2017, www.bain.com/insights/why-leading-medtech-companies-are-putting-customers-ahead/, accessed 11/11/19.

58. Ibid.

59. Ibid.

60. "Differentiating to Win Medical Device Marketing," Vennli, *Business Wire*, October 12, 2017, www.businesswire.com/news/home/20,171,012,005,211/en/60-Percent-Medical-Device-Brands-Meet-Healthcare, accessed 2/1/19.

61. Ibid.

62. Ibid.

63. Ibid.

64. "Premarket Approval (PMA)," Drugwatch, August 29, 2019, www.drugwatch.com/fda/premarket-approval/, accessed 11/16/19.

65. "The Impact of U.S. Regulation on Medical Device Innovation," MCRA, February 2018, www.mcra.com/news-publications/news/impact-us-regulation-medical-device-innovation, accessed 7/1/19.

66. *Pulse of the Industry EY 2018*, September 12, 2018, p. 2, www.ey.com/Publication/vwLUAssets/ey-pulse-of-the-industry-2018/$FILE/ey-pulse-of-the-industry-2018.pdf, accessed 7/12/19.

67. "FDA In Brief: FDA Proposes Improvements to the De Novo Pathway for Novel Medical Devices to Advance Safe, Effective, and Innovative Treatments for Patients," U.S. Food & Drug Administration, 12 April 2018, www.fda.gov/news-events/fda-brief/fda-brief-fda-proposes-improvements-de-novo-pathway-novel-medical-devices-advance-safe-effective-and, accessed 11/16/19.

68. "De Novo Classification Request, FDA," September 6, 2019, www.fda.gov/medical-devices/premarket-submissions/de-novo-classification-request, accessed 11/16/19.

69. "FDA Announces a New Digital Health Innovation Plan," *National Law Review*, July 7, 2017, www.natlawreview.com/article/fda-announces-new-digital-health-innovation-plan, accessed 7/15/19.

70. *Top Health Industry Issues of 2019: The New Health Economy Comes of Age*, PwC Health Research Institute, p. 9, www.pwc.com/us/en/industries/health-services/pdf/pwc-us-healthcare-top-health-industry-issues-2019.pdf, accessed 4/10/19.

71. Digital Health Software Precertification (Pre-Cert) Program, Software Precertification Program: Working Model—Version 1.0—January 2019, FDA, p. 14, www.fda.gov/media/119,722/download, accessed 4/10/19.

72. "Dartford and Gravesham NHS Home Health and Current Partner to Reduce Hospital Readmissions and Emergency Department Visits," April 11, 2019, http://currentmain.wpengine.com/dartford-and-gravesham-nhs-home-health-and-current-partner-to-reduce-hospital-readmissions-and-emergency-department-visits, accessed 7/18/19.

73. "The CHRONIC Care Act and Telehealth," American Well, June 20, 2018, www.americanwell.com/the-chronic-care-act-and-telehealth, accessed 7/26/19.

74. Synzi website, https://synzi.com/roi/, accessed 7/26/19.

75. "Telehealth Companies, Home Health Providers See Major Upside in CMS Proposal," *Home Health Care News*, November 11, 2018, https://homehealthcarenews.com/2018/11/telehealth-companies-home-health-providers-see-major-upside-in-cms-proposal/, accessed 7/26/19.

76. "Agetech has Potential to Transform Care for the Elderly, but Needs Buy-In from Older People," Jonathan Margolis, *Financial Times*, July 17, 2019, www.ft.com/content/ba4d0376-a7be-11e9-90e9-fc4b9d9528b4, accessed 7/22/19.

77. "CMS Expands COVID-19 Telehealth Reimbursement to Therapists, Phone Services," mHealth Intelligence, 5/1/20, https://mhealthintelligence.com/news/cms-expands-covid-19-telehealth-reimbursement-to-therapists-phone-services, accessed 7/22/20.

78. "How has Telehealth Utilization Changed from 2019 to 2020?" Definitive Healthcare, June 2020, https://blog.definitivehc.com/us-telehealth-adoption-2019, accessed 7/22/20.

79. "What Digital Health Challenges and Opportunities are 'Top of Mind' for Health System Leaders?" Center for Connected Medicine, 2018, https://connectedmed.com/blog/content/top-of-mind-2019-interoperability-cybersecurity-telehealth, accessed 8/6/19.

80. "The Big Five Tech Companies & Their Big Five Acquisition," Growth Rocks, April 2019, https://growthrocks.com/blog/big-five-tech-companies-acquisitions/, accessed 11/18/19.

81. *Digital Health Consumer Adoption Report 2019*, Rock Health and Stanford Center for Digital Health, p. 23, https://rockhealth.com/reports/digital-health-consumer-adoption-report-2019/, accessed 11/11/19.

82. "Health Sites Found to be Sharing Sensitive Data," *Financial Times*, November 13, 2019, www.ft.com/content/b1101836-063f-11ea-9afa-d9e2401fa7ca, accessed 11/14/19.

83. "Big Tech Companies Set their Sights on Health Care," *2019 Health Care IT Industry Trends*, Advisory Board Company, Health Care IT Advisor, slide 29, 2019.

84. "In Just Two Hours, Amazon Erased $30 Billion in Market Value for Healthcare's Biggest Companies," Quartz, January 30, 2018, https://qz.com/1,192,731/amazons-push-into-healthcare-just-cost-the-industry-30-billion-in-market-cap/, accessed 8/15/19.

85. "What 'Amazon Health Care' could look like in 5 years," Advisory Board Company, November 14, 2018, p. 2.

86. "Technology: Amazon Rolls Out Medical Services for Staff," *Financial Times*, September 27, 2019, www.ft.com/content/bc058a64-df11-11e9-9743-db5a370481bc, 9/27/19.

87. "The 3 Big Questions about Alexa's Future in Health Care (No.1: Will Anyone Actually Use It?)," Advisory Board Company, April 9, 2019.

88. "he 4 big ways Microsoft wants to change health care," Advisory Board Company, November 20, 2019, www.advisory.com/daily-briefing/2019/11/20/microsoft?WT.mc_id=Email|DailyBriefing+Headline|DB ECPost|DBA|DB|2019Nov20|ATestDB2019Nov20||||&elq_cid=388,721&x_id=003C000001GLiCcIAL, accessed 11/21/19.

89. Ibid.

90. "Digital Health: Surgical Intervention," *The Economist*, February 3, 2018, p. 54.

91. "Facebook Announces Preventive Health Tool," HealthExec, October 30, 2019, www.healthexec.com/topics/health-it/facebook-announces-preventive-health-tool, accessed 11/21/19.

92. www.zs.com/publications/articles/medtech-look-to-marketing-for-the-solutio, accessed 8/20/19.

93. "Proving and Improving Product Value," Healthcare IT Advisor, Advisory Board Company, 2016, pp. 10–12.

94. ProFlow is a pseudonym for an international company that manufactures infusion pumps.

95. "Drug Prices in 2019 are Surging, with Hikes at 5 Times Inflation," MoneyWatch, July 1, 2019, www.cbsnews.com/news/drug-prices-in-2019-are-surging-with-hikes-at-5-times-inflation/, accessed 11/28/19.

96. "Interventions to Improve Adherence to Self-administered Medications for Chronic Diseases in the United States: A Systematic Review," *Annals of Internal Medicine*, 157 (11), 2012, pp. 785–795; D. P. Goldman. "Pharmacy Benefits and the Use of Drugs by the Chronically Ill," *JAMA*, 291 (19), 2004, pp. 2344–2350.

97. "Chlorofluorocarbons (CFCs)," ToxTown, NIH, U.S. National Library of Medicine, https://toxtown.nlm.nih.gov/chemicals-and-contaminants/chlorofluorocarbons-cfcs, accessed 11/30/19.

98. "Sleep and Health," Division of Sleep Medicine at Harvard Medical School, January 16, 2008, http://healthysleep.med.harvard.edu/need-sleep/whats-in-it-for-you/health, accessed 12/6/19.

99. "Report: Sleep Deprivation Costs the U.S. Economy $400 Billion Every Year," *Forbes*, Niall McCarthy, December 1, 2016, www.forbes.com/sites/niallmccarthy/2016/12/01/report-sleep-deprivation-costs-the-u-s-economy-400-billion-every-year-infographic/#3abd56011998, accessed 12/6/19.

# CHAPTER 8

1. Despite this consolidation, they maintain separate trade organizations: PhRMA (Pharmaceutical Research and Manufacturers of America) www.phrma.org/en for traditional pharmaceuticals and Bio (Biotechnology Innovation Organization) www.bio.org/about. Bio membership covers all biotechnology (like agriculture), not just pharmaceuticals; all accessed 09/25/19.

2 A pharmacopeia is a "Collection of officially recognized standards for drugs, ingredients, dietary supplements, and herbal and/or other medicinal preparations." The US Pharmacopeia is the official source of this information in the U.S. See www.usp.org/, accessed 09/26/19.

3. 21 USC §321 Section 201(g)(1) Federal Food, Drug and Cosmetic Act [As Amended Through P.L. 116–22, Enacted June 24, 2019], https://legcounsel.house.gov/Comps/Federal%20Food,%20Drug,%20And%20Cosmetic%20Act.pdf, accessed 09/25/19.

4. "FDA 101: An Overview of FDA's Regulatory Review and Research Activities,"www.fda.gov/AboutFDA/WhatWeDo/ucm407684.htm, accessed 09/26/19.

5. While biologically derived drugs are generally covered by the drug definition, for historical reasons, they are regulated by public health laws. This fact came to light after it was necessary to create a pathway for generic biological medications in the ACA.

6. United States Code, 2011 Edition: Title 42—The Public Health and Welfare, Chapter 6A: Public Health Service Subchapter II—General Powers and Duties. Part F—Licensing of Biological Products and Clinical Laboratories subpart 1—biological products, Sec. 262—Regulation of biological products, www.gpo.gov/fdsys/pkg/USCODE-2011-title42/html/USCODE-2011-title42-chap6A-subchapII-partF-subpart1-sec262.htm, accessed 09/26/19.

7. Shalowitz, J., *The US Health Care System: Origins, Organization and Opportunities*, San Francisco, Jossey-Bass.

8. Abelson, R., "UnitedHealth Buys Large Doctors Group as Lines Blur in Health Care," *New York Times*, December 7, 2017. Section B page 3.

9. Numerous examples range from Partners Health Care in Boston to the Kaiser Permanente system.

10. https://www.projectrx.com, accessed 11/10/19.

11. https://civicarx.org, accessed 11/10/19.

12. The term "cost" is used here as the actual amount paid by a stakeholder. The cost of an episode of care depends on the medication's unit price, number of units, and the particular type of technology chosen for treatment (such as generic versus branded or class of anti-inflammatory, e.g., ibuprofen versus an immunomodulator such as Rituxan).

13. The term "efficacious" means the product does what it is supposed to do in controlled circumstances, such as clinical studies. It is often erroneously confused with the word "effective," which is a description of how well the product works under "real world" conditions after it is launched.

14. "FDA: The Drug Development Process," www.fda.gov/patients/learn-about-drug-and-device-approvals/drug-development-process, accessed 10/06/19.

15. A process is in place for those who urgently need medications in development. The traditional term for this process is "compassionate use;" recently, the FDA has changed the term to "expanded access." See "FDA: Expanded Access," www.fda.gov/news-events/public-health-focus/expanded-access, accessed 10/13/19.

16. "FDA: Development & Approval Process—Drugs," www.fda.gov/drugs/development-approval-process-drugs, accessed 10/06/19.

17. Weber, L., "Hurricane Maria's Effect on the Health Care Industry is Threatening Lives Across The U.S.," *Huffpost*, September 24, 2018, www.huffpost.com/entry/iv-bag-drug-shortage-puerto-rico-hurricane-maria_n_5ba1ca16e4b046313fc07a8b, accessed 10/15/19.

18. Rabin, R. C., "Faced With a Drug Shortfall, Doctors Scramble to Treat Children With Cancer," *New York Times*, October 15, 2019, www.nytimes.com/2019/10/14/health/cancer-drug-shortage.html, accessed 10/15/19.

19. Statistica: CMS (Office of the Actuary), www.statista.com/statistics/184914/prescription-drug-expenditures-in-the-us-since-1960/, accessed 12/31/19.

20. Kamal, R., Cox, C., and McDermott, D., "What are the Recent and Forecasted Trends in Prescription Drug Spending?" Kaiser Family Foundation, February 20, 2019, www.healthsystemtracker.org/chart-collection/recent-forecasted-trends-prescription-drug-spending/#item-start, accessed 12/31/19.

21. Bach, P. B. and Ohn, J., "Does the 6% in Medicare Part B Drug Reimbursement Affect Prescribing?" Drug Pricing Lab Policy Paper, Memorial Sloan Kettering, May 9, 2018. https://drugpricinglab.org/wp-content/uploads/2018/05/Part-B-Reimbursement-and-Prescribing.pdf, accessed 11/10/19.

22. "Pass-Through Payment Status and New Technology Ambulatory Payment Classification (APC)," CMS, www.cms.gov/Medicare/Medicare-Fee-for-Service-Payment/HospitalOutpatientPPS/passthrough_payment.html, accessed 11/26/19.

23. Sec. 340B Public Health Service Act. Limitation on Prices of Drugs Purchased by Covered Entities, HRSA, www.hrsa.gov/opa/programrequirements/phsactsection340b.pdf., accessed 12/29/19.

24. Further modifications were made by the Deficit Reduction Act (DRA) of 2005 and the ACA.

25. "340B Price/Covered Outpatient Drugs," Apexus, www.340bpvp.com/resource-center/faqs/340b-pricing-covered-outpatient-drugs/, accessed 12/29/19.

26. "340 B Eligibility," HRSA, www.hrsa.gov/opa/eligibility-and-registration/index.html, accessed 12/29/19.

27. Statement of Debra A. Draper (Director, Health Care) Before the Committee on Health, Education, Labor & Pensions, U.S. Senate: Drug Discount Program, Status of Agency Efforts to Improve 340B Program Oversight, United States Government Accountability Office, May 15, 2018, www.gao.gov/assets/700/691742.pdf, accessed 12/29/19.

28. "340B Office of Pharmacy Affairs Information System," HRSA, www.hrsa.gov/opa/340b-opais/index.html, accessed 12/29/19.

29. "Drug Discount Program: Federal Oversight of Compliance at 340B Contract Pharmacies Needs Improvement," United States Government Accountability Office, June 2018, www.gao.gov/assets/700/692697.pdf, accessed 12/29/19.

30. "Patient Definition," Apexus, www.340bpvp.com/resource-center/faqs/patient-definition, accessed 12/29/19.

31. "Republican Review of the 340B Drug Pricing Program," House Energy and Commerce Committee, January 2018, https://republicans-energycommerce.house.gov/wp-content/uploads/2018/01/20180110Review_of_the_340B_Drug_Pricing_Program.pdf, accessed 12/29/19.

32. Kamal, K., Fox, C., and McDermott, D., "What are the Recent and Forecasted Trends in Prescription Drug Spending?" Peterson-Kaiser Health System Tracker, February 20, 2019, www.healthsystemtracker.org/chart-collection/recent-forecasted-trends-prescription-drug-spending/#item-start, accessed 11/10/19.

33. Lorin, J., "The Pill That Made Northwestern Rich," *Bloomberg BusinessWeek*, August 18, 2016, www.bloomberg.com/news/articles/2016-08-18/the-pill-that-made-northwestern-rich, accessed 11/10/19.

34. U.S. National Library of Medicine. ClinicalTrials.gov—Clinical Trial Phases. www.clinicaltrials.gov, accessed 11/10/19.

35. www.fda.gov/Drugs/DevelopmentApprovalProcess/HowDrugsareDevelopedandApproved/ApprovalApplications/, accessed 11/10/19.

36. "Report to Congressional Requesters—Drug Industry, Profits, Research and Development Spending, and Merger and Acquisition Deals," GAO, November 2017, www.gao.gov/assets/690/688472.pdf, accessed 12/29/19.

37. "New Medicines in Development for Diabetes 2012," PhRMA, http://phrma-docs.phrma.org/sites/default/files/pdf/12-535phrmaoverviewdiabetes1109.pdf; also "Biopharmaceuticals in Perspective Spring 2017," PhRMA, http://phrma-docs.phrma.org/files/dmfile/Biopharmaceuticals-in-Perspective-2017.pdf, both accessed 07/05/18.

38. Vij, R., "Pharma Industry Merger and Acquisition Analysis 1995 to 2015," http://revenuesandprofits.com/pharma-industry-merger-and-acquisition-analysis-1995-2015/, R&P, accessed 07/05/18; www.genpact.com/insight/blog/how-can-pharma-companies-adapt-to-the-current-m-a-environment, accessed 11/10/19.

39. Farcas, C. and van Biesen, T., "The Real Reason Big Pharma Mergers Are Wise," *Forbes*, June 26, 2009, www.forbes.com/2009/06/26/big-pharma-mergers-leadership-governance-acquisitions.html, accessed 11/10/19.

40. Grabowski, H. and Kyle, M., "Mergers and Alliances in Pharmaceuticals: Effects on Innovation and R&D Productivity," in Klaus Gugler, K. and Burcin Yurtoglu, B. B. (eds), *Economics of Corporate Governance and Mergers*, Northampton, MA, Edward Elgar Publishing, Inc., pp. 262–287.

41. Danzon, P. M., "Economics of the Pharmaceutical Industry," NBER Reporter, Fall 2006, www.nber.org/reporter/fall06/danzon.html, accessed 12/29/19.

42. See, for example, Bounds, A., "Pharma Investors Put Less Skin in the Game as Risk Appetite Wanes—Focus is on Leaving Marketing, Manufacturing, and Global Distribution to Others," *Financial Times*, April 9, 2017, www.ft.com/content/f07ee806-1adf-11e7-bcac-6d03d067f81f?desktop=true, accessed 12/22/19.

43. Dunn, A., "Bankrupt Biopharmas Are Rare—2019 Has Some Worried That's Changing," *Biopharmadive*, November 19, 2019, accessed 12/26/19.

44. Ward, A., "GSK Spin-Off Gears Up for Possible Listing," *Financial Times*, June 15, 2014, www.ft.com/content/9bdf9b4a-f46a-11e3-a143-00144feabdc0, accessed 12/22/19.

45. "NYU Langone Creates Cutting-Edge Biotech 'Incubator' in Manhattan," Press Release, December 12, 2019, https://nyulangone.org/news/nyu-langone-creates-cutting-edge-biotech-incubator-manhattan, accessed 12/22/19.

46. "Duke University & Deerfield Management Announce Four Points Innovation," Press Release, December 18, 2019, https://olv.duke.edu/news/duke-deerfield-announce-four-points-innovation/, accessed 12/22/19.

47. Savlovschi-Wicks, T., "Top 10 Contract Research Organisations (CROs) to Watch in 2019," *Proclinical*, September 5, 2019, www.proclinical.com/blogs/2019-5/top-10-contract-research-organisations-cros-to-watch-in-2019, accessed 11/10/19.

48. Christiansen, C. et al., "The Big Idea: The New M&A Playbook," *Harvard Business Review*, March 1, 2011, pp. 49–57.

49. See, for example, Roland D., "Drug Firms Learn From Hollywood," *The Wall Street Journal* May 1, 2017. Page B3.

50. A good source for this information is the Regulatory Affairs Professionals Society, www.raps.org, accessed 12/29/19.

51. https://civicarx.org, accessed 12/22/19.

52. "Follow The Pill: Understanding the U.S. Commercial Pharmaceutical Supply Chain," Kaiser Family Foundation, February 28, 2005, http://kff.org/other/report/follow-the-pill-understanding-the-u-s/, accessed 11/10/19.

53. "World Preview 2019, Outlook to 2024," EvaluatePharma®, June, 2019, https://info.evaluate.com/rs/607-YGS-364/images/EvaluatePharma_World_Preview_2019.pdf?mkt_tok=eyJpIjoiWlRGbE1q VmpNV1kxTVRSayIsInQiOiIxb0JwRkE2VEdTTHhDR1VGVitnbUUyXC9pTUtRZGVaQTlGV0sx WDFHTzBnMklyeU9cLzcrRTdcL3MxTE5Qeml6OUNjQTZlTThOV1Eza0VpdVZzUFFjNTlp Rk9oMG1menlCY0poSml0aDRNY2hyS0orcmk3RjhqSjQrYzlha1BHbkdZTyJ9, accessed 12/01/19.

54. "Generic Competition and Drug Prices," FDA, December 13, 2019, www.fda.gov/about-fda/center-drug-evaluation-and-research-cder/generic-competition-and-drug-prices, accessed 12/29/19.

55. Kamalakaran, A., "Glaxo Chief Seeks Guidance from Health Systems," Reuters, July 7, 2008, www.reuters.com/article/glaxo-government/glaxo-chief-seeks-guidance-from-health-systems-wsj-idUSBNG12077820080707, accessed 12/01/19.

56. Bratulic, A., "Sanofi exits diabetes, CV research in strategy shake-up as it prioritises key growth drivers Dupixent, vaccines," *FirstWord Pharma*, December 9, 2019, www.firstwordpharma.com/node/1, 686,636?al=39df1a-bc0b8433cad60533f0c3519c1a24072b%5E%7C%5EMTA0NjA1Ng%3D%3D%5E%70 C%5ENQ%3D%3D&cp1=bmV3c2xldHRlcl9yZWdpc25faWQ9bGVhZF9hcnRpY2xl, accessed 12/15/19.

57. National Organization for Rare Disorders, https://rarediseases.org/about/, accessed 12/15/19.

58. Institute of Medicine (US) Committee on Accelerating Rare Diseases Research and Orphan Product Development, Field, M. J. and Boat, T. F. (eds.), *Rare Diseases and Orphan Products: Accelerating Research and Development*, Washington, DC, National Academies Press, 2010, www.ncbi.nlm.nih.gov/books/NBK56187/, accessed 12/15/19.

59. "Orphan Drug Act. Relevant Excerpts (Public Law 97–414, as amended), FDA, last updated August 2013,www.fda.gov/ForIndustry/DevelopingProductsforRareDiseasesConditions/Howtoapply forOrphanProductDesignation/ucm364750.htm, accessed 12/15/19.

60. "The Board shall be comprised of the Assistant Secretary for Health of the Department of Health and Human Services and representatives, selected by the Secretary, of the Food and Drug Administration, the National Institutes Health, the Centers for Disease Control, and any other Federal department or agency which the Secretary determines has activities relating to drugs and devices for rare diseases or conditions. The Assistant Secretary for Health shall chair the Board."SEC. 227 of the Public Health Service Act [42 USC 236].

61. Reichert, J. M., "Trends in Development and Approval Times for New Therapeutics in the United States," *Nature Reviews: Drug Discovery*, 2 (9), 2003, pp. 695–702.

62. Office of Orphan Products Development, FDA, www.fda.gov/AboutFDA/CentersOffices/Officeof MedicalProductsandTobacco/OfficeofScienceandHealthCoordination/ucm2018190.htm, accessed 12/15/19.

63. Search Orphan Drug Designations and Approvals, FDA,www.accessdata.fda.gov/scripts/opdlisting/ oopd/listResult.cfm, accessed 12/15/19.

64. "Drug Prices for Rare Diseases Skyrocket While Big Pharma Makes Record Profits," AHIP, September 10, 2019, www.ahip.org/drug-prices-for-rare-diseases-skyrocket-while-big-pharma-makes-record-profits/, accessed 12/15/19.

65. Frequently Asked Questions (FAQ)—Designating an Orphan Product, FDA, www.fda.gov/ ForIndustry/DevelopingProductsforRareDiseasesConditions/HowtoapplyforOrphanProduct Designation/ucm240819.htm, accessed 12/15/19.

66. Guidance from the FDA provides additional clarification of the MC to PC issue: "The following factors, when applicable to severe or life-threatening diseases, *may in appropriate cases be taken into consideration* [emphases added] when determining whether a drug makes a major contribution to patient care: convenient treatment location; duration of treatment; patient comfort; reduced treatment burden; advances in ease and comfort of drug administration; longer periods between doses; and potential for self-administration." Department of Health and Human Services, Food and Drug Administration, 21 CFR Part 316 [Docket No. FDA–2011–N–0583] RIN 0910–AG72 Orphan Drug Regulations: Final rule. Federal Register Vol. 78, No. 113 Wednesday, June 12, 2013, Rules and Regulations, pp. 35, 117–135, www.gpo.gov/fdsys/pkg/FR-2013-06-12/pdf/2013-13,930.pdf, accessed 12/15/19.

67. Daniel, M. G. et al., "The Orphan Drug Act: Restoring the Mission to Rare Diseases," *American Journal of Clinical Oncology*, 39 (2), 2016, pp. 210–213.

68. AHIP [originally called America's Health Insurance Plans]: Orphan Drug Utilization and Price Changes (2012–2014), Data Brief, October 2016, www.ahip.org/wp-content/uploads/2016/10/ OrphanDrug_DataBrief_10.21.16.pdf, accessed 12/15/19.

69. Blakeslee, S., "Scorned Thalidomide Raises New Hopes," *New York Times*, April 10, 1990, page C3.

70. "Drug Approval Package—Thalomid (Thalidomide) Capsules Approval Date, FDA, July 16, 1998, www.accessdata.fda.gov/drugsatfda_docs/nda/98/020785s000_ThalidomideTOC.cfm, accessed 12/15/19.

71. Fleming, N., "How Artificial Intelligence is Changing Drug Discovery," *Nature*, May 30, 2018, www.nature.com/articles/d41586-018-05267-x, accessed 12/22/19.

72. www.ibm.com/products/watson-drug-discovery, accessed 12/22/19.

73. Innovative Medicines Initiative: MELLODDY, www.imi.europa.eu/projects-results/project-factsheets/melloddy, accessed 12/22/19.

74. Japan provides an interesting international example with respect to off-label prescribing. If, for example, an oncologist uses one non-approved medication in the treatment regimen, the insurer will not pay for *any* of the drugs used.

75. EMD Serono Specialty Digest™ 14th Edition 2018, https://specialtydigestemdserono.com/?id=jklyHF lrXSCnRIblnaAzxNDRDA7t5GHAcXSLNxHXjojAQqBtjUXQ4JOTLM+uUJ+9k1FMhevkooeE qryQ8cklM7hIijMoiBtzUx3PSsGJNzU=, accessed 12/22/19.

76. Erman, M. and Humer, C., "Drugmakers Try Evasion, Tougher Negotiations to Fight New U.S. Insurer Tactic," *Reuters*, July 5, 2018, www.reuters.com/article/us-usa-healthcare/drugmakers-try-evasion-tougher-negotiations-to-fight-new-u-s-insurer-tactic-idUSKBN1JV1AX, accessed 12/22/19.

77. "Pfizer Settles With U.S. Over Practice of Using Charity to Pay Kickbacks to Medicare Patients," *Kasier Health News*, May 25, 2018, https://khn.org/morning-breakout/pfizer-settles-with-u-s-over-practice-of-using-charity-to-pay-kickbacks-to-medicare-patients/, accessed 12/22/19.

78. Pollack, Andrew., "Drug Deals Tie Prices to How Well Patients Do," *New York Times*, April 22, 2009. Page B1.

79. See, also, Rubenfire, A., "Pay-For-Performance Drug Pricing: Drugmakers Asked to Eat Costs When Products Don't Deliver," *Modern Health Care*, December 10, 2016, www.modernhealthcare.com/article/20,161,210/MAGAZINE/312,109,949?utm_source=modernhealthcare&utm_medium=email&utm_content=20,161,210-MAGAZINE-312,109,949&utm_campaign=dose, accessed 12/22/19.

80. "Drugs for Rheumatoid Arthritis," *The Medical Letter on Drugs Therapeutics*, 60 (1552), 2018, pp. 123–128.

81. Singh, S., "Basics About Biosimilars—The Savings Potential and the Challenges," CVSHealth, May 3, 2016, https://payorsolutions.cvshealth.com/insights/basics-about-biosimilars, accessed 12/22/19.

82. "Delivering on the Potential of Biosimilar Medicines: The Role of Functioning Competitive Markets," IMS Institute for Health Care Informatics [now part of IQVIA], March 2016, www.iqvia.com/-/media/iqvia/pdfs/institute-reports/delivering-on-the-potential-of-biosimilar-medicines.pdf?la=en&hash=030 18A6A86DED8F901DDF305BAA536FF0E86F9B4&_=1,530,986,176,970, accessed 12/22/19.

83. For a revealing, but unsuccessful, example of this tactic, see Carey, T., "Generic Manufacturers Gain Another Advantage in Disputing Drug Patents," December 24, 2009, http://pharmaceuticalcommerce.com/legal-regulatory/generic-manufacturers-gain-another-advantage-in-disputing-drug-patents/, accessed 12/22/19.

84. "Pay-for-Delay—When Drug Companies Agree Not to Compete," Federal Trade Commission, www.ftc.gov/news-events/media-resources/mergers-competition/pay-delay, accessed 12/31/19.

85. Bartz, D., "Controversial 'Pay-For-Delay' Deals Drop After FTC'S Win in Top Court," *Reuters Business News*, January 13, 2016, www.reuters.com/article/us-pharmaceuticals-patent-ftc-idUSKCN0UR2JA20160113, accessed 12/31/19.

86. Agreements Filed with the Federal Trade Commission under the Medicare Prescription Drug, Improvement, and Modernization Act of 2003. Overview of Agreements Filed in FY 2014. A Report

by the Bureau of Competition, www.ftc.gov/system/files/documents/reports/agreements-filled-federal-trade-commission-under-medicare-prescription-drug-improvement/160113mmafy14rpt.pdf, accessed 12/31/19.

87. Silverman, E., "Supreme Court Lets Pay-to-Delay Ruling Against Pharma Stand," *STAT*, November 7, 2016, www.statnews.com/pharmalot/2016/11/07/supreme-court-pay-delay-glaxo-teva, accessed 12/26/19,

88. Blankenship, Kyle., "California Bans Pharma's Infamous 'Pay-for-Delay' Deals," *FiercePharma*, October 8, 2019, www.fiercepharma.com/pharma/california-governnor-inks-bill-banning-pay-for-delay-deals-pharma?mkt_tok=eyJpIjoiTkRoa09XWmtObVF3TldVNCIsInQiOiJadVwvVGd5ZzFjVXRnVkNEOWU3aTNMczNSZWZ2RHdVVnFXOTlBZ0pKbmpCd3duUlJVSlwvUnhyOTVoXC9uaVpEU09za0pJemFFIcDVPc0l0REYreVZXWFBDDdzM5WWhjSjZ3eWtIUTVEb1FJcUhOSzNGMk9kMitPTlZHbUZsTXVTSEhaTiJ9&mrkid=936,233, accessed 12/26/19.

89. Feldman, Robin, "May Your Drug Price Be Evergreen," *Oxford Journal of Law and the Biosciences*, 2018, available at SSRN: https://ssrn.com/abstract=3,061,567, accessed 12/27/19.

90. National Asthma Education and Prevention Program, Third Expert Panel on the Diagnosis and Management of Asthma. Guidelines for the Diagnosis and Management of Asthma: Section 4, Stepwise Approach for Managing Asthma in Youths≥12 years of Age and AdultsBethesda (MD): National Heart, Lung, and Blood Institute; August 2007, www.ncbi.nlm.nih.gov/books/NBK7222/figure/A2212/?report=objectonly, accessed 12/22/19. Also see, Global Initiative for Asthma—2018 Pocket Guide for Asthma Management and Prevention, https://ginasthma.org/download/836/, accessed 12/22/19.

91. Firozi, P., "The Health 202: 'Gag Clauses' Mean You Might Be Paying More For Prescription Drugs Than You Need To," *Washington Post*, July 5, 2018, www.washingtonpost.com/news/powerpost/paloma/the-health-202/2018/07/05/the-health-202-gag-clauses-mean-you-might-be-paying-more-for-prescription-drugs-than-you-need-to/5b3a36ca1b326b3348addc4a/?noredirect=on&utm_term=.714601c14174, accessed 12/31/19.

92. Armour, S. and Burton, T. M., "U.S. Advances Plan to Allow Imports of Some Drugs in Bid to Cut Prices," *Wall Street Journal*, December 18, 2019, www.wsj.com/articles/u-s-advances-plan-to-allow-imports-of-certain-drugs-in-bid-to-cut-prices-11,576,676,700, accessed 12/27/19.

93. DTC advertising to the public (such as television ads) of branded pharmaceuticals is only legal in the U.S. and New Zealand.

94. Centers for Medicare & Medicaid Services—Medicare and Medicaid Programs; Regulation To Require Drug Pricing Transparency, May 5, 2019, www.federalregister.gov/documents/2019/05/10/2019-09655/medicare-and-medicaid-programs-regulation-to-require-drug-pricing-transparency, accessed 12/27/19.

95. Waddill, K., "Federal Judge Strikes Down New Drug Price Transparency Rule," *HealthPayer Intelligence*, July 10, 2019, https://healthpayerintelligence.com/news/federal-judge-strikes-down-new-drug-price-transparency-rule, accessed 12/27/19.

96. For a well-written summary of this issue, see, Van Groningen, N., "Big Pharma Gives Your Doctor Gifts—Then Your Doctor Gives You Big Pharma's Drugs," *The Washington Post*, June 13, 2017, www.washingtonpost.com/opinions/big-pharma-gives-your-doctor-gifts-then-your-doctor-gives-you-big-pharmas-drugs/2017/06/13/5bc0b550-5045-11e7-b064-828ba60fbb98_story.html, accessed 12/27/19.

97. "Code on Interactions With Health Care Professionals," PhRMA, www.phrma.org/codes-and-guidelines/code-on-interactions-with-health-care-professionals, accessed 12/27/19.

98. Medicare, Medicaid, Children's Health Insurance Programs; Transparency Reports and Reporting of Physician Ownership or Investment Interests, CMS, February 8, 2013, www.federalregister.gov/

documents/2013/02/08/2013-02572/medicare-medicaid-childrens-health-insurance-programs-transparency-reports-and-reporting-of, accessed 12/27/19. The ACA provision is sometimes called The Sunshine Act.

99. "Open Payments," CMS, www.cms.gov/openpayments/, accessed 12/27/19.

100. Loftus, P. and Hopkins, J. S., **"Drugmakers Overhaul the Sales Pitch Amid Coronavirus Lockdowns,"** *Wall Street Journal*, May 11, 2020, www.wsj.com/articles/drugmakers-overhaul-the-sales-pitch-amid-coronavirus-lockdowns-11,589,194,800, accessed 05/13/20.

101. Schnipper, L. E. et al., "Updating the American Society of Clinical Oncology Value Framework—Revisions and Reflections in Response to Comments Received," *Journal of Clinical Oncology*, 34 (24), 2016, pp. 2925–2934.

102. DrugPricingLab, Memorial Sloan Kettering: Drug Abacus, https://drugpricinglab.org/tools/drug-abacus/, accessed 12/27/19.

103. The Office of Prescription Drug Promotion (OPDP),www.fda.gov/about-fda/center-drug-evaluation-and-research-cder/office-prescription-drug-promotion-opdp, accessed 03/06/20. The reader is referred to this site for the details of governmental approvals.

104. "Drug Advertising: A Glossary of Terms," FDA,www.fda.gov/drugs/prescription-drug-advertising/drug-advertising-glossary-terms, accessed 03/06/20.

105. "PhRMA Code on Interactions with Health Care Professionals," www.phrma.org/-/media/Project/PhRMA/PhRMA-Org/PhRMA-Org/PDF/A-C/Code-of-Interaction_FINAL21.pdf, accessed 03/08/20. The updated Code took effect January 2009 and was last revised September 2019.

106. "Open Payments," CMS, www.cms.gov/OpenPayments Last Modified:01/15/2020, accessed 03/08/20.

107. SUPPORT for Patients and Communities Act: Public Law 115–271 October 24, 2018, www.congress.gov/bill/115th-congress/house-bill/6, accessed 03/08/20.

108. Carey, C. et al., "Drug Firms' Payments and Physicians' Prescribing Behavior in MedicarePart D," NBER Working Paper No. 26,751, issued in February 2020, www.nber.org/papers/w26751.pdf, accessed 03/10/20.

109. IMS Health Inc. v. Sorrell, 630 F.3d 263 (2d Cir. 2010).

110. See Ventola, C. L., "Off-Label Drug Information—Regulation, Distribution, Evaluation, and Related Controversies," *Pharmacy and Therapeutics*, 34 (8), 299, pp. 428–440; Lama, C., "Addressing the Threshold—Regulating Off-Label Drug Promotion," *Washington University Journal of Law & Policy*, 60, 2019, pp. 359–393, https://openscholarship.wustl.edu/law_journal_law_policy/vol60/iss1/19, accessed 03/12/20.

111. Scott, D., "The Untold Story of TV's First Prescription Drug Ad," *StatNews*, December 11, 2015, www.statnews.com/2015/12/11/untold-story-tvs-first-prescription-drug-ad/, accessed 03/12/20.

112. "PhRMA Guiding Principles Direct to Consumer Advertisements About Prescription Medicines," http://phrma-docs.phrma.org/sites/default/files/pdf/phrmaguidingprinciplesdec08final.pdf, accessed 03/12/20.

113. Bulik, B. S., "The Top 10 Ad Spenders in Big Pharma for 2019," *FiercePharma*, February 19, 2020, www.fiercepharma.com/special-report/top-10-advertisers-big-pharma-for-2019?mkt_tok=eyJpIjoiT0RNNVl6Z3pPR0U0WlRjeSIsInQiOiJZUVJBa210RVhuZXXJKRTd4N3JMSmhsakp4anlrVDJsNDRJM1owN2dVRjk0TkV3K3JhTWVQbmJHVG8yM2dPcDVMeWdCRTE4K3ZBV1JCbkpBalhBSkdTYTRlV0F1YVNyaWhGSm9YeTBKOVhpMjFibmZ6Y2tKc0FjVzYrZkxsTEdzTyJ9&mrkid=936,233, accessed 03/12/20.

114. Bulik, B. S., "AbbVie, Lilly, Pfizer Lead Pharma TV Spending to Roaring Start in 2020," *FiercePharma*, March 9, 2020, www.fiercepharma.com/special-report/top-10-advertisers-big-pharma-for-2019?mkt_tok

=eyJpIjoiT0RNNVl6Z3pPR0U0WlRjeSIsInQiOiJZUVJBa210RVhuZXJKRTd4N3JMSmhsak
p4anlrVDJsNDRJM1owN2dVRjk0TkV3K3JhTWVQbmJHVG8yM2dPcDVMeWdCRTE4K3
ZBV1JCbkpBalhBSkdTYTR1V0FlYVNyaWhGSm9YeTBKOVhpMjFibmZ6Y2tKc0Fj
VzYrZkxsTEdzTyJ9&mrkid=936233, accessed 03/12/20.

115. Ibid.

116. "TV Ads Dominate Pharma DTC Budgets, But Online Ads Prove Effective at Prompting Patients to 'Ask Your Doctor,'" *PRNewswire*, www.prnewswire.com/news-releases/tv-ads-dominate-pharma-dtc-budgets-but-online-ads-prove-effective-at-prompting-patients-to-ask-your-doctor-300,696,746. html., accessed 03/14/20.

117. Alpert, A. et al., "Prescription Drug Advertising and Drug Utilization—The Role of Medicare Part D," NBER Working Paper No. 21,714, issued in November 2015, www.nber.org/papers/w21714, accessed 03/14/20.

118. For details of DTC spending in different media outlets and disease categories, see Schwartz, L. M. and Woloshin, S., "Medical Marketing in the United States, 1997–2016," *JAMA*, 321 (1), 2019, pp. 80–96.

119. Liu, Q. et al., "'See Your Doctor': The Impact of Direct-to-Consumer Advertising on Patients with Different Affliction Levels," *Marketing Letters*, February 13, 2020, https://link.springer.com/article/10.1007%2Fs11002-020-09514-y, accessed 03/14/20.

120. Tiku, N., "Facebook Has a Prescription—More Pharmaceutical Ads," *The Washington Post*, March 4, 2020, www.washingtonpost.com/technology/2020/03/03/facebook-pharma-ads/?utm_campaign=wp_the_health_202&utm_medium=email&utm_source=newsletter&wpisrc=nl_health202, accessed 03/17/20.

121. Aikin, K. J. et al., "Consumer Tradeoff of Advertising Claim versus Efficacy Information in Direct-to-Consumer Prescription Drug Ads," *Research in Social and Administrative Pharmacy*, 15, 2019, pp. 1484–1488.

122. DeFrank, J. T. et al., "Direct-to-Consumer Advertising of Prescription Drugs and the Patient–Prescriber Encounter: A Systematic Review," *Health Communication*, 35 (6), 2019, pp. 739–746.

123. "Patient-Focused Drug Development—Methods to Identify What Is Important to Patients," FDA, October 2019, www.fdanews.com/ext/resources/files/2019/09-30-19-DraftPatientFocusedDrugDevelop. pdf?1,569,867,993, accessed 12/31/19.

124. Van Zee, A., "The Promotion and Marketing of OxyContin: Commercial Triumph, Public Health Tragedy," *American Journal of Public Health*, 99 (2), 2009, 221–227. The early history of OxyContin is taken from this source. While this case focuses on one company, Purdue Pharma, it certainly was not alone in causing the opioid epidemic. For example, see Estes, C., "Insys Founder, John Kapoor, Sentenced To 66 Months in Fentanyl Bribery Case," *Forbes*, January 23, 2020, www.forbes.com/sites/claryestes/2020/01/23/insys-founder-john-kapoor-sentenced-to-66-months-in-fentanyl-bribery-case/#26465b6d4533, accessed 02/22/20. For a highly fictionalized, fantasy version of that fentanyl story (despite the author's disclaimer), see Rushdie, S., *Quichotte*, New York, Random House.

125. For an excellent review of this issue, see Baker, D. W. *The Joint Commission's Pain Standards: Origins and Evolution*, Oakbrook Terrace, IL: The Joint Commission, 2017, https://cergm.carter-brothers.com/wp-content/uploads/2019/03/2019-03-07-Joint-Commission-on-Pain-2017.pdf, accessed 02/11/20.

126. James N. Campbell, "Presidential Address—American Pain Society," November 12, 1995. Reproduced in *Journal of Pain* 5 (1), 1996, pp. 85–88.

127. OxyContin® is a registered trademark of Purdue Pharma. For ease of presentation the "®" will be omitted and Purdue Pharma will be referred to as Purdue.

128. Chakradhar, S. and Ross, C., "The History of OxyContin, Told Through Unsealed Purdue," *Stat News*, December 3, 2019, www.statnews.com/2019/12/03/oxycontin-history-told-through-purdue-pharma-documents/, accessed 02/15/20.

"Purdue conducted a clinical trial in elderly patients with osteoarthritis to test the safety and efficacy of OxyContin. It enrolled 133 patients, but only 63 completed the trial. About 82% of the patients had some sort of adverse event related to the treatment. Yet Purdue concluded that the study 'demonstrated that [controlled-release] Oxycodone is a safe and effective analgesic for the control of osteoarthritis-related pain.'"

129. While perfectly acceptable and common practice in the industry at the time, as mentioned elsewhere in this chapter, such giveaways are now considered unethical.

130. The program was launched in 1993 and eventually was put online. The site no longer exists but the program is described at: Partners Against Pain's Pain Management Kit, www.mdmag.com/journals/pain-management/2008/sep2008/partners_against_pain, accessed 02/15/20.

131. Egilman, DS et al., "The Marketing of OxyContin®: A Cautionary Tale," *Indian Journal of Medical Ethics*, https://ijme.in/articles/the-marketing-of-oxycontin-a-cautionary-tale/?galley=html, accessed 02/16/20.

132. Van Zee, A., "The Promotion and Marketing of OxyContin: Commercial Triumph, Public Health Tragedy," *American Journal of Public Health*, 99 (2), 2009, 221–227.

133. Chakradhar, S. and Ross, C., "The History of OxyContin, Told Through Unsealed Purdue," *Stat News*, December 3, 2019, www.statnews.com/2019/12/03/oxycontin-history-told-through-purdue-pharma-documents/, accessed 02/15/20.

134. Geriatrics and Extended Care Strategic Healthcare Group, National Pain Management Coordinating Committee, Veterans Health Administration—*Pain as the 5th Vital Sign Toolkit*, revised October 2000, www.va.gov/PAINMANAGEMENT/docs/Pain_As_the_5th_Vital_Sign_Toolkit.pdf, accessed 02/11/20.

135. "Kentucky OxyContin Task Force Recommendations," August 3, 2001, www.documentcloud.org/documents/6,562,756-14-Purdue-Docs-2-81-to-88.html, accessed 02/15/20.

136. It is noteworthy that the generic form was available only in 80 mg doses while the branded drug came in 10, 20, 40 and 80 mg strengths; the potential for overdose and addiction was therefore greater with the generic.

137. Crow, D., "How Purdue's 'One-Two' Punch Fuelled the Market for Opioids," *Financial Times*, September 9, 2018, www.ft.com/content/8e64ec9c-b133-11e8-8d14-6f049d06439c, accessed 02/16/20.

138. Van Zee, A., "The Promotion and Marketing of OxyContin: Commercial Triumph, Public Health Tragedy," *American Journal of Public Health*, 99 (2), 2009, 221–227.

139. Crow, D., "How Purdue's 'One-Two' Punch Fuelled the Market for Opioids," *Financial Times*, September 9, 2018, www.ft.com/content/8e64ec9c-b133-11e8-8d14-6f049d06439c, accessed 02/16/20.

140. The suit was settled in 2015 but the compensation payout was still not accomplished by early 2020.

141. Ibid.

142. For example, researchers found in a review of patients from 2011 to 2016 that some "surgeons wrote prescriptions for more than 100 opioid pills in the week following the surgery, often with instructions to take one to two pills every four to six hours, as needed. The total amounts frequently exceeded current guidelines from several academic medical centers, which call for zero to 10 pills for many of the procedures in the analysis, and up to 30 for cardiac bypass surgery."
Appleby, J. and Lucas, E., "While Addiction Crisis Raged, Many Surgeons Overprescribed Opioids, Analysis Shows," *Stat News*, June 21, 2019, www.statnews.com/2019/06/21/surgeons-overprescribed-opioids-analysis-shows/, accessed 02/17/20.

143. Spector, M. and Hals, T., "OxyContin Maker Purdue is 'Pharma Co X' in U.S. Opioid Kickback Probe—Sources," *NASDAQ*, January 28, 2020, www.nasdaq.com/articles/exclusive-oxycontin-maker-purdue-is-pharma-co-x-in-u.s.-opioid-kickback-probe-sources-2020, accessed 02/18/20.

144. National Institute on Drug Abuse: Opioid Crisis, revised January 2019, www.drugabuse.gov/drugs-abuse/opioids/opioid-crisis, accessed 02/11/20.

145. The new questions on the written form are:

   ▪ During this hospital stay, did you have any pain?

   ▪ During this hospital stay, how often did hospital staff talk with you about how much pain you had?

   ▪ During this hospital stay, how often did hospital staff talk with you about how to treat your pain?

   See: Hospital Inpatient Prospective Payment Final Rule, https://s3.amazonaws.com/public-inspection.federalregister.gov/2017-16,434.pdf, accessed 02/11/20.

146. The Joint Commission Report, *Requirement, Rationale, Reference—Pain Assessment and Management Standards for Hospitals*, August 29, 2017, www.jointcommission.org/assets/1/18/R3_Report_Issue_11_Pain_Assessment_8_25_17_FINAL.pdf, accessed 02/17/20.

147. Hoffman, J., "Payout From a National Opioids Settlement Won't Be as Big as Hoped," *New York Times*, February 17, 2020, www.nytimes.com/2020/02/17/health/national-opioid-settlement.html, accessed 02/22/20.

148. Bernstein, L., "Major Drugstore Chains Sue Doctors in Sprawling Federal Opioid Case," *The Washington Post*, January 8, 2020, www.washingtonpost.com/health/major-drugstore-chains-sue-doctors-in-sprawling-federal-opioid-case/2020/01/07/3ac9cd70-317d-11ea-9313-6cba89b1b9fb_story.html, accessed 02/22/20.

149 Goldberg, D., "FDA Says 'No' to Another New Opioid," *Politico*, January 16, 2020, www.politico.com/newsletters/politico-pulse/2020/01/16/fda-says-no-to-another-new-opioid-784,430, accessed 02/22/20.

# CHAPTER 9

1. Philip Kotler and Gerald Zaltman, "Social Marketing: An Approach to Planned Social Change," *Journal of Marketing*, 35 (3), 1971, pp. 3–12.

2. "Reducing Tobacco Use in the United States: A Public Health Success Story ... So Far," in Cheng, H., Kotler, P., and Lee, N. R. (eds.), *Social Marketing for Public Health: Global Trends and Success Stories*, Sudbury, MA, Jones and Barlett, 2011, chapter 2, pp. 31–55.

3. Philip Kotler, Nancy Lee, and Michael Rothschild, *Social Marketing: Influencing Behaviors for Good*, Thousand Oaks, CA, Sage, 2006.

4. Philip Kotler and Nancy Lee, *Social Marketing: Behavior Change for Social Good*, 6th ed.,Thousand Oaks, CA, Sage, 2019, p. 8.

5. David J. Tenenbaum, "Tackling the Big Three (Air and Water Pollution, and Sanitation)," *Environmental Health Perspectives*, 106 (5), 1998, n.p.

6. "Ethnographic Research to Study the Use of Water Treatment Devices in Andhra Pradesh, India: PATH's Safe Water Project (2006–2011)," in Lee, N. R. and Kotler, P. (eds.), *Social Marketing: Influencing Behaviors for Good*, 4th edition, Thousand Oaks, CA, Sage, 2011, pp. 257–260.

7. Paper contributed by Dr. K Vijaya, Director, Corporate Marketing & Communications Division and Mr. Johnson Seah, Deputy Director, Corporate Marketing Department, Health Promotion Board, Singapore.

8. Jones, L., "AIDS in New York City," LaGuardia Community College/CUNY: La Guardia and Wagner Archives, July 12, 1987, Edward I. Koch Collection, Koch Collection Subject Files, https://en.wikipedia.org/wiki/HIV/AIDS_in_New_York_City, accessed 7/22/20.

9. See "Be Where Your Target Audience Hangs Out—Example: HIV/AIDS Tests in Gay Bathhouses," in Lee, N. R. and Kotler, P. (eds.), *Social Marketing: Influencing Behaviors for Good*, 4th edition, Thousand Oaks, CA, Sage, 2011, pp. 300–301.

10. Lee, N. R. and Kotler, P., *Social Marketing: Influencing Behaviors for Good*, 4th edition, Thousand Oaks, CA, Sage, 2011, p. 327.

11. Kotler, P. and Lee, N., *Social Marketing: Influencing Behaviors for Good*, 3rd ed., Thousand Oaks, CA, Sage, 2008.

12. Haughey, D., "Smart Goals," Project Smart, http://www.projectsmart.co.uk/smart-goals.html, accessed 04/08/09.

13. Coreil, J., Bryant, C. A., and Henderson, J. N. (with contributions from M. S. Forthofer and G. P. Quinn), *Social and Behavioral Foundations of Public Health*, Thousand Oaks, CA, Sage, 2001, p 231.

# INDEX

Note: Page numbers in *"fig"* refer to figures and *"t"* refer to tables.